# Statements: Diagnostics and Therapy in Dental Medicine Today and in the Future

Jean-François Roulet and Heinrich F. Kappert

# Statements:
## Diagnostics and Therapy in Dental Medicine Today and in the Future

Edited by

### Jean-François Roulet
and
### Heinrich F. Kappert

With contributions from:

Ken Anusavice
Thomas Attin
Hans-Peter Bantleon
Marcio Vivan Cardoso
Alessandro Devigus
Josephine F. Esquivel-Upshaw
Horst Fischer
Josef Freudenthaler
Hans Geiselhöringer
Reinhard Hickel
Stefan Holst
Nicoleta Ilie
Søren Jepsen
Matthias Kern

Claus Löst
Bart van Meerbeek
Ina Nitschke
Mutlu Özcan
Sandro Palla
Bjarni E. Pjetursson
Bernhard Christian Seiner
Franz-Xaver Reichl
Giovanni E. Salvi
Patrick R. Schmidlin
Roberto Spreafico
Svante Twetman
David Watts
Yasuhiro Yoshida

Quintessenz Verlags-GmbH
Berlin, Chicago, Tokio, Barcelona, Istanbul, London, Mailand, Moskau,
Neu-Delhi, Paris, Peking, Prag, São Paulo und Warschau

Quintessenz

British Library Cataloguing in Publication Data

Statements : diagnostics and therapy in dental medicine
 today and in the future
 1. Dentistry
 I. Roulet, Jean-Francois II. Kappert, Henrich F.
 617.6

ISBN-13: 9781850971825

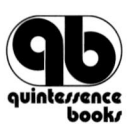

© 2009 Quintessence Publishing Co, Ltd
Quintessence Publishing Co, Ltd,
Grafton Road, New Malden, Surrey KT3 3AB,
Great Britain
www.quintpub.co.uk

Editing: Quintessence Publishing Co, Ltd, London
Layout and production: Quintesssenz Verlags-GmbH, Berlin
Printing and binding: fgb freiburger graphische betriebe, Freiburg
Printed in Germany
ISBN: 978-1-85097-182-5

# Preface

Today's science is the basis for tomorrow's products. To be successful, research and development departments must deal with the science and also be active in the field of basic research. The R&D division of Ivoclar Vivadent, headed by Dr. Volker Rheinberger, has lived by and cultivated these rules for many years. It became a tradition that every year a scientific congress took place, where scientists and researchers from all over the world were invited to Liechtenstein to present and discuss their research with our scientific staff. In 2008, we chose to expand this idea by reviewing the current state of the art of dentistry. We've looked back in order to be able to look forward. We asked many researchers and clinicians to answer important questions in today's dentistry, which is in a phase of major change. Minimally invasive dentistry, the ability to imitate the true aspect of teeth (esthetics), implantology, and digital dentistry are changing the face of today's and tomorrow's dentistry. Realizing the importance of the topic, the decision was taken to ask the participants to formulate their views and results in advance of the congress as review papers in order to summarize the content of the Ivoclar Vivadent Scientific Congress 2008 in the present book, which is dedicated to Dr. Volker Rheinberger for his 60th birthday.

This book is divided into three parts. The first is a trip through dentistry. We start with diagnosis and causal therapy (prevention). We critically assess the options for restoring decayed teeth, and the question of which way to go is debated. Furthermore, we need to understand the role of esthetics as a driving force for restoration. When it comes to replacing teeth, implants have led to completely new routes. However, it should be assessed how successfully they may replace standard therapies, and whether they may become the new standard. Dentures and orthodontics have also been influenced by the changes not only in technology, but also in perception. In the second part, the focus is on technologies. Very often they are the driving force for future application techniques. The third and final part is a look into the future, seen from a technological stance and from a broader, more generalized perspective.

Last but not least we wish to thank to all the contributors who have spontaneously agreed to put time and effort into this project. It was a pleasure to work together. We are grateful to Quintessence Publishing Company, who took on the risk and burden to produce such a high-quality book within an extremely short period.

*Professor Jean-François Roulet*
*and Professor Heinrich F. Kappert*

# Contributors

Kenneth J. Anusavice, PhD, DMD
Distinguished Professor and Chairman
Department of Dental Biomaterials, Associate Dean for
Research, University of Florida, Gainesville, Florida, USA
e-mail: kanusavice@dental.ufl.edu

Prof. Dr. med. dent. Thomas Attin
Chairman
Clinic for Preventive Dentistry, Periodontology and
Cariology,
University Zurich, Zurich, Switzerland
e-mail: thomas.attin@zzmk.unizh.ch

O. Univ.-Prof. Dr.med. dent. Hans-Peter Bantleon,
MDDentD
Chairman
Deptartment of Orthodontics
Bernhard Gottlieb University Clinic of Dentistry, Vienna,
Austria
e-mail: hans-peter.bantleon@meduniwien.ac.at

Dr. Marcio Vivan Cardoso DDS, MSc, PhD
Postdoctoral Research Fellow
Leuven BIOMAT Research Cluster, Department of
Conservative Dentistry, School of Dentistry, Oral
Pathology and Maxillo-Facial Surgery, Catholic University
of Leuven, Leuven, Belgium
e-mail: marcio.vivancardoso@med.kuleuven.be

Dr. med. dent. Alessandro Devigus
Private Practice, Bülach, Switzerland
e-mail: devigus@dentist.ch

Josephine F. Esquivel-Upshaw D.M.D., M.S.
Associate Professor and Interim Chair
College of Dentistry Department of Prosthodontics,
University of Florida
Gainesville, Florida, USA
e-mail: jesquivel@dental.ufl.edu

Prof. Dr.-Ing. Horst Fischer
Team Leader of the Section Bioceramics and Materials of
Medical Technology
Department of Ceramics and Refractory Materials, Institute
of Mineral Engineering, RWTH Aachen University,
Aachen, Germany
e-mail: h.fischer@rwth-aachen.de

Ao. Univ. Prof. Josef Freudenthaler MDDentD
Assistant Head of the Deptartment of Orthodontics
Bernhard Gottlieb University Clinic of Dentistry, Vienna,
Austria
e-mail: josef.freudenthaler@meduniwien.ac.at

Hans Geiselhöringer, ZTM
Dental X´ GmbH & Co. KG, Munich, Germany
e-mail: Verwaltung@dentalx.de

Univ.-Prof. Dr. med.dent. Reinhard Hickel
Chairman
Department of Restorative Dentistry, Dental School of the
Ludwig-Maximilians-University, Munich, Germany
e-mail: reinhard.hickel@dent.med.uni-muenchen.de

Priv.-Doz. Dr. med. dent. Stefan Holst
Associate Professor and Senior Lecturer
Dental Clinic 2 -Department of Prosthodontics
University Clinic Erlangen, Erlangen, Germany
e-mail: stefan.holst@uk-erlangen.de

Dr. rer. hum. biol. Dipl.-Ing. Nicoleta Ilie
Assistant Professor
Department of Restorative Dentistry, Dental School of the
Ludwig-Maximilians-University, Munich, Germany
e-mail: nilie@dent.med.uni-muenchen.de

Univ.-Prof. Dr. med. Dr. med. dent. Søren Jepsen, M.S.
Chairman
Dept. of Periodontology, Operative and Preventive
Dentistry, University of Bonn, Germany
e-mail: jepsen@uni-bonn.de

Univ.-Prof. i.R., Dr.rer.nat. Heinrich F. Kappert
Director Research & Development / technical
Ivoclar Vivadent, Schaan, Liechtenstein
e-mail: heinrich.kappert@ivoclarvivadent.com

Univ. -Prof. Dr. med. dent. Matthias Kern
Chairman
Department of Prosthodontics, Propaedeutics and Dental
Materials,
School of Dentistry, Christian-Albrechts University at Kiel,
Kiel, Germany
e-mail: mkern@proth.uni-kiel.de

Univ. Prof. Dr. med. dent. Claus Löst
Chairman
Department of Conservative Dentistry, School of Dental
Medicine, University Hospital, Tübingen, Germany
e-mail: claus.loest@med.uni-tuebingen.de

Prof. Dr. Bart van Meerbeek DDS, PhD
Professor of Biomaterials Science
BIOMAT Research Cluster, Department of Conservative
Dentistry, School of Dentistry, Oral Pathology and Maxillo-
Facial Surgery, Catholic University of Leuven, Leuven,
Belgium
e-mail: bart.vanmeerbeek@kuleuven.be

PD Dr. med. dent. Ina Nitschke, MPH
Head of the Clinic of Gerodontology and Special Care
Dentistry
Clinic for Masticatory Disorders, Removable
Prosthodontics and Special Care Dentistry, University of
Zurich, Zurich, Switzerland
e-mail: ina.nitschke@zzmk.uzh.ch

Prof. Dr. med. dent. Mutlu Özcan, PhD
Professor of Clinical Dental Biomaterials,
Center for Dentistry and Oral Hygiene, University Medical
Center Groningen, Groningen, The Netherlands
e-mail: mutluozcan@hotmail.com

Prof. Dr. med. dent. Sandro Palla
Chairman
Clinic for Masticatory Disorders, Removable
Prosthodontics and Special Care Dentistry, University of
Zurich, Zurich, Switzerland
e-mail: sandro.palla@zzmk.uzh.ch

Dr. med. dent. Bjarni E. Pjetursson, DDS, MAS.
Professor and Head of Reconstructive Dentistry Faculty of
Odontology, Reykjavík, Iceland
e mail: bep@hi.is

Dr. med. dent. Bernhard Christian Pseiner
Department of Orthodontics
Bernhard Gottlieb University Clinic of Dentistry, Vienna,
Austria
e-mail: bernhard.pseiner@meduniwien.ac.at

Univ.-Prof. Dr. rer. nat. Dr. rer. hum. biol. Franz-Xaver Reichl
Head of the Department of Dental Toxicology,
Department of Restorative Dentistry, Dental School of the
Ludwig-Maximilians-University, Munich, Germany
e-mail: reichl@lmu.de

Prof. Dr. med. dent. Jean-François Roulet
Director Research & Development / clinical
Ivoclar Vivadent, Schaan, Liechtenstein
e-mail: jean-francois.roulet@ivoclarvivadent.com

PD Dr. med. dent. Giovanni E. Salvi
Department of Periodontology
School of Dental Medicine, University of Bern,
Bern, Switzerland
e-mail: giovanni.salvi@zmk.unibe.ch

PD Dr. med. dent. Patrick R. Schmidlin
Senior Research Fellow
Clinic for Preventive Dentistry, Periodontology and
Cariology, University of Zurich, Zurich, Switzerland
e-mail: patrick.schmidlin@zzmk.uzh.ch

Dott. Roberto Spreafico
Private Practice
Busto Arsizio (Varese), Italy
e-mail: robertosprea@tiscalinet.it

Prof. Dr. Svante Twetman
Chairman
Department of Cariology and Endodontics, Faculty of
Health Sciences, University of Copenhagen, Copenhagen,
Denmark
e-mail: stw@odont.ku.dk

Prof. Dr. David C Watts, PhD, DSc, FRSC, FInstP, FADM
Professor of Biomaterials Science
Biomaterials Research Group, School of Dentistry and
Photon Science Institute, The University of Manchester.
Manchester, United Kingdom.
e-mail: david.watts@manchester.ac.uk

Dr. Yasuhiro Yoshida DDS, PhD
Associate Professor
Department of Biomaterials, Okayama University Graduate
School of Medicine, Dentistry and Pharmaceutical Sciences,
Okayama, Japan
e-mail: yasuhiro@md.okayama-u.ac.jp

# Table of Contents

# Diagnostics of Dental Diseases – How do we Distinguish Ourselves from our Grandparents?

Thomas Attin and Patrick R. Schmidlin

## Introduction

Dental diseases can be classified into two main types, namely the diseases of the dental hard tissues (enamel and dentin) and the diseases of the soft tissue (gingiva and periodontium). Several methods have been described and are used to exclude, detect, monitor and classify dental diseases – these might be distinguished from traditional methods, such as the visual-tactile method for detection of carious lesions and novel methods that have emerged in recent decades. The novel methods are often designed to allow for detection of the respective disease at a very early stage. This feature allows already mild forms of the disease to be treated, thus preventing further tissue damage or destruction.[1] The development of novel methods may also reflect changes in the prevalence and severity of dental disease over the years, thus rendering detection methods with improved sensitivity more necessary. However, it should be noted that the advent and use of new, more sophisticated methods does not automatically lead to a better and more reliable diagnosis of a disease. It has been shown that the error rates for the correct diagnosis of a disease depend on the one hand on the familiarity of the clinican with the diagnostic tool, and on the other

hand on overconfidence of practitioners.[2] The latter means that practitioners under appreciate the likelihood that their diagnoses are wrong. This estimation often occurs when clinicians are highly experienced or lack knowledge. In this sense it was, for example, shown that radiographs are judged differently by radiologists than by other physicians.[2]

In the present chapter the terms sensitivity and specificity are used to describe the reliability of the different methods. The ability of a method to detect a truly existing pathology is described by its sensitivity and the ability to identify the existing absence of pathology is given by its specificity. Thus, a high sensitivity is needed for detection of a disease and to initiate an appropriate therapy and a high specificity is needed to prevent unnecessary and incorrect treatments. As a control, so-called gold standard methods are needed, such as histological assessments of caries lesions. Other important issues are the positive and negative predictive values, which indicate the probability that, for example, a tooth with a positive (or negative) finding in the test method really does show the disease (or not). These values have to be considered and mathematically adjusted for the prevalence of the disease in the examined population. This means that (under the premise of a defined sensitivity and specificity) with an increasing prevalence the positive predictive value also increases, whereas the negative predictive value decreases.

In the following chapters, traditional and novel developments for diagnosis of oral soft and hard tissue diseases are described and judged. Thereby, focus is placed on the most common hard tissue diseases, such as caries and erosion, and soft tissue diseases, such as gingivitis and periodontitis. The overview of the diagnosis methods is intended to primarily focus on methods often described in the literature. Thus, future trends and methods rarely described or used are not explicitly included.

# Hard Tissue Diseases
## Dental Caries

### Definition

Dental caries is the result of a chemical dissolution of the dental hard tissues, induced by metabolic components such as acids and enzymes generated in the dental bacterial plaque (biofilm) covering the affected area of the tooth. Dental caries may appear clinically in different ways and severities, from a mild dissolution of the outermost enamel to the complete destruction of the organic and inorganic components of the hard tissues. In the very early stages, the caries lesion resembles the appearance of an acid-induced enamel erosion. At this stage the lesion may be categorized as subclinical, being in a dynamic state of progression and regression. In later stages, the caries process will lead to a so-called white-spot lesion (initial lesion), which is more or less limited to the enamel and shows a subsurface mineral loss below a mildly demineralized enamel surface, clinically (i.e. with naked eyes) often showing no or barely visible cavitation. When the carious process progresses, it will reach the dentin of the tooth, where enzymatic degradation of the organic components will take place. When the dentin (and especially deeper parts of the dentin) is involved, the carious affected enamel surface

will often break down, clinically resulting in a cavity. The term 'hidden caries' describes the situation, where the enamel seems to be clinically intact above the carious destruction in dentin.

### Epidemiology

Although dental caries, for example, fissure caries, is an ancient disease, the current patterns of caries onset occur with the increased consumption of processed food and the greater availability of sugar. The prevalence of dental caries in high-income countries has declined for all age groups since the mid-1980s.[3] This fact may have implications on the positive and negative predictive values of certain tests, as mentioned above. In those countries, an uneven distribution of caries especially in the younger population has been noted, meaning that the proportion of children with low decayed, missing, filled (DMF)- scores has increased, whereas the percentage of children with high caries scores has decreased. However, it should be noticed that in epidemiological studies most clinically or radiographically detectable dentinal lesions with cavitation are categorized as 'caries', whereas teeth with enamel lesions (with or without cavitation) are often considered as 'caries free'. This means that the diagnostic threshold levels have an impact on epidemiological data, and also on the decision of how to treat the patient.

Epidemiological data also give a hint to the site-specificity of caries in distinct age groups. Estimates indicate that especially in children about 90% of dental caries occurs in pits and fissures.[4] In the elderly population the number of root caries lesions is higher compared with younger patients groups.[5]

### Methods for Detection, Monitoring and Classification of Dental Caries

An overview of the accuracy of the data for the methods most often described in the literature are given in Table 1-1. The data presented are based on the excellent overviews written by Bader et al.[6] and Bader and Shugar[7].

All methods for caries detection should help the practitioner to obtain information about the simple existence of caries or a caries risk, in order to elaborate a treatment plan for the patient. With respect to initiation of restorative approaches it is necessary to know, whether or not the lesion is cavitated, and whether or not progression of the lesion is (highly) probable. A feature lacking in many studies is the fact that a real clinical gold standard is missing and that only *in vitro* or *ex vivo* studies using histological examination as the gold standard provide most appropriate conditions to validate a method for caries detection. Thus, studies comparing two or more methods under the *in vivo* situation are not very helpful in showing the limitations of either of the methods applied.

## Traditional Methods

### Visual, Visual-Tactile and Radiographic Methods and Fiber-Optic Transillumination

The visual-tactile method relies on a combined visual and tactile examination of the tooth using a probe for searching of the carious lesion. In former times the dental probe was used to decide whether or not a non-continuous surface with a cavity existed. By doing so, the sharp probe was forced onto the surface leading to damage of the fragile demineralized surface layer of a lesion. It is generally thought that remineralization of caries lesion depends on the existence of a non-cavitated surface. To avoid this undesired event, it is nowadays recommended to refrain from using a sharp probe and to use a blunt probe for careful cleaning of pits and fissures during visual examination. The traditional visual and visual-tactile methods focused on the detection of cavitated lesions only in a dichotomous pattern (yes/no). Thus, early enamel lesions were not recorded, and monitoring of a caries development was not possible. Moreover, caries lesions at proximal sites, which have not caused cavitation of the occlusal surface, could only be guessed by the greyish discoloration of the cariously undermined proximal tooth area, or after separa-

tion of the teeth with, for example, orthodontic rubber rings. The visual inspection mostly shows a fair accuracy to detect sound hard tissue, but has shortcomings in detection of caries sites (low sensitivity). The same is also true for bitewing radiography.

The periodic examination using bitewing radiography for monitoring of proximal and occlusal caries was introduced by Raper in 1925,[8] who had already pointed out that this tool may encounter some difficulties, such as a frequent underestimation of the depth of caries lesion. Moreover, approximately 30 to 60% of the mineral has to be lost before the caries process will be visible as a dark shadow on the radiograph.[9] Some other shortcomings are: the tendency to misinterpret radiolucencies (e.g. triangular shaped radiolucencies at the cervical area), the low validity to diagnose early lesions, differences in successive bitewings owing to different angles of projections, and overlapping of adjacent proximal sites or restoratives. The depths of the proximal radiolucencies are most commonly classified into five degrees, with a higher risk of lesion progression and cavitation when dentin is affected.[10,11] Although uncertainty of the real depth and status of cavitation exists and despite the shortcomings mentioned, bitewing radiography is still one of the main tools for caries diagnosis.

Fiber-optic transillumination (FOTI) is a qualitative method for caries evaluation, which was introduced in the 1970s. With FOTI, a tooth is illuminated with white light from a cold-light source, often described as an alternative to bitewing radiography owing to the absence of radiation. The specificity of the method is high, especially for proximal lesions.[12] However, FOTI shows a rather low sensitivity for both occlusal dentinal and enamel lesions and also for proximal cavitated caries. This renders the method not suitable as a true alternative to bitewing radiography.[13]

### Developments Based on Traditional Methods

In order to better discriminate between different stages of occlusal caries, Ekstrand et al[14] introduced more detailed criteria for the visual inspection. `Using these criteria the sensitivity (0.92 to 0.97) and specificity

**Table 1-1** Median prevalence, sensitivity and specificity of different diagnostic tools for caries assessment in studies using histology as the gold standard, adopted from Bader et al.[6] and calculated according to values given by Bader and Shugars[7]

| Method | Surface: Extent of lesion | Prevalence (%) | Sensitivity (%) | Specificity (%) |
|---|---|---|---|---|
| Visual | occlusal surface | | | |
| | cavitated | 51 | 51 | 89 |
| | dentinal | 44 | 25 | 91 |
| | enamel | 21 | 66 | 69 |
| | any | 75 | 62 | 74 |
| | proximal surfaces | | | |
| | cavitated | nr** | 94* | 92* |
| Visual-tactile | occlusal surfaces | | | |
| | cavitated | nr** | 92* | 85* |
| | dentinal | 29 | 19 | 97 |
| | any | 40 | 39 | 94 |
| | proximal surfaces | | | |
| | cavitated | 6 | 32 | 99 |
| | dentinal | nr** | 50* | 71* |
| Radiographic | occlusal surfaces | | | |
| | dentinal | 55 | 54 | 85 |
| | enamel | 18 | 28 | 76 |
| | any | 84 | 27 | 95 |
| | proximal surfaces | | | |
| | cavitated | 9 | 66 | 97 |
| | dentinal | 25 | 40 | 96 |
| | enamel | 25 | 41 | 78 |
| | any | 66 | 49 | 88 |
| Electric conductance | occlusal surfaces | | | |
| | dentinal | 37 | 91 | 80 |
| | enamel | 24* | 65* | 73* |
| | any | 64 | 70 | 85 |
| Fiber-optic transillumination | occlusal surfaces | | | |
| | dentinal | 36* | 14* | 95* |
| | enamel | 24* | 21* | 88* |
| | proximal surfaces | | | |
| | cavitated | 6* | 4* | 100* |
| Diagnodent | occlusal surfaces | | | |
| | enamel | 35 | 67 | 83 |
| | dentinal | 29 | 81 | 86 |
| | any | 32 | 93 | 50 |

**      not reported
*       mean value is given, as only 1 study was available

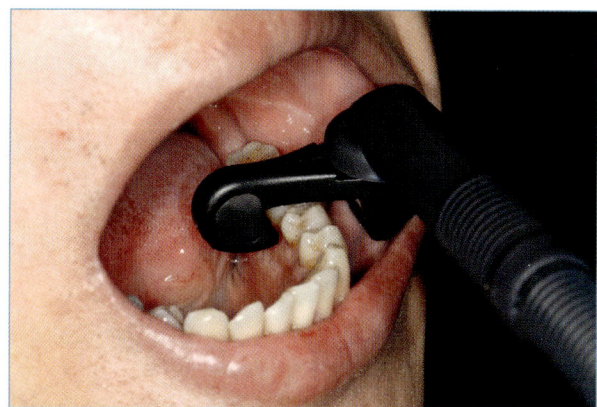

Fig 1-1a  Intraoral application of the digital imaging fiber optic transillumination (DIFOTI) for detection of proximal caries. *(Courtesy of Prof Dr Karl-Heinz Kunzelmann, Munich).*

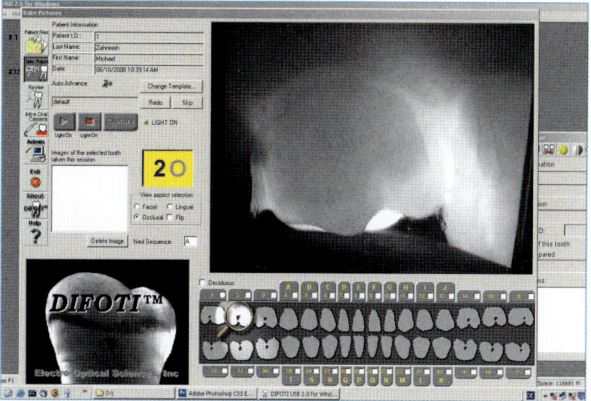

Fig 1-1b  Screen-shot of an image generated by DIFOTI for caries examination. *(Courtesy of Prof Dr Karl-Heinz Kunzelmann, Munich).*

(0.85 to 0.93) to detect dentinal lesions could be increased, compared with the classical dichotomous approach.

With respect to radiography, digital intraoral radiography, which was introduced in the 1980s, allows the application of computer-automated algorithms to generate subtraction images useful for monitoring caries processes.[15] Moreover, the digital image can be further processed (adjustment of contrast or brightness) to improve the quality of the radiograph image for caries detection. This might help to identify caries more easily, compared with using conventional film-based radiographs. However, studies comparing the efficacy of digital imaging versus film-based (traditional) imaging revealed that both tools are not significantly different in their ability to record dental disease states. Radiation dose and, thus, X-ray exposure of the patient, is lower when performing digitally processed images. However, this advantage is limited, as due to the ease and speed of producing digital images, clinicians tend to retake digital images more than conventional ones in cases of problems occurring, such as wrong angulation or missing of anatomical regions on the image.[16,17]

Digital imaging fiber-optic transillumination (DIFOTI) is a more recent development combining FOTI with a digital intraoral camera (Fig 1-1a). The

images are captured and displayed on a computer screen, which allows the observer to interpret the image subjectively. As the images are stored on a computer, the method allows monitoring of a clinical situation (Fig 1-1b). In an *in vitro* study, DIFOTI was indicated to have a higher sensitivity than radiographic assessment for detecting lesions on interproximal, occlusal and smooth surfaces.[18] However, data using this new method is scarce in the literature. Moreover the method needs to be developed further before it can be applied routinely in clinical situations.[19]

## Novel Developments

### *Electrical Impedance-based Method*

These devices are based on the theory that sound dental hard tissue, especially enamel, shows higher electrical resistance than demineralized, porous enamel. As the pores are filled with liquid from saliva, the electrical conductance increases with increasing enamel porosity. The electrical resistance of teeth was already used in 1978 for monitoring occlusal caries. Further developments have brought the ECM device (Electrical Caries Monitor, Lode Diagnostics BV, The Netherlands) (Figs. 1-2a and b), and its suitability for assessing occlusal surfaces has been evaluated since the 1990s in a number of

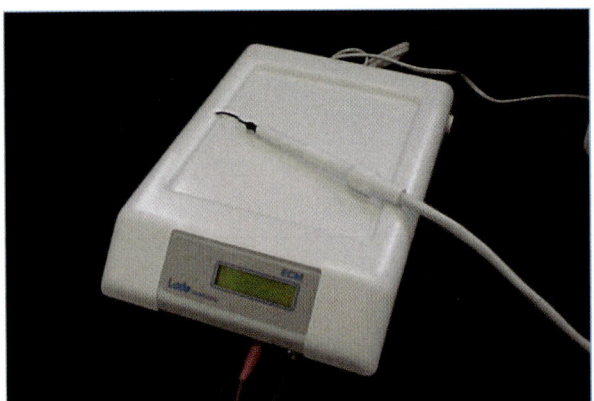

**Fig 1-2a** Electrical conductance measurement (ECM). *(Courtesy of PD Dr Rainer Haak, Cologne).*

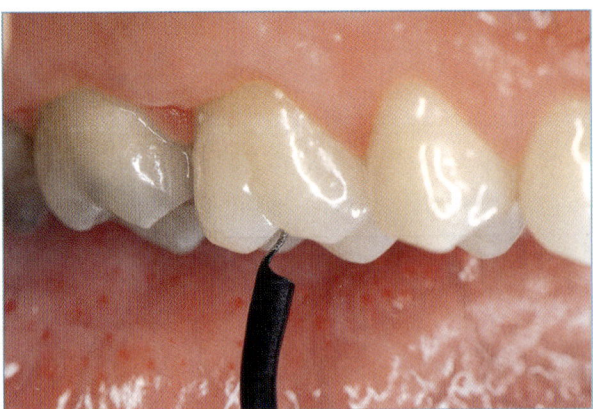

**Fig 1-2b** Intraoral application of tip of the ECM for spot measurement. *(Courtesy of PD Dr Rainer Haak, Cologne).*

studies.[20-22] The sensitivity for site-specific detection of dentinal caries ranged from 0.67 to 0.96 with specificity from 0.71 to 0.98, which could be regarded as acceptable.[22,23] However, some conditional factors, such as degree of dehydration of tooth tissue, the maturation of the enamel and temperature variations affected the accuracy of the measurements. Thus, until now, the use of ECM is not well established in clinical practice and needs more research and development to make the procedure less delicate to environmental and technical influences.

### Optically Based Methods

#### ♦ *Visible light fluorescence*

In brief, quantitative visible light fluorescence (QLF, Inspektor Research Systems, The Netherlands) was developed as a non-destructive diagnostic method for the longitudinal assessment of early caries lesions.[24] The method applies a xenon gas discharge lamp to illuminate a tooth with filtered blue–violet light to provoke its natural fluorescence. It is assumed that the natural fluorescence is caused by fluorophores, which are predominately located at the dentin–enamel junction (DEJ) and in the dentin. Due to higher scattering in carious enamel, less excitation light reaches the fluorescing DEJ and underlying dentin and less fluorescence from the

DEJ and dentin is able to find its way back through the carious lesion. Therefore, the lesion appears dark in contrast to the surrounding, fluorescing area of the tooth. The area of interest is imaged by a CCD-video camera through an optical high-pass filter that blocks the excitation light and allows only the fluorescing light to pass. When the tooth dries out, the enamel fluorescence becomes stronger. Additionally, the scattering effects of porosities also become stronger due to a more rapid loss of water from the sites with open porosities, for example of active lesions. This allows for discrimination of arrested lesions and active enamel lesions.[25,26] Due to high inter- and intra-examiner agreements, and good sensitivity and specificity values, the method is suitable for monitoring early lesions very well.[27] However, the system is still not suitable to control proximal lesions, although some developments are focused in solving this problem.

#### ♦ *Laser fluorescence - Diagnodent*

The Diagnodent (KaVo, Germany) device is a small laser system that produces an excitation light with a 655nm wavelength. In its first launch, Diagnodent was designed to mainly detect hidden caries of the fissure system. A small tip transports the light to the tooth surface and re-collects the resultant fluorescence of the caries lesion. The fluorescence is induced in several

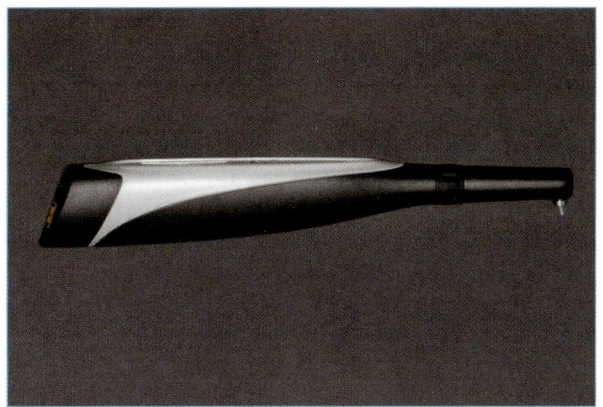

Fig 1-3a  The Diagnodent Pen.

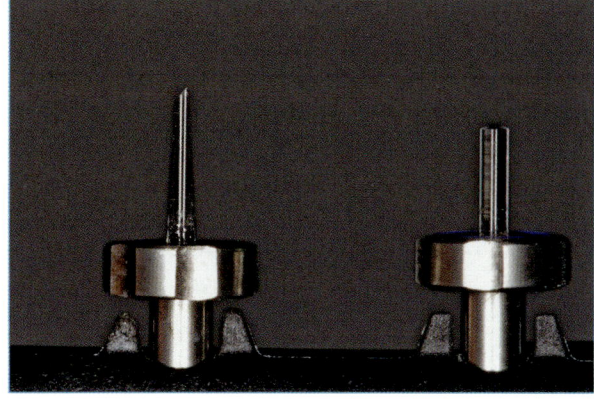

Fig 1-3b  Close-up of the tips for detection of proximal (**left**) and occlusal (**right**) caries.

ways, including the presence of porphyrins in the lesion generated by bacteria. The inter- and intra-examiner readings are in good agreement, so that the system is useful for monitoring. A systematic review has emphasized that Diagnodent is more sensitive than traditional methods. However, it has an increased likelihood of false-positive diagnoses, which limits its routine use in dental practice.[7] Due to a smaller design of the tip, the further development of the method (Diagnodent Pen) (Fig 1-3a) now allows for assessing both proximal and fissure lesions (Fig 1-3b). Using the more recent Diagnodent Pen for assessing occlusal surfaces leads to results that are comparable with the classical Diagnodent.[28] However, only a few studies are available using the Diagnodent Pen for detection of proximal lesions, so no judgement on this particular use is waranted.

# Erosion

## Definition

Erosion has been described as 'the physical result of a pathologic, chronic, localized loss of dental hard tissue that is chemically etched away from the tooth surface'.[29] This chemical attack may be induced by acidic substances and/or chelation without bacterial involvement.

Therefore, dietary acids or gastric acid are common causes of dental erosion. The irreversible loss of dental hard tissue induced by the acids is accompanied by a demineralization and softening of the tooth surface. During the first stages only the enamel is affected, later the dentin is exposed, often leading to hypersensitivity of the teeth.

## Epidemiology

Most of the epidemiological studies previously carried out did not focus on the presence of dental erosions. Since the 1990s, more epidemiological studies have started to collect data on tooth erosion. Some of these studies hint that an increasing trend in the prevalence of erosions in all age groups exists.[30] However, this trend is not clearly shown in all epidemiological surveys.

## Methods for Detection, Monitoring and Classification

There are distinctly fewer methods described for detection of erosion compared with those described for caries. This is especially true for clinical applications, whereas for *in vitro* assessment of hard tissue loss various techniques are described.[31] Traditionally, like other signs of hard tissue loss (abrasion, attrition), erosions are assessed by visual examination and classified by index systems, which allow for a rough discrimination with regard to the amount of the hard tissue lost.[32] Higher scores are given when dentin is exposed. It was recently shown that these classifications are poorly reproducible, and further grading procedures are necessary.[33-35] However, with the visual method it is difficult to detect the very early signs of erosion or to monitor erosive lesions properly, even if new indices intend to better discriminate between the different degrees of erosions.

Some methods originally designed for caries monitoring (e.g. QLF) have also been used in experimental studies for erosion assessment.[31] On the other hand, computer-based techniques have been developed presenting a method to obtain digital surface models using electroconductive replicas generated from silicone impressions of teeth taken at different time points.[36] However, none of these new approaches has gained entrance into a routine dental examination.

## Diagnosis of Hard Tissue Diseases – How do we Distinguish ourselves from our Grandparents?

There is no easy answer to this provocative question. On the one hand, various new and validated methods are described and have been developed for better detection and monitoring of dental hard diseases, especially of early caries lesions. This would mean that we distinguish ourselves from our grandparents at least by having access to more sophisticated methods. On the other hand, the use of some of these techniques is still limited to application in scientific and experimental studies. This might be due to the fact that the devices are more expensive and that their additional value for gaining a more precise diagnosis is not given or accepted by the practitioners. Little is known about the methods and techniques really applied in routine dental examinations in dental practices. This lack of information refers to the more sophisticated methods using new technologies, but also to further developments of traditional

methods, such as the better discrimination of the early caries by using the Ekstrand-classification for the visual examination – a method that could be easily implemented without buying any additional tools and only by spending some more time and awareness during examination. However, it should be appreciated that various methods for detection of the early signs of caries have been developed (and are still to come). This might give a hint that in the mind of the modern clinician the concept of understanding caries as a process starting from superficial mineral dissolution to cavitation as a final result is anchored. Accepting this view of the caries process has led to elaborate concepts to treat the various appearances of caries differently, either preventive or restorative, and to place more focus on implementation of preventive care. This might be the main issue modern clinicians that distinguishes from more traditional clinicians.

# Periodontal Diseases
## Definitions and Clinical Signs

Healthy gingiva acts as a sealing soft tissue collar around the tooth. Bacteria (plaque or biofilm) can cause inflammation and lead to gingivitis, which represents the primary form of periodontal diseases. This infection process results in classical cardinal symptoms of inflammation-like redness, swelling, bleeding, exudation, but rarely pain.

The term periodontitis literally means 'inflammation around the tooth'. It is a complex infectious disease modulated by several host and environmental factors, leading to more severe tissue inflammation, attachment fiber loss and bone resorption. Disease progression can be chronic, aggressive or acute. Clinically, the marginal gingiva usually shows classical signs of inflammation. At later stages, teeth may secondarily become loose and start to migrate. In most cases, it is painless.

# Pathogenesis

During the last 50 years, the prevailing clinical concept of pathogenesis of chronic periodontitis included: (a) the marginal accumulation and maturation of plaque and the development of gingivitis,[37] (b) the apical migration of bacteria and the associated inflammation process associated with connective tissue destruction[38] and (c) the apical extension of the epithelium, the formation of a periodontal pocket and loss of marginal bone.[39]

Periodontitis represents a mixed infection. However, it is associated with relatively specific groups of indigenous oral bacteria.[40] Susceptibility seems variable and depends on host responses to periodontal pathogens.[41] Progression and clinical features are influenced by both acquired and genetic factors.

# Epidemiology

Data show that gingivitis is sometimes found in early childhood, is more prevalent and severe in adolescence, and then tends to level off in older age groups, but still remains highly prevalent.[42]

The percentage of the population aged 35 to 44 years with periondontitis with shallow pockets of 4 to 5 mm probing depth(Community Periodontal Index of Treatment Needs [CPITN] code 3); in Europe is 37% (95% confidence interval [CI] 31 to 42%). In non-European countries, the mean values range from 33 to 40%.[42] The number of subjects with deep pockets (CPITN 4; > 6 mm probing pocket depth) accounts for 14% (95% CI: 11 to 17%) in Europe. In non-European countries, this value ranges from 9 to 36%.

Based on the evaluation of archaeological material in Britain, it was found that the prevalence of periodontitis appears to have remained virtually constant during the past 3000 years.[43] However, it was suggested that a periodontitis epidemic fuelled by smoking remained hidden for most of the 20th century.[44]

# Current Clinical Methods for Periodontal Diagnosis

## Self-Reported Diagnosis

A primary sign of inflammation is bleeding of the gums. Self-reported gingivitis based on gingival bleeding seems to correlate with clinical examinations.[45] However, self-reporting of periodontal disease in general is not successful, as many people with some indications of periodontal disease appear to be unaware of the disease.[45,46]

Secondary signs of periodontitis, such as increased tooth mobility and migration, also have limited value for self-diagnosis, although this is controversial.[45]

## Clinical Diagnosis

Diagnosis and classification of periodontal diseases is still based almost entirely on traditional clinical assessments as follows[47,48]: (a) presence or absence of clinical signs of inflammation (e.g. bleeding upon probing); (b) probing depths; (c) extent and pattern of loss of clinical attachment and bone; (d) patient's medical and dental histories; and (e) presence or absence of miscellaneous signs and symptoms, including pain, ulceration, and amount of observable plaque and calculus.[49,50]

### Visual Signs of Causative Factors of Inflammation

Primary causative factors, that is, bacterial hard and soft deposits, can be assessed using several indices: oral hygiene index[51], plaque index[52], calculus index and the plaque control report.[53] However, these indices are applied in patient motivation and hygiene control rather than as a diagnostic tool.

Characteristics of the inflamed soft tissues, in contrast, may indicate disease, for example, swelling, color and surface texture (Fig 1-4a). However, per se, they also do not allow the detection and diagnosis of the actual amount of tissue destruction.

### Periodontal Probing

The periodontal probe was introduced in 1925 (Simonton) and is still the prevailing and indispensable

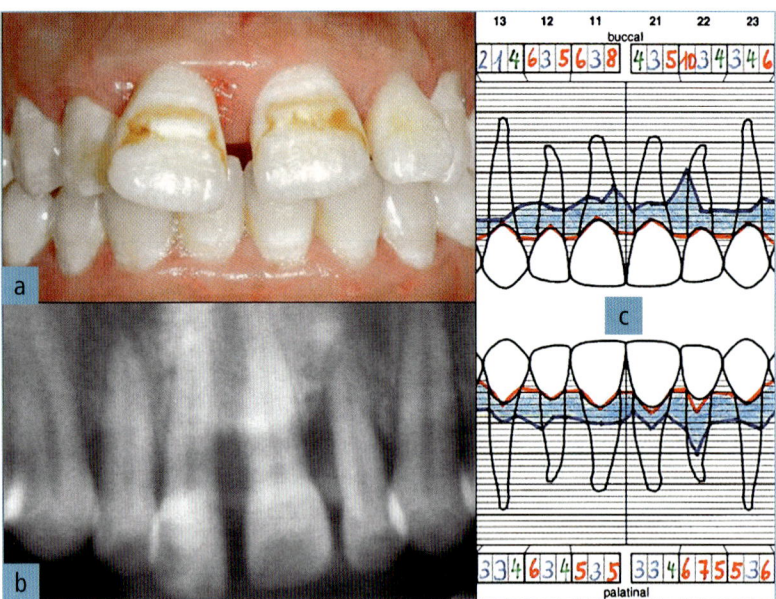

**Fig1-4a–c** Intraoral frontal view of a 22-year-old female patient (systemically healthy, non-smoker) with distinct local signs of gingival inflammation (redness, swelling and ulceration) and tooth migration (**a**). Only radiographs (**b**) and probing (**c**) revealed the severe bone resorption, periodontal pocket formation and attachment loss, especially in the maxillary. The case was diagnosed as generalized aggressive periodontitis.

tool for daily clinical periodontal examination. Its primary purpose is to measure the level of pocket formation, attachment level (Fig 1-4c) and, very importantly, bleeding as a major indicator for inflammation.

The diagnostic accuracy of probing depth depends on several factors: probe geometry, probing force and direction. Penetration of the probe largely depends on the inflammatory status of the tissues and the histological attachment is not directly comparable with the clinical attachment levels.[54,55] Several automated probes have been introduced to improve accuracy of the measurements. Automated probes have been developed and marketed, such as the Florida,[56] the Toronto probe[57] or others. They are especially useful when conducting longitudinal studies as they have an accuracy of greater than 0.2 mm. However, these devices also have their limitations and offer little advantage for general practice.[58]

Several indices to assess the inflammatory activity of the pockets have been introduced: gingival sulcus bleeding index,[59] papilla bleeding index[60] and 'bleeding on probing'. The gingival bleeding index by Löe and Silness is a combination of visual and bleeding aspects.[61]

## Conventional Radiographs

Radiographs are commonly used in addition to the clinical examination. They aim to visualize the bony component and offer a two-dimensional view. An accurate projection technique is inevitable to avoid distortion of the obtained images. Radiographs have low sensitivity, but higher specificity, particularly as the use of non-standardized radiographs tends to underestimate the clinical results as they do not register alveolar bone loss until 30 to 50% of the bone mineral are destroyed.[62]

Subtraction radiography offers the possibility of monitoring changes in bone morphology. Using standardized and digitized images, they can identify bone loss (or gain) with rather high sensitivity and specificity.[63] This method can additionally help to minimize intra-examiner errors.[64] However, the technique is challenging, especially when obtaining perfectly aligned images under clinical routine conditions. The technique also requires additional hardware and software.

## Supplemental Diagnostic Methods

### Microbiological Evaluation

Bacteria play a pivotal role in the etiology of periodontal disease as mentioned above. There has been a great debate whether or not the mass of unspecific bacteria or rather specific pathogens play a causative role in the development of chronic and aggressive forms of periodontitis. However, a great body of literature exists implicating bacteria such as *Porphyromonas gingivalis*, *Tannerella forsythensis*, and *Treponema denticola* (red complex), and others in the development of chronic periodontitis.[40,65] The presence of *Aggregatibacter actinomycetemcomitans* (formerly known as *Actinomyces actinomycetemcomitans*) has been implicated as an etiological factor in aggressive forms of periodontitis.[66] Microbiological testing could, therefore, be used for diagnosis or treatment (i.e. adequate use of antibiotics) of periodontal disease. These issues have also been controversially discussed. In terms of periodontal diagnosis, such a test should be able to accurately identify the presence or absence of disease and eventually discern between chronic and aggressive forms. However, it has been shown that the presence of the above-mentioned specific bacteria complexes does not necessarily lead to periodontitis and could not discriminate between subjects with aggressive or chronic forms.[67] The difference between health and disease seems to relate to the proportions and to some extent the levels of *Aggregatibacter actinomycetemcomitans* and other complex species.[68]

### Biomarkers

Supplemental tests aim to measure: (a) substances associated with putative pathogens, (b) host-derived enzymes, (c) tissue breakdown products or d) inflammatory mediators.[69]

The so-called benzoyl-DL-arginine-naphthylamide (BANA) test measures indirectly the production of trypsin-like enzymes by periodontal pathogens capable of hydrolyzing β-naphtylamide derivatives, mainly BANA. However, this test produces a high proportion of false positive results in healthy sites.[70]

Host-derived enzymes, tissue breakdown products, and inflammatory mediators can also be collected in the crevicular fluid. They are released from host cells and tissues during the development and progression of periodontal infections. Some of these substances have been suggested as possible markers for the detection of progressing periodontal lesions for chair-side tests. As one example, the β-glucuronidase (BG) diagnostic kit has been developed with a sensitivity and specificity of 89%, each. Several other test kits, for example for prostaglandin E2 as an inflammatory mediator, have also been developed.[71] Most of these have not been commercialized.

### IL-1 Polymorphism

A host-based test for susceptibility to periodontitis is currently available to practitioners in the form of a genetic test for polymorphisms in the interleukin-1 (IL-1) gene cluster.[72] Approximately 30% of Caucasians are positive for a composite genotype of IL1A and IL1B polymorphisms consisting of allele 2 of both IL1A + 4845 (or the concordant -889) and IL1B + 3954. Subjects having this composite genotype may be at an increased risk of periodontal disease,[72-74] probably due to a hypersecretion of IL1B in response to inflammation-inducing stimuli. In contrast, there is insufficient evidence that a positive IL1 genotype status contributes to progression of periodontitis and/or treatment outcomes.[75]

## Measurement of Pocket Temperature, pH and Blood Perfusion

It has been shown that there is a positive correlation between elevated subgingival temperature and inflammation in infection status.[76-78] However, measurement of temperature alone has a low sensitivity of 31%, but a high specificity of 97%. Discriminant analysis using the percentage of sites with suppuration and redness, loss of attachment level of > 3 mm and mean site temperature, 'predicted' disease activity more correctly with a sensitivity, specificity and overall agreement of roughly 75%. There are studies, which have evaluated the gingival crevicular fluid pH changes that can occur during the progression of periodontitis.[79,80] Although the techniques may have applications in screening for disease activity in clinical practice, additional work to confirm the observations is necessary to corroborate these associations.[81]

In addition, inflammation changes the microcirculatory and micromorphological dynamics of human gingiva.[82] Laser Doppler flow registrations have shown to positively correlate with the degree of gingival inflammation. However, modifications of the probe are needed to enhance its clinical applicability in clinical examination of periodontal diseases.[83]

## Current Periodontal Diagnosis, Past and Future: How do we Distinguish ourselves from our Grandparents?

Since ancient medicine, gingival inflammation and periodontitis have mainly been recognized by changes in tooth mobility, gingival architecture or color and bad breath.[84] The examination of occlusion and the measuring as well as the recording of tooth mobility were a great part of diagnosis of periodontal disease in the first half of the 20th century. With this approach, teeth affected by periodontitis were identified at a very late stage in the process of periodontal destruction. However, in the last few decades, this topic has lost much of its attraction and nowadays traditional periodontal diagnostic methods mainly include assessment of clinical parameters and radiographs. Measuring pockets and bleeding still remain the primary tools in daily clinical practice allowing for rapid screening, diagnosis and monitoring of periodontal disease. This method is simple and cost effective and, therefore, represents the basis for comparison against any of the proposed diagnostic tests. Though efficient, these conventional techniques are inherently limited in that only a rather historical perspective and not a current appraisal, of disease status and etiology can be determined.

The complexity of the disease, including several bacterial and host defense mechanisms will lead to the development of additional, more sophisticated diagnostic methods and tools. To date, no test has entered the periodontal market that has broad acceptance among practitioners and gained ultimate evidence to have higher sensitivity/specificity and being more reliable. However, new tests will be developed in the near future to detect biomarkers in other oral fluids (e.g. saliva) representing inflammatory mediators and several specific collagen degradation and bone turnover-related molecules, which may have emerging potential as possible measures of periodontal disease activity.[85]

## References

1. Zandona AF, Zero DT. Diagnostic tools for early caries detection. J Am Dent Assoc 2006;137:1675–84;quiz 1730.
2. Berner ES, Graber ML. Overconfidence as a cause of diagnsotic error in medicine. Am J Med 2008;121:S2–S23.
3. Bratthall D, Hansel-Petersson G, Sundberg H. Reasons for the caries decline: what do the experts believe? Eur J Oral Sci 1996;104:416–422.
4. Kaste LM, Selwitz RH, Oldakowski RJ, Brunelle JA, Winn DM, Brown LJ. Coronal caries in the primary and permanent dentition of children and adolescents 1-17 years of age: United States, 1988-1991. J Dent Res 1996;75 Spec No;631–641.
5. Hahn P, Reinhardt D, Schaller HG, Hellwig E. Root lesions in a group of 50-60 year-old Germans related to clinical and social factors. Clin Oral Invest 1999;3:168–174.
6. Bader JD, Shugars DA, Bonito AJ. Systematic reviews of selected dental caries diagnostic and management methods. J Dent Educ 2001;65:960–968.
7. Bader JD, Shugars DA. A systematic review of the performance of a laser fluorescence device for detecting caries. J Am Dent Asso 2004;135:1413–1426.
8. Raper HR. Practical clinical preventive dentistry based upon periodic roentgen-ray examinations. J Am Dent Assoc 1925;12:1084–1100.
9. Topazian RG, Goldberg MN. Oral and maxillofacial infections. Philadelphia: Saunders, 1987.p. 208–209.
10. Mejare I, Kallest l C, Stenlund H. Incidence and progression of approximal caries from 11 to 22 years of age in Sweden: A prospective radiographic study. Caries Res 1999;33:93–100.
11. Stenlund H, Mejare I, Kallestal C. Caries rates related to approximal caries at ages 11-13: a 10-year follow-up study in Sweden. J Dent Res 2002;81:455–458.

12. van Rijkom HM, Verdonschot EH. Factors involved in validity measurements of diagnostic tests for approximal caries—a meta-analysis. Caries res1995;29:364–370.

13. Young DA, Featherstone JD. Digital imaging fiber-optic trans-illumination, F-speed radiographic film and depth of approximal lesions. J Am Dent Assoc 2005;136:1682–1687.

14. Ekstrand KR, Ricketts DN, Kidd EA. Reproducibility and accuracy of three methods for assessment of demineralization depth of the occlusal surface: an in vitro examination. Caries Re 1997;31:224–231.

15. Parks ET, Williamson GF. Digital radiography: an overview. J Contemp Dent Pract 2002;3:23–39.

16. Wenzel A, Moystad A. Decision criteria and characteristics of Norwegian general dental practitioners selecting digital radiography. Dentomaxillofac Radiol 2001;30:197–202.

17. Berkhout WE, Sanderink GC, Van der Stelt PF. Does digital radiography increase the number of intraoral radiographs? A questionnaire study of Dutch dental practices. Dentomaxillofac Radiol 2003;32:124–127.

18. Schneiderman A, Elbaum M, Shultz T, Keem S, Greenebaum M, Driller J. Assessment of dental caries with Digital Imaging Fiber-Optic TransIllumination (DIFOTI): in vitro study. Caries Res 1997;31:103–110.

19. Tranaeus S, Shi XQ, Angmar-Mansson B. Caries risk assessment: methods available to clinicians for caries detection. Community Dent Oral Epidemiol 2005;33:265–273.

20. Huysmans MC, Longbottom C, Hintze H, Verdonschot EH. Surface-specific electrical occlusal caries diagnosis: reproducibility, correlation with histological lesion depth, and tooth type dependence. Caries Res 1998;32:330–336.

21. Wicht MJ, Haak R, Stutzer H, Strohe D, Noack MJ. Intra- and interexaminer variability and validity of laser fluorescence and electrical resistance readings on root surface lesions. Caries Res 2002;36:241–248.

22. Huysmans MCDNJM. Electrical measurements for early caries detection. In: Stookey GK, editors. Early detection of dental caries II. Indianapolis, USA: Indiana School of Dentistry, 2000.p. 123–142.

23. Pretty IA. Caries detection and diagnosis: novel technologies. J Dent 2006;34:727–739.

24. Stookey GK. Quantitative light fluorescence: a technology for early monitoring of the caries process. Dent Clin North Am 2005;49:753–70, vi.

25. van der Veen MH, de Josselin de Jong E, Al-Kkateeb S. Caries activity detection by dehydration with quantitative light fluorescence In· Stookey GK, editors. Early detection of dental caries II. Indianapolis, USA: Indiana University School of Dentistry, 2000.p. 251–260.

26. van der Veen,M.H., de Josselin de Jong,E. Application of quantitative light-induced fluorescence for assessing early caries lesions. Monogr Oral Sci 2000. p 144–162.

27. ten Bosch JJ. Summary of research of quantitative light induced fluorescence. In: Stookey GK, editors. Early detection of caries II. Indianapolis: Indiana School of Dentistry, 2000.p. 261–277.

28. Kühnisch J, Bucher K, Henschel V, Hickel R. Reproducibility of DIAGNOdent 2095 and DIAGNOdent Pen measurements: results from an in vitro study on occlusal sites. Eur J Oral Sci 2007;115:206–211.

29. ten Cate JM, Imfeld T. Dental erosion, summary. Eur J Oral Sci 1996;104:241–244.

30. Putz B, Attin T. Die Prävalenz von Erosionen. Dtsche Zahnärzt Z 2002;57:637–643.

31. Attin T. Methods for assessment of dental erosion. Monogr in Oral Sci 2006;20:152–172.

32. Lussi A, Hellwig E, Zero D, Jaeggi T. Erosive tooth wear: diagnosis, risk factors and prevention. Am J Den 2006;19:319–325.

33. Bartlett D, Ganss C, Lussi A. Basic Erosive Wear Examination (BEWE): a new scoring system for scientific and clinical needs. Clinl Oral Invest 2008;12 Suppl 1;S65–8.

34. Ganss C, Lussi A. Current erosion indices—flawed or valid? Clin Oral Invest 2008;12 Suppl 1;S1–3.

35. Young A, Amaechi BT, Dugmore C, Holbrook P, Nunn J, Schiffner U, Lussi A, Ganss C. Current erosion indices-flawed or valid? Summary. Clin Oral Investig 2008;12 Suppl 1;S59–63.

36. Chadwick RG, Mitchell HL, Cameron I, Hunter B, Tulley M. Development of a novel system for assessing tooth and restoration wear. J Dent 1997;25:41–47.

37. Löe H, Theilade E, Jensen SB. Experimental gingivitis in man. J Periodontol 1965;36:177–187.

38. Lindhe J, Hamp SE, Loe H. Plaque induced periodontal disease in beagle dogs. A 4-year clinical, roentgenographical and histometrical study. J Periodontal Res 1975;10:243–255.

39. Waerhaug J. The gingival pocket;anatomy, pathology, deepening and elimination. Odontol Tidskr 1952;60:1–186.

40. Socransky SS, Haffajee AD. Periodontal microbial ecology. Periodontol 2000 2005;38:135–187.

41. Kornman KS, Page RC, Tonetti MS. The host response to the microbial challenge in periodontitis: assembling the players. Periodontol 2000 1997;14:33–53.

42. Sheiham A, Netuveli GS. Periodontal diseases in Europe. Periodontol 2000 2002;29:104–121.

43. Kerr NW. The prevalence and natural history of periodontal disease in Britain from prehistoric to modern times. Br Dent Jl 1998;185:527–535.

44. Hujoel PP, del Aguila MA, DeRouen TA, Bergstrom J. A hidden periodontitis epidemic during the 20th century? Community Dent Oral Epidemiol 2003;31:1–6.

45. Airila-Mansson S, Bjurshammar N, Yakob M, Soder B. Self-reported oral problems, compared with clinical assessment in an epidemiological study. Int J of Dent Hyg 2007;5:82–86.

46. Gilbert AD, Nuttall NM. Self-reporting of periodontal health status. Br Dent J 1999;186:241–244.

47. Armitage GC. Periodontal diseases: diagnosis. Ann Periodontol 1996;1:37–215.

48. Armitage GC. Development of a classification system for periodontal diseases and conditions. Ann Periodontol 1999;4:1–6.

49. Lang NP, Joss A, Tonetti MS. Monitoring disease during supportive periodontal treatment by bleeding on probing. Periodontol 2000 1996;12:44–48.

50. Greenstein G. Contemporary interpretation of probing depth assessments: diagnostic and therapeutic implications. A literature review. J Periodontol 1997;68:1194–1205.

51. Rodrigues CR, Ando T, Guimaraes LO. [Simplified oral hygiene index for ages 4 to 6 and 7 to 10 (deciduous and mixed dentition)]. Rev Odontol Univ São Paulo 1990;4:20–24.

52. Silness J, Löe H. Periodontal dieseases in pregnancy. II Correlation between oral hygiene and periodontal condition. Acta Odontol Scand 1964;22:121–135.

53. O'Leary TJ, Drake RB, Naylor JE. The plaque control record. J Periodontol 1972;43:38.

54. Caton J, Greenstein G, Polson AM. Depth of periodontal probe penetration related to clinical and histologic signs of gingival inflammation. J Periodontol 1981;52:626–629.

55. van der Velden U, Jansen J. Probing force in relation to probe penetration into the periodontal tissues in dogs. A microscopic evaluation. J Clin Periodontol 1980;7:325–327.

56. Gibbs CH, Hirschfeld JW, Lee JG, Low SB, Magnusson I, Thousand RR, Yerneni P, Clark WB. Description and clinical evaluation of a new computerized periodontal probe—the Florida probe. J Clin Periodontol 1988;15:137–144.

57. Birek P, McCulloch CA, Hardy V. Gingival attachment level measurements with an automated periodontal probe. J Clin Periodontol 1987;14:472–477.

58. Pihlstrom BL. Measurement of attachment level in clinical trials: probing methods. J Periodontol 1992;63:1072–1077.

59. Mühlemann HR, Son S. Gingival sulcus bleeding—a leading symptom in initial gingivitis. Helv Odontol Acta 1971;15:107–113.

60. Mühlemann HR. [Gingival inflammation]. Dental Cadmos 1977;45:18–28.

61. Silness J, Löe H. Periodontal disease in pregnancy. 3. Response to local treatment. Acta Odontol Scand 1966;24:747–759.

62. Jeffcoat MK. Radiographic methods for the detection of progressive alveolar bone loss. J Periodontol 1992;63:367-372.

63. Brägger U, Pasquali L, Rylander H, Carnes D, Kornman KS. Computer-assisted densitometric image analysis in periodontal radiography. A methodological study. J Clin Periodontol 1988;15:27–37.

64. Benn DK. A computer-assisted method for making linear radiographic measurements using stored regions of interest. J Clin Periodontol 1992;19:441–448.

65. Haffajee AD, Socransky SS. Microbial etiological agents of destructive periodontal diseases. Periodontol 2000 1994;5:78–111.

66. Albandar JM, Brown LJ, Loe H. Putative periodontal pathogens in subgingival plaque of young adults with and without early-onset periodontitis. J Periodontol 1997;68:973–981.

67. Mombelli A, Casagni F, Madianos PN. Can presence or absence of periodontal pathogens distinguish between subjects with chronic and aggressive periodontitis? A systematic review. J Clin Periodontol 2002;29 Suppl 3:10–21;discussion 37–8.

68. Ximenez-Fyvie LA, Haffajee AD, Socransky SS. Comparison of the microbiota of supra- and subgingival plaque in health and periodontitis. J Clin Periodontol 2000;27:648–657.

69. Position Paper. Diagnosis of periodontal diseases. J Periodontol 2003;74:1237–1247.

70. Loesche WJ, Giordano J, Hujoel PP. The utility of the BANA test for monitoring anaerobic infections due to spirochetes (Treponema denticola) in periodontal disease. J Dent Res 1990;69:1696–1702.

71. Nelson SL, Hynd BA, Pickrum HM. Automated enzyme immunoassay to measure prostaglandin E2 in gingival crevicular fluid. J Periodontal Res 1992;27:143–148.

72. Kornman KS, Crane A, Wang HY, di Giovine FS, Newman MG, Pirk FW, Wilson TGJ, Higginbottom FL, Duff GW. The interleukin-1 genotype as a severity factor in adult periodontal disease. J Clin Periodontol 1997;24:72–77.

73. McGuire MK, Nunn ME. Prognosis versus actual outcome. IV. The effectiveness of clinical parameters and IL-1 genotype in accurately predicting prognoses and tooth survival. J Periodontol 1999;70:49–56.

74. Lang NP, Tonetti MS, Suter J, Sorrell J, Duff GW, Kornman KS. Effect of interleukin-1 gene polymorphisms on gingival inflammation assessed by bleeding on probing in a periodontal maintenance population. J Periodontal Res 2000;35:102–107.

75. Huynh-Ba G, Lang NP, Tonetti MS, Salvi GE. The association of the composite IL-1 genotype with periodontitis progression and/or treatment outcomes: a systematic review. J Clin Periodontol 2007;34:305–317.

76. Haffajee AD, Socransky SS, Goodson JM. Subgingival temperature (I). Relation to baseline clinical parameters. J Clin Periodontol 1992;19:401–408.

77. Haffajee AD, Socransky SS, Goodson JM. Subgingival temperature (II). Relation to future periodontal attachment loss. J Clin Periodontol 1992;19:409–416.

78. Haffajee AD, Socransky SS, Smith C, Dibart S, Goodson JM. Subgingival temperature (III). Relation to microbial counts. J Clin Periodontol 1992;19:417–422.

79. Eggert FM, Drewell L, Bigelow JA, Speck JE, Goldner M. The pH of gingival crevices and periodontal pockets in children, teenagers and adults. Arch Oral Biol 1991;36:233–238.

80. Watanabe T, Soeda W, Kobayashi K, Nagao M. The pH value changes in the periodontal pockets. Bull Tokyo Med Dent Univ 1996;43:67–73.

81. Galgut PN. The relevance of pH to gingivitis and periodontitis. J Int Acad Periodontol 2001;3:61–67.

82. Kerdvongbundit V, Vongsavan N, Soo-Ampon S, Hasegawa A. Microcirculation and micromorphology of healthy and inflamed gingivae. Odontology 2003;91:19–25.

83. Gleissner C, Kempski O, Peylo S, Glatzel JH, Willershausen B. Local gingival blood flow at healthy and inflamed sites measured by laser Doppler flowmetry. J Periodontol 2006;77:1762–1771.

84. Gold SI. Diagnostic techniques in periodontology: a historical review. Periodontol 2000 1995;7:9–21.

85. Kinney JS, Ramseier CA, Giannobile WV. Oral fluid-based biomarkers of alveolar bone loss in periodontitis. Ann NY Acad Sci 2007;1098:230–251.

# Caries Prevention and Caries Control – Two Sides of the Same Coin?

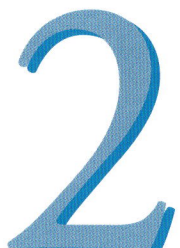

Svante Twetman

## Introduction

The semantic meaning of the word 'prevention' is 'action taken in order to avoid an event occurring'. In medicine, prevention has been classified as primary, secondary and tertiary. Primary prevention comprises procedures taken to stop the initiation of a disease and this can be made on both the individual and the community level. Secondary prevention aims to hinder progression of an already existing disease or to reverse its natural course, whereas tertiary prevention is normally used for limiting the damage caused by the disease and preventing further infections. The corresponding levels in cariology are as follows: measures to reduce the risk for caries-free individuals to become decayed are termed primary prevention; secondary prevention is the non-operative (non-invasive) treatment provided in order to control existing caries lesions; and tertiary prevention is used for operative and restorative care such as fillings, pulp therapy and extractions. Another name commonly used for secondary prevention/caries control in childhood is interceptive caries treatment, meaning techniques aiming at the postponement, arrest or reversal of the caries process. It is important to keep in mind that only the primary and secondary prevention deals with the disease itself. There is a strong tradition in dentistry of associating caries management with restorative and endodontic treatment procedures and one important reason for this is that the same word is used for the disease itself and for its clinical symptoms. A parallel would be that a physician would use the same name for high blood cholesterol, high blood pressure and heart failure. There is a severe drawback with the traditional view on caries treatment because it promotes non-biological mechanical thinking, rather than a causative common risk factor approach.

This chapter discusses preventive strategies and examines the current evidence for caries prevention and caries control, and focuses on the methods with the highest evidence.

## Preventive Strategies

Different strategies can be applied in order to prevent a disease.[1] The population strategy means that measures are taken for everybody, irrespective of risk and age. This approach is highly applicable for frequently occurring diseases and the advantage is that a healthy message or intervention can be organised on a community level with a great potential to reduce the risk for the majori-

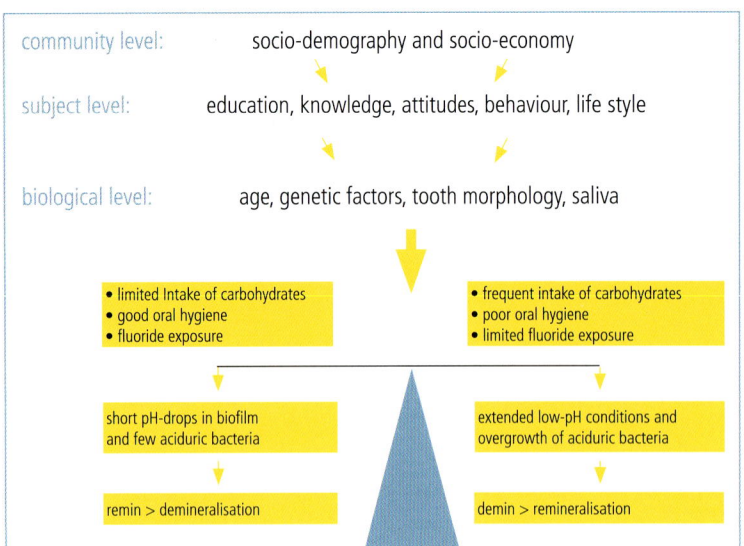

Fig 2-1 Factors on different levels are influence the caries balance. A lesion will occur when demineralization is greater than remineralization (right side) over a period of time (*modified from SBU, 2007*[19]).

ty of the population – just like 'speed bumps' on the road force all drivers to reduce speed when passing. The obvious disadvantage is over-treatment, especially in the case of rare conditions or diseases with an uneven distribution such as dental caries. Therefore, the high-risk strategy has gained interest within cariology, meaning that the preventive resources should be directed to those with the highest need. However, prerequisites for this strategy are reliable methods for caries risk assessment and effective ways to manage caries risk. The fact that there are no current tests available with sufficient predictive power to identify individuals at high risk is certainly a concern. The main advantage of the high-risk strategy is that the cost may be reduced by a more effective allocation of available resources. However, this may occur at the expense of a certain under-treatment of those wrongly considered at low risk. Thus, both strategies must go hand-in-hand and a golden mix is a high-risk group strategy (or directed population strategy) that focuses on groups of people with common risk factors, such as immigrants and residents in low socioeconomic areas. This concept has been implemented and evaluated in several field trials with the aim to bridge the gap of health inequalities in socially disadvantaged groups.[2,3] However, it is important to stress that the different strategies differ in terms of cost-effectiveness and

outcome. It is always more cost-effective and beneficial for health to reduce the risk to some extent in a large population (the population strategy) rather than to dramatically reduce the risk in a few individuals (the high-risk strategy). A consequence is that the collective measures are taken care of by society through community health, whereas the latter is managed by the dental professionals in an individual setting. However, this does not relieve the clinicians from the responsibility of being health advocates to politicians and decision makers in government, communities and media.

# The Caries Balance and the Ecological Plaque Hypothesis

Dental caries forms through a complex interaction over time between acid-producing bacteria, fermentable carbohydrates and many host factors including teeth and saliva.[4] During recent decades, the process has been explained by the ecological plaque hypothesis.[5] In a simple way, this can be described as an imbalance

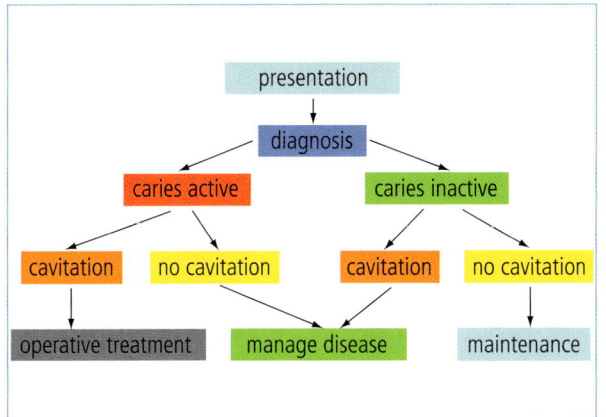

Fig 2-2 Flow-chart showing the medical management of dental caries *(modified from Edelstein, 1994[28])*.

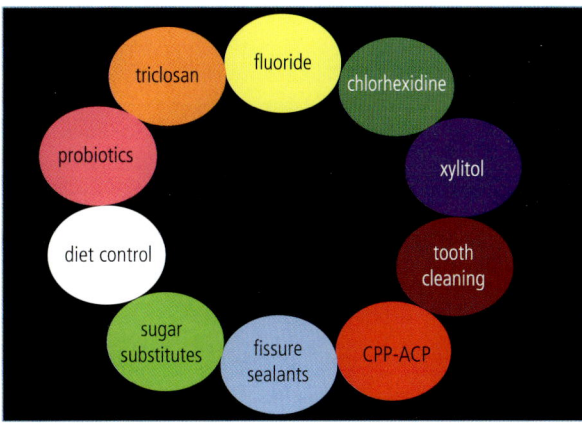

Fig 2-3 The preventive palette consists of professional measures that could be used to influence the caries balance.

between re- and demineralization; if more minerals are lost than gained from the hard tissues over time, a lesion will occur (Fig 2-1). The reason for this imbalance is a broken homeostasis in the oral ecosystem driven by low pH. For example, frequent small eating or a reduced saliva flow will increase the time with low pH and favor the growth of aciduric bacterial species and strains that are normal inhabitants of the oral biofilm (dental plaque). Highly aciduric strains simply get an ecological advantage over the less aciduric strains and a selection of bacteria such as the mutans streptococci group and lactobacilli will occur. These aciduric strains are also highly acidogenic and the extended pH-drop will promote an even faster overgrowth, which enhances a down-going spiral with an increased cariogenic challenge. However, it is important to stress that there are no specific bacteria, for example *Streptococcus mutans*, that are directly causative for caries according to Koch's classical postulate; it is a variety of bacteria with specific aciduric properties that are linked to the initiation of the disease. The fact that *S. mutans* is a marker organism for caries, but not the sole cause, explains why caries-preventive actions directed to eliminate this specific bacterium seldom meet the expectations.[6]

# The Preventive Palette

The ecological plaque hypothesis has brought new thinking to the science of preventive dentistry. The formation of plaque is a natural process that cannot be prevented *per se*, so it is the ecological shift that should be prevented. If nature is used as an allegory, caries is a result of an 'ecological catastrophe'. However, such disasters can be reversed and a long-term healing and equilibrium can be achieved once the reason is identified and appropriate actions are taken. There are numerous examples of re-established ecosystems in nature from all over the world and this can also be achieved in the oral cavity. The key elements are, of course, detection of early caries lesions and a comprehensive caries activity assessment, which together are decisive for the further management, as illustrated in Fig 2-2. When the individual cause or causes for the caries imbalance is disclosed, there is a palette of non-operative preventive maneuvers to choose from in order to restore the oral ecosystem and some examples are given in Fig 2-3. Although the level of evidence for efficacy may vary between the various measures, the most important factors are the experience, skill and knowledge of the caregiver. Also the patient's preferences and willingness and

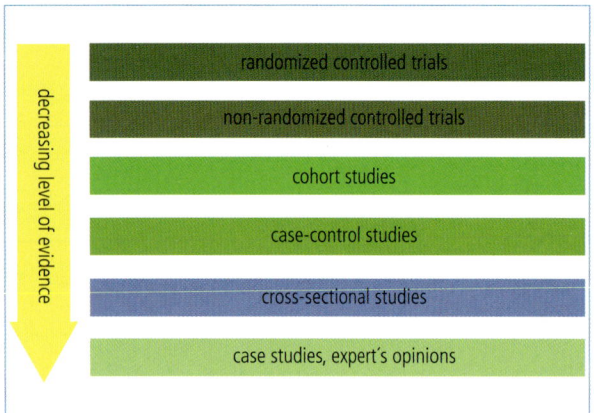

**Fig 2-4** The hierarchy of clinical trials in evidence-based dentistry. In systematic reviews evaluating the outcome of interventions, only prospective randomized or quasi-randomized controlled trials are normally taken into account.

means to pay must be taken into account. The palette can, therefore, be used as a starting point to explain, plan and discuss the treatment options together with the patient in order to improve compliance.

To summarize, caries management must include consideration of the patient at risk, the status of each lesion, patient and clinical management followed by monitoring.

## Evidence-Based Dentistry

In the era of evidence-based medicine, the systematic review of literature is the core tool to evaluate the efficacy, effectiveness and efficiency of various treatments. Several national health technology assessment agencies such as the Cochrane Collaboration in the UK (www.cochrane.org) and the Swedish Council on Health Technology Assessment (www.sbu.se) publish systematic and updated reviews on the management of various medical and dental conditions. A systematic review contains a systematic search for and inclusion of relevant literature after predetermined criteria, as well as a critical appraisal with a quality assessment of the included trials. The hierarchy of clinical trials is illus-

trated in Fig 2-4. Randomized controlled trials (RCT) of moderate and high quality with a low chance of bias or confounding influences are compiled in evidence tables, graphically indicating a beneficial or non-beneficial treatment effect. Thereafter, a formal grading of the level of evidence is provided. However, it must be strongly emphasized that insufficient or inclusive evidence for a method or treatment does not necessarily mean that it does not work or should be abandoned. The reason could simply be that high quality clinical trials are lacking or that the method or technique is impossible to evaluate in a RCT design. One example of this is water fluoridation. All clinical experience and results from cohort field studies indicate a beneficial effect on caries, but it has never been proved in a high-hierarchy study design. In addition, as fluoride exposure is regarded as 'best clinical practice' today, it would no longer be ethically acceptable to omit fluoride in a RCT.

## Evidence-Based Caries Prevention

The evidence grade for various self-applied and professional measures to prevent caries are defined and displayed in Table 2-1. As a full discussion of each measure is beyond the limits of this chapter, only the methods with the highest evidence grade are further commented on below.

### Fluoride Dentifrice

There is strong scientific evidence that tooth brushing twice daily with fluoride dentifrice is the most cost-effective and feasible way to prevent caries in patients of all ages, irrespective of caries level and dental care system.[7] The number needed to treat (NNT), which is defined as the number of patients who need to be treated in order to prevent one additional bad outcome, varies with the level of disease in the population and is

Table 2-1   Level of evidence for the caries-preventive effect of selected preventive maneuvers according to the Swedish Council on Technology Assessment in Health Care *(SBU,[22] 2003)*.

| Measure | Evidence grade (1-4)* |
|---|:---:|
| Fluoride supplements | |
|     Fluoride dentifrice | 1 |
|     Fluoride varnish | 2 |
|     Fluoride rinse | 3 |
|     Fluoride supplements (tablets, gums, drops) | 4 |
| Antibacterial measures | |
|     Fissure sealants | 2 |
|     Oral hygiene instruction | 4 |
|     Professional tooth cleaning (without fluoride) | 4 |
|     Chlorhexidine (topical rinses, gel, varnish) | 4 |
| Diet control | |
|     Dietary counselling | 4 |
|     Sugar substitutes (sorbitol, xylitol etc) | 4 |
| Dental health education | 4 |

- *Evidence grade 1 = strong scientific evidence. Conclusion supported by ≥ 2 RCTs with high study quality and relevance and with a low probability of bias and confounding factors.
- Evidence grade 2 = moderately strong scientific evidence. Conclusion supported by at least one RCT of high study quality and relevance as well as ≥ 2 RCTs with medium study quality and moderate risk of bias and confounding factors.
- Evidence grade 3 = limited scientific evidence. Conclusion supported by ≥ 2 RCTs of medium study quality and relevance and a moderate risk for bias and confounders.
- Evidence grade 4 = insufficient or inconclusive scientific evidence. No studies meet the inclusion criteria or studies of equal study quality and relevance generates conflicting results.

most favourable (NNT=1.6) in communities with a high incidence of caries.[8] Some key features concerning fluoride dentifrice and its caries-preventive effect are summarized in Table 2-2. There is a global consensus for recommending the use of fluoride dentifrice according to the '2-2-2' rule; 2 cm of dentifrice, 2 times a day (morning and evening) and 2 minutes of brushing. The remaining controversies deal with the optimal fluoride concentration in the dentifrice and at which age parents should start to brush their children's teeth with fluoride dentifrice. In Europe, 1500 ppm fluoride is the upper limit in over-the-counter products, whereas high-fluoride dentifrices with up to 5000 ppm are available on prescription in some countries for high-risk patients such as teenagers and elderly patients suffering from dry

Table 2-2   Summary of factors influencing the caries-preventive effect of fluoridated dentifrice.[7,8]

- Daily brushing with fluoride dentifrice is the most cost-effective way of preventing caries
- Increasing effect with increasing fluoride concentration up to 2800 ppm
- Increased effect by moving from once to two times brushing per day
- Better effect in high-caries communities
- Better effect when tooth brushing is supervised by teachers in school-based programs
- Limited evidence from studies of the primary dentition
- No evidence for low-fluoride (≥ 500ppm ) dentifrice

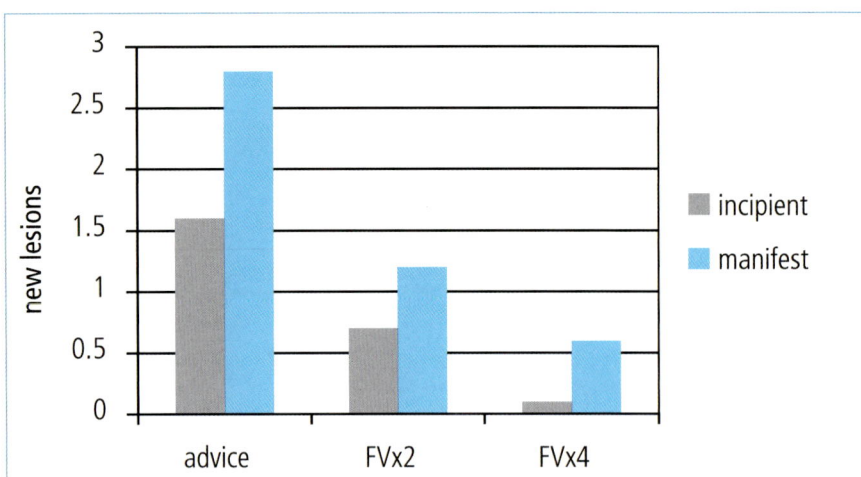

Fig 2-5  Caries incidence in three groups of initially caries-free toddlers from low-income families. All groups received basic dental health education and the experimental groups were additionally treated with fluoride varnish applications on two or four occasions, respectively, during the 2-year study period.[11]

mouth. Concerning the age for the first introduction of fluoridated toothpaste, the recommendations do vary from county to country, but most guidelines advocate parents to start with a normal fluoridated dentifrice from the eruption of the first primary molar and adjust the amount of dentifrice according to the size of the child, beginning with a smear layer.

*Fluoride Varnish*

Fluoride varnish has a strong tradition of use in Germany and the Scandinavian countries, whereas fluoride gels have been the treatment of choice elsewhere. A current understanding is that professional topical fluoride varnish applications at least twice yearly results in a prevented fraction of 30% compared with untreated controls.[9] However, a number of recent RCTs have reinforced the effectiveness of fluoride varnish applications in different settings. Moberg-Sköld and co-workers[10] found that regular fluoride varnish applications could dramatically reduce the incidence of proximal caries in adolescents over a 3-year period, and that the treatment was most effective in the study population within the lowest socioeconomic group. The aim of this novel approach was to utilize the school as an arena for intervention and the applications were conducted in the classroom by dental assistants without high-tech equipment (which increased compliance and reduced the costs). A more traditional concept adapted for a differ-

ent age group was presented by Weintraub et al.[11] who selected initially caries-free toddlers from low-income families. The children were randomized into three groups with one or two fluoride varnish applications per year on top of traditional dental health education (control group). The results after 2 years showed a strong preventive effect on early childhood caries that was clearly directly dependent on the number of professional treatments (Fig 2-5). A third, recent placebo-controlled double-blind study conducted on orthodontic patients revealed that fluoride varnish applications around the bracket base could prevent the incidence of white spot lesions during treatment with fixed appliances.[12] As the body of evidence concerning fluoride varnish is gathering,[13] the American Dental Association has added fluoride varnish to their treatment guidelines.[14] In fact, it was stated that it has been proved effective, not only in the young permanent dentition, but in contrast to fluoride gel, also in primary teeth. Furthermore, fluoride varnish takes less time, creates less patient discomfort, and achieves greater patient acceptability compared with fluoride gel, especially in preschool children.[14]

In recent years, there has been a formal explosion in the number of different fluoride varnishes that have entered the market, but it should be emphasized that practically all clinical trials have been carried out using only two: Duraphat (Colgate Duraphat, UK) and Fluor

Protector (Ivoclar Vivident, Liechtenstein). However, the yellow color of the former brand is often perceived as a shortcoming from a compliance point of view. Therefore, the current trend is moving towards transparent varnishes with user-friendly single applicators.

### Fissure Sealants

The application of fissure sealants is a cornerstone in the management of caries and sealing with resin-based sealants is a recommended procedure to prevent caries of the occlusal surfaces of permanent molars.[15] An illustration is shown in Fig 2-6. The prevented fractions in first permanent molars averaged 76 and 65%, 4 and 9 years after initial treatment when the sealants were checked, maintained or reapplied as and when needed.[16] Fissure sealants play a unique double role, as recent evidence indicates that sealants can be used effectively to prevent both the initiation[17] and the progression of non-cavitated fissure caries.[18] The current debate concerns the indications on which the sealants should be placed. As the application procedure of fissure sealants is highly technique sensitive and thereby costly, the general understanding is that sealants should be considered only when it is determined that the tooth, or the patient, is at risk of experiencing caries. The best preventive effect in permanent molars is achieved when the treatment is performed within 4 years of eruption, whereas a reduced progression rate of early non-cavitated lesions can be achieved at any age and also in adults. Finally, it is important to stress that the evidence clearly suggests that resin-based sealants are the first choice of material.

A frequently asked question is whether or not cavitated molars with dentin involvement could also be fissure-sealed with subsequent caries arrest, and there is not yet a definite evidence-based answer to this issue.[18] One barrier is that the identification methods for early occlusal dentine caries are not accurate.[19] The need for further studies that meet standards of quality in design, conduct and reporting is obvious, but, until then, a simple rule would be to encourage the placement of fissure sealants for surfaces where the caries status is uncertain.

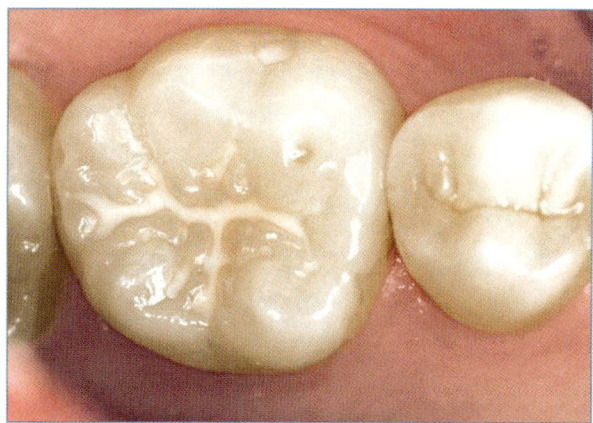

**Fig 2-6**  Fissure sealants constitute a cornerstone in comprehensive preventive dentistry. There is firm evidence showing that fissure caries can not only be prevented, but also controlled by placing sealants in non-cavitated lesions of permanent molars (evidence grade 2).

# Evidence-Based Caries Control

In contrast to caries prevention, surprisingly few controlled studies have been performed to evaluate the effectiveness of non-operative (non-invasive) methods to control caries. The exception is the abovementioned studies of fissure sealants. One reason for this lack of investigations is probably due to the fact that caries has traditionally been diagnosed on the cavity level and that validated methods for early caries detection, arrest and regression have been lacking. Another reason for the small amount of data is that clinical trials have not been designed to answer the 'control question' and surfaces with very early lesions are rarely quantified at baseline. In a recent systematic review of the literature, it was concluded that there is insufficient scientific support for any conclusion as to whether or not early caries lesions can be treated effectively by non-invasive methods.[19] Forty-eight studies were identified, 12 of them fulfilled the inclusion criteria, but only two of them were assessed as being of medium quality. One study was conducted in Denmark and demonstrated a similar proximal progression rate after fortnightly fluoride rinses compared with biannual Fluor Protector applications in school children over a 3-year period.[20] The second paper investigated the effect of fluoride varnish in Swedish schoolchildren over a 3-year period – the conclusion was that the proximal progression rate was significantly reduced in the test group.[21] However, it should be underlined that the general caries activity in both investigations was low.

The issue of caries control has more frequently been investigated concerning root caries in frail elderly patients. Although most results point in the same direction, suggesting that high fluoride dentifrice and other topical fluoride supplements are associated with root caries arrest, the identified studies presented methodological problems with a considerable risk for bias and confounders.[22] For example, a short study duration (<1 year), extensive attrition (dropouts), low diagnostic validity of 'changes in lesion texture' and missing data on progression/regression were common problems that diminished the level of evidence. However, an interesting observation was that a combination of professional fluoride- and chlorhexidine-varnish treatments could improve active root caries lesions to a slightly larger extent compared with the use of fluoride varnish applications alone.[23]

Summarizing the paragraphs above, at the moment there is insufficient scientific evidence for non-invasive measures to control caries in children as well as in adults, and this must be a high priority challenge to elucidate among dental researchers in the near future.

# What Can be Done with Caries-Active Patients?

This question has gained surprisingly little attention in dental research and most guidelines emanate from clinical experience and common sense. However, a research group from the University of Oulu in Finland has conducted a series of clinical trials on high-risk school children and not surprisingly, a number of the trials have displayed rather discouraging results. The most recent study focused on adolescents selected with active caries lesions and randomized to either a comprehensive anticaries program based on non-invasive measures or to routine basic prevention provided by the public dental clinics in the area.[24] Adolescents in the experimental group were offered an individually designed patient-centered preventive program aimed at identifying and eliminating factors that had led to the presence of active caries. The program included counselling sessions with emphasis on enhancing the subject's own resources in everyday life. The staff were specially trained in empowerment techniques and provided with personal coaches and the participants were frequently recalled. Toothbrushes, fluoride dentifrice and fluoride and xylitol lozenges were distributed to the adolescents. They also received repeated applications of fluoride- and chlorhexidine-containing varnishes. After 3 years, a prevented fraction of 44% was obtained, but the authors stated that a 'huge effort was made to achieve the results' and, so far, no cost-effective analysis has been presented. Nevertheless, the study is important because it demonstrates that it is possible to combat dental decay among caries-active patients by combining multiple measures, when the patient can take own responsibility and when manpower and sufficient economical resources are available.

# What's in the Future?

As has been previously pointed out, restorative dentistry is slowly moving towards the non-invasive era. At first, a development within the field of caries risk assessment led by the introduction of novel and rapid techniques in saliva diagnostics can be foreseen. It is only a matter of time until molecular biological techniques such as polymerase chain reactions (PCR) and DNA-hybridization will enter the dental office enabling analyses of predisposing genes and specific bacteria involved in the caries process. Secondly, the possibilities for early caries detection will be improved by a further chairside development of digital imaging fiber-optic transillumination (DIFOTI), laser fluorescence and quantitative light-induced fluorescence (QLF). Thirdly, the ecological approaches to interfere with the oral biofilm will open new possibilities for caries prevention. For example, the use of probiotic bacteria is a hot topic because it has become increasingly clear that strategies directed at eliminating specific caries-associated microorganisms, which are members of the endogenous microflora, have not only been proved to be difficult, but perhaps also unwise. Probiotics are live microbial feed supplements, which beneficially affect the host animal by improving its intestinal microbial balance as documented in clinical trials.[25] The background thinking is that the harmless bacteria, such as species of *lactobacilli* and *bifidobacteria*, may compete with bacteria that are injurious to health and occupy a space in the biofilm that would otherwise be colonized by a pathogen. The research within dentistry is still in its infancy, but the findings so far are promising and encourage further studies.[26,27] Other possible areas for improvement in prevention in the near future are fluoride-releasing appliances and dental materials, the use of ozone, novel sugar substitutes (erythritol and xylitol) and remineralization enhancement through the presence of casein phospho-peptide-amorphous calcium phosphate (CPP-ACP) nanocomplexes. However, the future for replacement therapy with gene-modified bacteria and caries immunization is questionable.

# Conclusions

The answer to the question stated in the title of this chapter is 'no' - from an evidence point of view there are two different sides. Caries prevention is most effective on a population basis and caries control is based on identifying and eliminating factors that have led to the presence of active caries on the individual level. While the scientific evidence is strong for some self-applied and non-invasive professional measures to prevent caries in childhood, the body of evidence for professional non-invasive methods to control caries is insufficient. This is most likely one of the reasons that preserves the conservative restorative thinking and holds back the management of caries as a disease. Thus, the urgent challenge for the future is to conduct RCT of high quality with evaluations of novel anti-caries measures in patients with existing, active lesions.

# References

1. Rose G. Sick individuals and sick populations. Int J Epidemiol 1985;14:32–38.
2. Watt R, Sheiham A. Inequalities in oral health: a review of the evidence and recommendations for action. Br Dent J 1999;187:6-12.
3. Wennhall I, Matsson L, Schröder U, Twetman S. Outcome of an oral health outreach programme for preschool children in a low socioeconomic multicultural area. Int J Paediatr Dent 2008;18:84–90.
4. Selwitz RH, Ismail AI, Pitts NB. Dental caries. Lancet 2007;369:51–59.
5. Marsh PD. Are dental diseases examples of ecological catastrophes? Microbiology 2003;149:279–294.
6. Twetman S. Antimicrobials in future caries control? A review with special reference to chlorhexidine treatment. Caries Res 2004;38:223–229.
7. Twetman S, Axelsson S, Dahlgren H, Holm AK, Källestål C, Lagerlöf F, Lingström P, Mejàre I, Nordenram G, Norlund A, Petersson LG, Söder B. Caries-preventive effect of fluoride toothpaste: a systematic review. Acta Odontol Scand 2003;61:347–355.
8. Marinho VC, Higgins JP, Logan S, Sheiham A. Topical fluoride (toothpastes, mouthrinses, gels or varnishes) for preventing dental caries in children and adolescents. Cochrane Database Syst Rev 2003;4:CD002782.
9. Petersson LG, Twetman S, Dahlgren H, Norlund A, Holm AK, Nordenram G, Lagerlöf F, Söder B, Källestål C, Mejàre I, Axelsson S, Lingström P. Professional fluoride varnish treatment for caries control: a systematic review of clinical trials. Acta Odontol Scand 2004;62:170–176.
10. Moberg-Sköld U, Petersson LG, Lith A, Birkhed D. Effect of school-based fluoride varnish programmes on approximal caries in adolescents from different caries risk areas. Caries Res 2005;39:273–279.
11. Weintraub JA, Ramos-Gomez F, Jue B, Shain S, Hoover CI, Featherstone JD, Gansky SA. Fluoride varnish efficacy in preventing early childhood caries. J Dent Res 2006;85:172–176.
12. Stecksén-Blicks C, Renfors G, Oscarson ND, Bergstrand F, Twetman S. Caries-preventive effectiveness of a fluoride varnish: a randomized controlled trial in adolescents with fixed orthodontic appliances. Caries Res 2007;41:455–459.
13. Azarpazhooh A, Main PA. Fluoride varnish in the prevention of dental caries in children and adolescents: a systematic review. J Can Dent Assoc 2008;74:73–79.

14. American Dental Association Council on Scientific Affairs. Professionally applied topical fluoride: evidence-based clinical recommendations. J Dent Educ 2007;71:393–402.

15. Ahovuo-Saloranta A, Hiiri A, Nordblad A, Worthington H, Mäkelä M. Pit and fissure sealants for preventing dental decay in the permanent teeth of children and adolescents. Cochrane Database Syst Rev 2004;(3):CD001830.

16. Beauchamp J, Caufield PW, Crall JJ, Donly K, Feigal R, Gooch B, Ismail A, Kohn W, Siegal M, Simonsen R. American Dental Association Council on Scientific Affairs. Evidence-based clinical recommendations for the use of pit-and-fissure sealants: a report of the American Dental Association Council on Scientific Affairs. J Am Dent Assoc 2008;139:257–268.

17. Azarpazhooh A, Main PA. Pit and fissure sealants in the prevention of dental caries in children and adolescents: a systematic review. J Can Dent Assoc 2008;74:171–177.

18. Griffin SO, Oong E, Kohn W, Vidakovic B, Gooch BF; CDC Dental Sealant Systematic Review Work Group, Bader J, Clarkson J, Fontana MR, Meyer DM, Rozier RG, Weintraub JA, Zero DT. The effectiveness of sealants in managing caries lesions. J Dent Res 2008;87:169–174.

19. The Swedish Council on Technology Assessment in Health Care (SBU). Caries – diagnosis, risk assessment and non-invasive treatment. A systematic review. The Swedish Council on Technology Assessment in Health Care. Report No. 188, ISBN:978-91-85413-21-8 2007. www.sbu.se

20. Bruun V, Bille J, Hansen KT, Kann J, Qvist V, Thylstrup A. Three-year caries increment after fluoride rinses or topical applications with a fluoride varnish. Community Dent Oral Epidemiol 1985;13:299-303.

21. Modéer T, Twetman S, Bergstrand F. Three-year study of the effect of fluoride varnish (Duraphat) on proximal caries progression in teenagers. Scand J Dent Res 1984;92:400–407.

22. The Swedish Council on Technology Assessment in Health Care (SBU). Prevention of dental caries. A systematic review. The Swedish Council on Technology Assessment in Health Care. Report No. 510-19 2002. www.sbu.se

23. Brailsford SR, Fiske J, Gilbert S, Clark D, Beighton D. The effects of the combination of chlorhexidine/thymol- and fluoride-containing varnishes on the severity of root caries lesions in frail institutionalised elderly people. J Dent 2002;30:319–324.

24. Hausen H, Seppä L, Poutanen R, Niinimaa A, Lahti S, Kärkkäinen S, et al. Noninvasive control of dental caries in children with active initial lesions. A randomized clinical trial. Caries Res 2007;41:384-391.

25. Doron S, Gorbach SL. Probiotics: their role in the treatment and prevention of disease. Expert Rev Anti Infect Ther 2006;4:261–275.

26. Meurman JH. Probiotics: do they have a role in oral medicine and dentistry? Eur J Oral Sci 2005;113:188–196.

27. Twetman S, Stécksen-Blicks C. Probiotics and oral health effects in children. Int J Paediatr Dent 2008;18:3–10.

28. Edelstein BL. The medical management of dental caries. J Am Dent Assoc 1994;125 Suppl:31S-39S.

# Adhesion to Tooth Enamel and Dentin – A View on the Latest Technology and Future Perspectives

Marcio Vivan Cardoso, Yasuhiro Yoshida and Bart van Meerbeek

## Introduction

The fast progress that is occurring in dental adhesive technology has extensively influenced modern restorative dentistry. The mechanical approach of 'extension for prevention' introduced by GV Black[1] in 1917 is no longer justifiable, and has been replaced by the concept of 'minimal-invasive dentistry'.[2] This concept dictates a more conservative cavity design, basically providing sufficient access to the lesion in order to completely eliminate the diseased tissue, along with the use of a dental adhesive to bond the restorative composite to the remaining sound tissue.[3]

Although decayed or fractured teeth can be reconstructed with minimal invasion and almost invisibly using adhesive technology (Fig 3-1), the clinical longevity of composite restorations today is still too short.[4,5] This forces the clinician to replace restorations too soon, leading to further weakening of the patient's tooth with each new intervention and also to higher public health costs.

Despite the enormous advances made in adhesive technology during the last 50 years, the bonded interface itself remains the Achilles heel of an adhesive filling.[6,7] Mainly water sorption is thought to destabilize the adhesive-tooth bond, though the actual interfacial

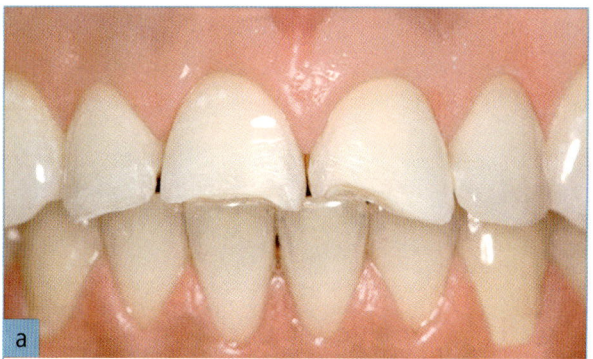

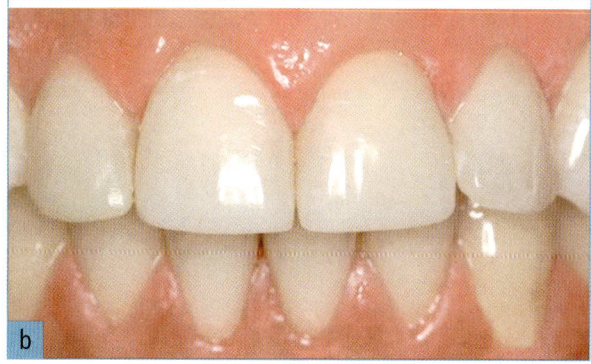

**Fig 3-1a–b** Clinical example illustrating the potential of minimally-invasive and nearly invisible tooth reconstruction using adhesives and restorative composites. **(a)** Preoperative situation. **(b)** Reconstruction with composite and adhesive technique.

degradation mechanisms are far from understood. In this context, several aspects should be considered with regard to the strength and durability of the bond to

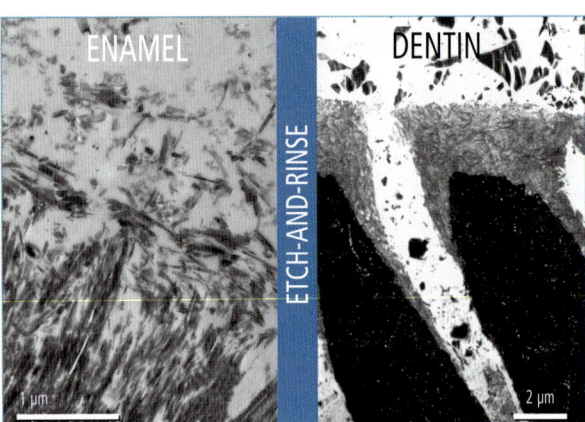

**Fig 3-2** Collage of TEM photomicrographs illustrating the interfacial ultra-structure of an etch-and-rinse adhesive at enamel and dentin.

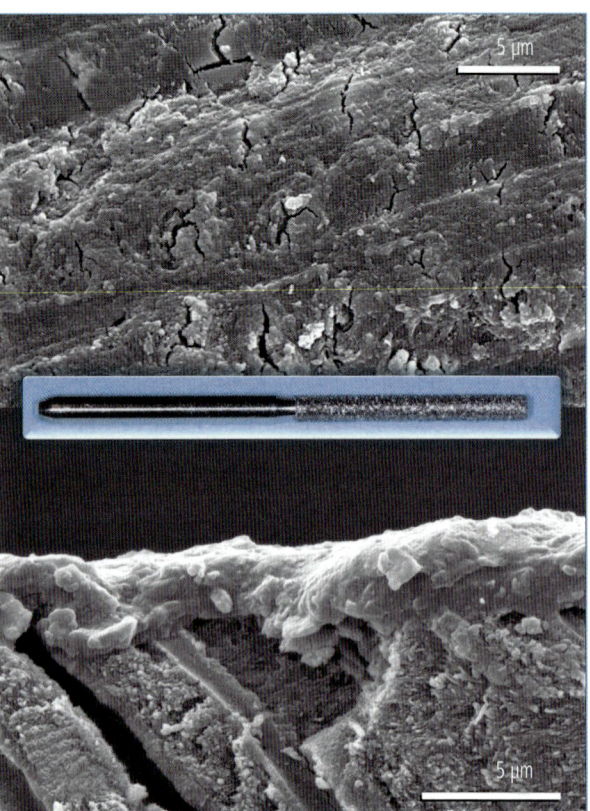

**Fig 3-3** Field-emmission gun scanning electron microscopy (Feg-SEM) photomicrographs of a typically thick and compact dentinal smear layer prepared by a 100-grit diamond bur.

both dental hard tissues, enamel and dentin. These include the heterogeneity of tooth structure and composition, the features of the dental surface exposed after cavity preparation, and the characteristics of the adhesive itself, such as its strategy of interaction with both substrates and its basic physicochemical properties. Furthermore, all sorts of chemical and mechanical challenges that are inherent to the oral environment should be taken into account, such as moisture, masticatory stresses, changes in temperature and pH, and dietary and chewing-related habits.[8]

## Interaction with Dental Hard Tissues

The fundamental mechanism of bonding to enamel and dentin is essentially based on an exchange process, in which minerals removed from the dental hard tissues are replaced by resin monomers that upon polymerization become micromechanically interlocked in the created porosities.[3,9]

Dissolution of superficial dental hard tissue is conventionally achieved by phosphoric-acid etching, one of the major breakthroughs in adhesive technology introduced by Buonocore more than 50 years ago.[10] On

enamel, acid-etching selectively dissolves the enamel rods, thereby providing micro-etch pits that increase the surface energy so much that an ordinary hydrophobic bonding agent is readily sucked in by capillary attraction[11] (Fig 3-2). Without doubt, this micro-mechanical interlocking of tiny resin tags within the acid-etched enamel surface is still today the best achievable bond to enamel.[9] It not only effectively seals the restoration margins in the long term, but also protects the more vulnerable dentin bond against degradation.[12]

However, the more reliable adhesion to enamel is, the less predictable and durable bonding to dentin today still is. The main hindrance is dentin's mixed inorganic–organic nature with dentinal hydroxyapatite deposited on a mesh of collagen, essentially providing dentin with its hardness, but also its toughness.[3] In addition, dentin is intimately connected with pulpal tissue by means of numerous fluid-filled tubules, which transverse through dentin from the dentino–enamel junction to the pulp. Once under constant outward pressure, this fluid renders the exposed dentin surface naturally moist and, thus, intrinsically hydrophilic.[13] This hydrophilic character definitely represents one of the major challenges for modern adhesives to durably interact with dentin, and has, in essence, led to the different bond strategies that are available.

The presence of cutting debris on instrumented dental surfaces in the form of a smear layer, and smear plugs that obstruct the dentin tubules (Fig 3-3), is also a primary co-factor that should not be underestimated.[14-16] Considering the evolution in adhesive technology, surface-smear precluded interaction of early 'dentin bonding agents' with the underlying tooth tissue, leading to low bond strengths and unsatisfactory clinical performances in the 1980s.[3,17,18] The first bonding protocol that revealed a clinically acceptable outcome involved complete removal of the smear layer by a 'total-etch' and now the better termed 'etch-and-rinse' approach.[3,9] These multi-step dental adhesives have been marketed since the early 1990s and can still today be considered as the 'gold standard' adhesives. In order to deal with the organic collagen mesh exposed following acid-etching dentin, these 'adhesive systems' provide a separate adhesion promoter or 'primer' that contains hydrophilic functional monomers dissolved in an organic solvent.[3]

The market-driven demand for simplified adhesive procedures has rapidly led to the introduction of the alternative, so-called 'self-etch' (or 'etch-and-dry') approach, which was first in Japan in the mid 1990s. This bond strategy only dissolves the smear layer (but does not remove it, as there is no rinse phase) and embeds the dissolved calcium phosphates within the interfacial transition zone[19] (Fig 3-4). Especially for the relatively high-pH self-etch adhesives, rather thick and compact smear layers may negatively influence their bonding effectiveness.[16,20]

Despite the major difference in etching technique between etch-and-rinse and self-etch adhesives, other

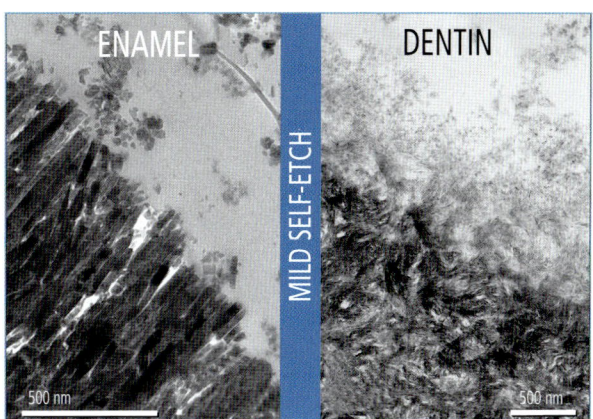

**Fig 3-4** Collage of TEM photomicrographs illustrating the interfacial ultra-structure of a 'mild' self-etch adhesive at enamel and dentin.

fundamental steps for adhesion, namely the 'priming' and 'bonding' phase, can be either carried out separately or combined.[3] Etch-and-rinse adhesives then require either three or two steps depending on whether the primer and bonding agent are separated or combined in a single bottle. Similarly, self-etch adhesives can be either two- or one-step systems depending on whether or not the self-etching/primer solution is separated from the bonding agent or combined with it, enabling a single application procedure of a so-called 'all-in-one' adhesive.

# Latest Advances in Etch-and-Rinse Technology

Acid-etching demineralises dentin over a depth of 3 to 5 µm, thereby exposing a scaffold of collagen fibrils that is nearly totally depleted of hydroxyapatite (Fig 3-2).[21–23] According to the three-step procedure, the subsequently applied primer contains specific monomers with hydrophilic properties, such as HEMA (2-hydroxyethyl methacrylate), that with help of organic solvents (acetone, ethanol and/or water), can diffuse rapidly into the micro-porous collagen network to individually envelope collagen fibrils with resin.[24,25] The functional monomers within etch-and-rinse primers basically need good diffusion potential, whereas the primer solvent functions as a carrier to bring the monomers deep within the collagen network, but needs to evaporate as much as possible afterwards. In this way, the primer prepares the acid-etched dentin for the final infiltration of the solvent-free adhesive resin in the third and last application step. Micro-mechanical interlocking is then achieved through the 3 to 5 μm hybrid-layer formation in combination with resin tags inside the dentin tubules (Fig 3-2). Interestingly, neither the thickness of the hybrid layer, nor the length of the resin tags seems to influence the bonding effectiveness to dentin.[26] Separate polymerization of the adhesive resin stabilizes the interface, after which the restorative composite is applied and coupled via co-polymerization with the adhesive.[3]

Simplified two-step adhesives combine primer and adhesive resin, but although they are slightly more user-friendly, they tend to perform inferiorly when compared with their three-step counterparts.[27,28] Besides sub-optimal hybridization owing to blending primer and bonding components into a single solution,[3,9] the solvent-rich and hydrophilic nature of these simplified two-step etch-and-rinse adhesives render them more susceptible to water sorption and consequently to hydrolytic bond degradation processes.[6,7] The solvent provided at the interface with these 'one-bottle' adhesives is also more difficult to evaporate, and, therefore remains entrapped within the hybrid and adhesive layer upon polymerization more easily.[28]

In general, the major weakness of the etch-and-rinse approach is that dentinal collagen is nearly completely depleted from hydroxyapatite. Collagen fibrils keep extracellular fluid bonded, whereby acid-etched dentin gets its highly hydrophilic state. Therefore, although primary chemical bonding as the most stable form of intermolecular interaction is highly desirable, an intrinsically hydrophobic medium such as the methacrylate-based dental adhesive cannot chemically link to this hydrophilic dentinal surface. Therefore, replacement of the mineral content that was etched away, as complete

as possible with resin is the best action to achieve long-term bond durability.

It is obvious that especially the post-etching handling of surface water is crucial for the success of the etch-and-rinse protocol. Ideally, the etched collagen network must be kept loosely arranged during adhesive procedures in order to allow proper resin-monomer infiltration.[29] Actually, a certain amount of surface water is needed to prevent the collagen network from collapsing, a methodology commonly referred to as (water) 'wet bonding'.[30] An excessively wet surface will keep water at the interface and, thus, negatively influence bonding.[31,32] In the latter over-wet condition, the residual water will cause phase separation between hydrophobic and hydrophilic components of the adhesive, resulting in the formation of water-filled blisters at the adhesive–dentin interface that definitely weakens the interfacial strength.[33,34] Furthermore, excess moisture decreases resin-polymerization conversion, and, thereby reduces the mechanical properties of the adhesive layer.[34-36] This need for a wet-bonding application procedure definitely makes the etch-and-rinse approach a rather technique-sensitive clinical technique.

Adhesive systems containing hydrophilic monomers dissolved in acetone were found to produce higher bond strengths when acid-conditioned dentin was left visibly moist.[37,38] Owing to their relatively high volatility, solvents such as acetone and to a lesser degree ethanol, displace the surface water that was left after etching, allowing the primer monomers to effectively fill the 20 to 30 nm interfibrillar spaces within the exposed collagen network.[29] Although sufficient surface moisture clinically manifests as a uniformly shiny dentin surface, the 'window of opportunity' between over-dry and over-wet conditions is narrow; in clinical circumstances and especially in complex cavity configurations, pooling of water might be difficult to avoid.[33]

Interestingly, water-based primers have shown a potential self-rewetting effect on gently air-dried dentin.[29] Their water content rehydrates the air-dried and, thus, collapsed collagen network, transforming it into a loosely arranged structure that allows the hydrophilic primer monomers to infiltrate it. Over-drying where the acid-etched dentin surface gets severely dehydrated should naturally be avoided at any time during the clinical application procedure. Therefore, the surface should be gently dried until the etched enamel presents its white-frosted appearance and the dentin looses its shine and turns dull. The major drawback of this (gently) 'dry-bonding' technique is that additional water is delivered to the interface with the water-based primers. Self-evidently, it should ideally be removed as much as possible in a 15 sec time period, once its job of re-wetting agent and monomer carrier is completed and before the adhesive resin is light-cured. To facilitate solvent-evaporation in water-based adhesives, ethanol and acetone can be used in conjunction with water as co-solvents, resulting in an azeotropic mixture.[39] This implies the formation of hydrogen bonds between water and ethanol/acetone molecules, resulting in a solvent that is easier to evaporate.[40] In this way, multi-step 'etch-and-rinse' adhesives that provide water-based primers are less technique-sensitive to variations in the bonding protocol as far as the wetness of the acid-etched dentinal surface is concerned.[29] Applied following the classic three-step 'etchant-primer-bonding' procedure, the repeatedly documented superior performance of adhesives such as OptiBond FL (KerrHawe, Orange, USA) and Syntac Classic (Ivoclar-Vivadent, Schaan, Liechtenstein) in a multitude of laboratory studies as well as in clinical trials at world-wide independent research institutes, has granted them the gold standard label.

Unfortunately, 'complete' hybridization of the exposed collagen network seems practically unattainable, even with these three-step etch-and-rinse adhesives. Numerous papers have reported on 'nano-leakage,' as the presence of nanometer-sized voids within and/or beneath the hybrid layer.[41-45] They originate from spaces around collagen fibrils that were not completely enveloped by resin, and/or from discrepancies between the etching and subsequent resin-infiltration depth.

Recent attempts to improve infiltration efficiency involve the use of a new solvent known as 'tert-butanol',

resulting in an innovative two-step etch-and-rinse adhesive, commercialized by Dentsply (Konstanz, Germany) as an extra performance (XP)-Bond. This adhesive is much less technique sensitive with regard to maintaining the appropriate surface wetness after etching, compared with its acetone-based precursors. The results obtained so far with this adhesive appear promising, potentially thanks to the new solvent presenting an ethanol-like vapor pressure, along with better stability towards chemical interference with the functional monomers.[46] Long-term data, gathered in the laboratory after ageing and especially in clinical studies, definitely need to confirm if this new adhesive solvent technology is a step forward towards more stable bonding.

It is clear that the current etch-and-rinse bonding protocol requires adhesive systems that are hydrophilic enough to interact with the intrinsically moist acid-etched dentin. This prerequisite is somewhat contradictory with the need for more hydrophobic adhesives in order to extend the bond longevity. In this way, less water will be absorbed from both the host dentin and the oral environment, and render the interface more resistant to water-degradation effects.[47] One interesting attempt by Tay, Pashley and colleagues to optimize infiltration of more hydrophobic resins into acid-etched dentin has recently been introduced as an 'ethanol wet-bonding' technique.[48] It basically involves an intermediate ethanol step to replace most water within the exposed collagen fibril network, thereby dehydrating the acid-etched dentin as well as transforming it into a more hydrophobic state. In this way, the acid-etched dentinal substrate is better prepared to receive more hydrophobic and, thus, less water absorbing resin monomers.[49] The actual experimental protocol aimed to infiltrate acid-etched dentin with bisphenol-A-diglycidyl methacrylate (BisGMA) by decreasing the hydrophilic nature of the dentin surface as water is replaced by ethanol, and by increasing the hydrophilicity of BisGMA as it is solvated in ethanol. In this way, the dentin primer falls within the miscibility range of the ethanol-saturated collagen matrix, allowing more effective infiltration of hydrophobic resin monomers.

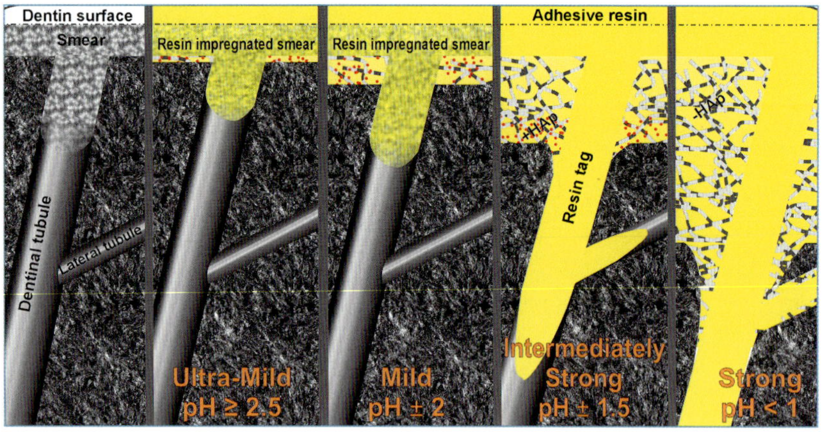

**Fig 3-5** Schematic illustrating the differential interaction of self-etch adhesives with dentin depending on the pH of the self-etching solution.

Concurrently, as water is replaced by ethanol, it has been suggested that some interpeptide hydrogen bonds develop within collagen, stiffening the matrix in such a way that it does not collapse.[50] After infiltration of the collagen matrix and evaporation of ethanol, a more hydrophobic resin–dentin interface is formed that is expected to absorb less water over time and provide better resistance against degradation.[51] This unfortunately laborious and, therefore, perhaps clinically less practical technique found its origin in the lab-processing of samples for electron microscopy, in particular for transmission electron microscopy (TEM) that typically undergo a gradual and, thus, slow dehydration process using ascending concentrations of ethanol prior to embedding procedures with highly hydrophobic epoxy resins.[52] As mentioned by the proponents of this technique, 'the bonding of BisGMA to acid-etched dentin should be viewed as a proof-of-concept for hydrophobic dentin-bonding, rather than as the development of a clinically applicable bonding technique'.[49] The similar performance of this experimental ethanol wet-bonding technique, combined with the application of a hydrophobic adhesive formulation, with that of the abovementioned gold standard three-step etch-and-rinse adhesive OptiBond FL (KerrHawe) with its ethanol/water-based primer is striking, and confirms the overall superior effectiveness of the latter adhesive.

# Latest Advances in Self-Etch Technology

Differently from etch-and-rinse adhesives, self-etch adhesives do not require a separate etching step, as they contain acidic monomers that simultaneously condition and prime the dental substrate.[3] Consequently, this approach has been claimed to be more user-friendly and less technique-sensitive, thereby resulting (though very product dependent) in a clinically reliable performance.[5,53] Some self-etch adhesives have indeed proved to perform quite satisfactorily, both *in vitro* and *in vivo*, leading to a growing popularity of self-etch adhesives in modern dental practices.[3,9]

The morphological features of the adhesive-tooth interface produced by self-etch adhesives depends to a great extent on the manner in which functional monomers interact with the dental substrate (Fig 3-5). In part depending on the pH of the self-etch solutions, the actual interaction depth of self-etch adhesives at dentin differs from: (a) a few hundreds of nanometers following an 'ultra-mild' self-etch approach (pH > 2.5), sometimes being referred to as 'nano-interaction',[54] including AdheSE One (Ivoclar-Vivadent) (Fig 3-6), Clearfil S3 Bond (Kuraray, Tokyo, Japan), G-Bond (GC, Tokyo,

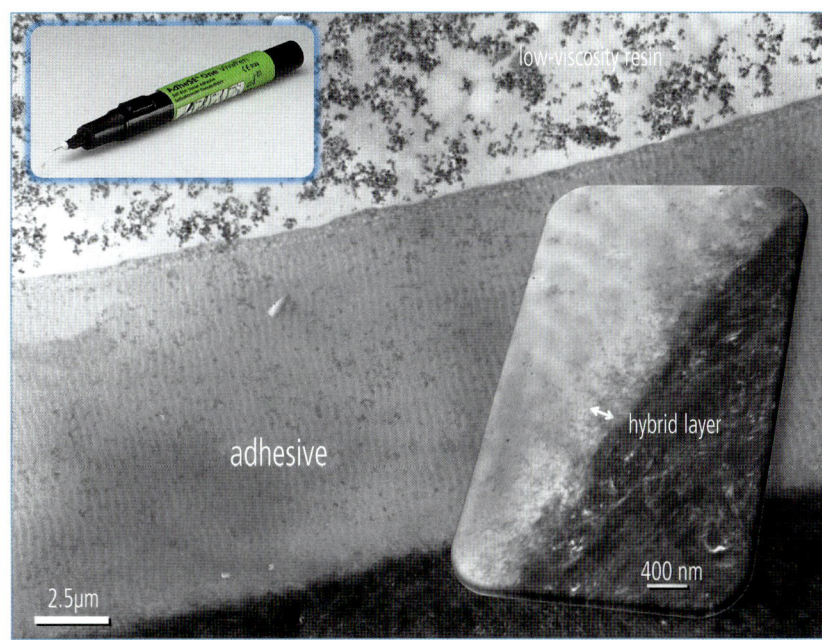

**Fig 3-6** TEM photomicrographs illustrating the interfacial ultra-structure of the 'ultra-mild' one-step self-etch adhesive AdheSE One (Ivoclar-Vivadent) at dentin.

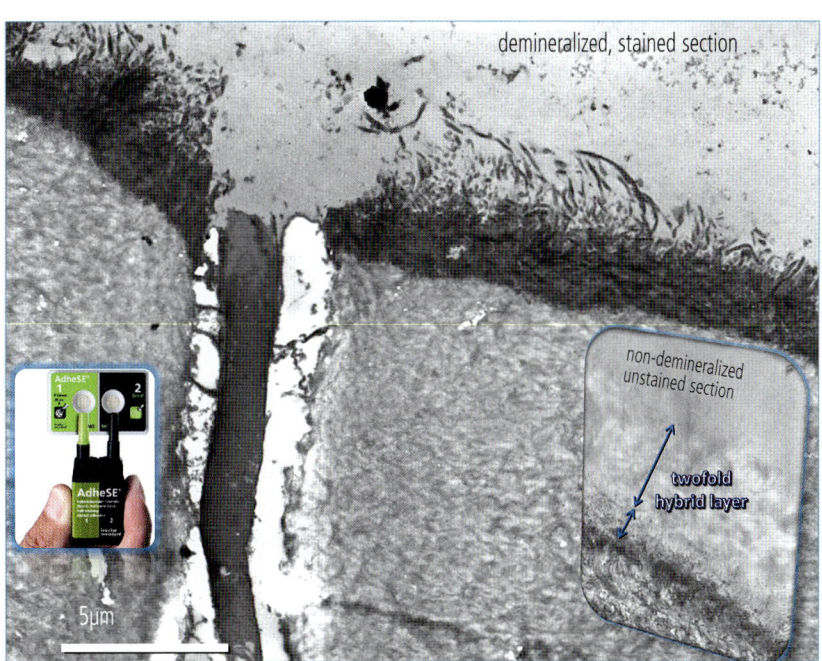

**Fig 3-7** TEM photomicrographs illustrating the interfacial ultra-structure of the 'intermediately strong' two-step self-etch adhesive AdheSE (Ivoclar-Vivadent) at dentin.

Japan) and Bond Force (Tokuyama, Tsukuba, Japan); (b) an interaction depth of around 1 μm or a 'mild' self-etch approach (pH ≈ 2) such as Clearfil SE (Kuraray) (Fig 3-4); (c) an interaction depth between 1 and 2 μm for an 'intermediately strong' self-etch approach (pH between 1 and 2) such as AdheSE (Ivoclar-Vivadent) (Fig 3-7); and (d) to an interaction of several micrometers deep for a 'strong' self-etch approach (pH ≤ 1) such as Adper Prompt L-Pop (3M ESPE, Seefeld, Germany).[3]

In general, self-etch adhesives have the advantage of demineralizing and infiltrating the tooth surface simultaneously to the same depth, theoretically preventing incomplete penetration of the adhesive. With increasing depth, the acidic monomers are gradually buffered by the mineral content of the substrate, losing their ability to further etch the dentin. Typical resin tags are formed only with the strong self-etch adhesives whereas with the mild and ultra-mild self-etch adhesives resin tags are hardly formed, or at maximum the smear plugs get slightly demineralised and subsequently resin-infiltrated. This effect is to a great extent believed to contribute to the significantly lower risk on post-operative sensitivity of mild self-etch adhesives, compared with being regularly reported for etch-and-rinse adhesives.

'Strong' self-etch adhesives present rather deep demineralization effects in both enamel and dentin. The interfacial ultrastructure produced by these adhesives resembles that of etch-and-rinse systems (relatively deep etch pits at enamel, along with deep 2 to 3 mm hybrid layers at dentin), with the difference being that the dissolved calcium phosphates are not rinsed away. It is currently not known how stable these embedded calcium phosphates are and, when they are not very dissolution resistant, to what extent they may weaken the interfacial integrity. Laboratory as well as clinical data have shown that, despite their rather reasonable bonding potential to enamel, they generally under-perform at dentin, in particular with regard to bond durability and restoration longevity.[55,56] This could be attributed to the low hydrolytic stability of the embedded calcium phosphates along with the lack of chemical bonding potential to the exposed collagen.

On the other hand, 'mild' self-etch adhesives only partially demineralize dentin, leaving a substantial amount of hydroxyapatite crystals around the collagen fibrils (Fig 3-4). These residual mineral crystals remain available for possible additional chemical interactions,[3,57] by which their two-fold bonding mechanism (i.e. micro-mechanical and chemical adhesion) closely resembles that of glass-ionomers.[3,9,58-63] The latter also typically present with a submicron hybrid layer that still contains substantial hydroxyapatite that was not dissolved by the polyalkenoic-acid surface treatment. In this respect, glass-ionomers could even be regarded as a kind of mild self-etch adhesives. Glass-ionomers do have the lowest annual failure rate with regard to class-V adhesive restorations,[5] proving that they possess a unique mechanism of self-adhesiveness.

The additional chemical bonding of glass-ionomers and mild self-etch adhesives is believed to be advantageous in terms of bond durability.[57,58,64] The desirable chemical bonding documented with some self-etch adhesives is related to the presence of specific functional monomers in their composition, such as 10-MDP (10-methacryloyloxydecyl dihydrogen phosphate), 4-MET (4-methacryloxyethyl trimellitic acid) and phenyl-P (2-methacryloxyethyl phenyl hydrogen phosphate). These monomers contain carboxylic or phosphate groups that are able to ionically bond with calcium in hydroxyapatite, as was proved by X-ray photoelectron spectroscopy (XPS).[57] However, chemical bonding potential on its own is insufficient; the formed ionic bonds should also be stable in an aqueous environment. In this sense, the chemical bonding promoted by 10-MDP is not only more effective, but also more stable in water than that provided by 4-MET and phenyl-P, in this order.[57] The dissolution rate of the respective calcium salts of these three monomers, as measured by atomic absorption spectroscopy (AAS), was inversely related to their chemical bonding potential as revealed by XPS; the more intense the chemical bonding potential, the less the resultant calcium salt could be dissolved. This finding was further explained in the adhesion-decalcification (AD) concept that dictates whether molecules will either adhere to or decalcify mineralized tissues (Fig 3-8).[65,66]

Confirming the AD-concept, the bond strength to dentin of the 10-MDP-based mild two-step self-etch adhesive Clearfil SE remained high after long-term thermo-cycling, whereas that of Unifil Bond (GC) that contains 4-MET, significantly dropped (but only after 100,000 cycles) and that of Clearfil Liner Bond II (Kuraray) that contains phenyl-P, gradually decreased the longer the bond was exposed to thermo-cycling.[64] The improved resin-tooth interaction provided by 10-MDP definitely enhances its interface-sealing ability, playing an

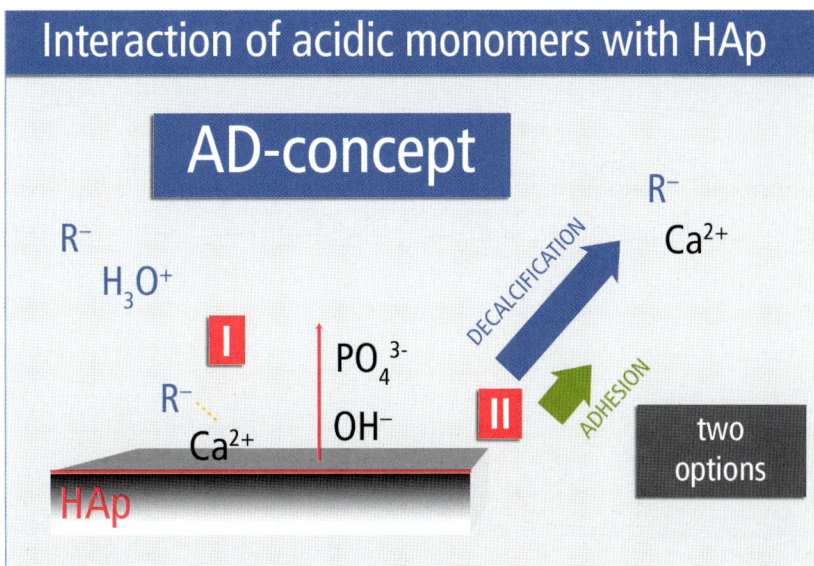

**Fig 3-8** Schematic illustrating the AD-concept, dictating whether molecules either adhere to or decalcify hydroxyapatite-based hard tissues.

important role with regard to bond durability.[67] Clearfil SE has been proven to yield reliable results in terms of bonding effectiveness and durability when compared to other commercially available self-etch adhesives, this in laboratory as well as clinical research.[5,6,53,55,56]

The pKa value of the acid was generally considered as the major parameter in determining the decalcification process of mineralized tissues.[68] However, this does not fully explain the mechanisms for adhesion to and decalcification of hydroxyapatite.[65,66] For example, 1M oxalic acid ($pK_1$ = 1.27, $pK_2$ = 4.28) with a pH of 0.6 is more acidic than 10% maleic acid ($pK_1$ = 1.94, $pK_2$ = 6.23), which has a pH of 0.9. Nevertheless, oxalic acid chemically bonds to hydroxyapatite, whereas maleic acid decalcifies it. That such acids either adhere to or decalcify hydroxyapatite is dependent according to the AD-concept (Fig 3-8) on the dissolution rate of their respective calcium salts in the acid solution; calcium maleate is more soluble than calcium oxalate.[65,66] More specifically, molecules such as phosphoric acid, but also functional monomers including phenyl-P and HEMA-phosphates, will initially bond to calcium of hydroxyapatite. However, this bond (or formed calcium salt) will easily dissociate in the own acidic solution, with the negatively loaded phosphate ions (or carboxyl groups

for carboxyl-based monomers/acids) taking the positively loaded (and, thus, electrostatically attracted) calcium ions with them. This results in a severe decalcification or etching effect, as is the basis of the etch-and-rinse approach when phosphoric acid as etchant is applied, but this also occurs when strong self-etch adhesives are used. Consequently, deep (3 to 5 µm) hybrid layers are formed at the dentin and do not contain any hydroxapatite crystals (Fig 3-2).

On the contrary, molecules such as 10-MDP, but also polyalkenoic acids (as the functional molecules in glass-ionomers), will readily chemically bond to calcium of hydroxyapatite with only a limited decalcification effect, as the formed calcium salt is stable in its own acidic solution and only weakly dissociates. Thin, submicron, hybrid layers that still contain abundant hydroxyapatite are consequently formed at the dentin (Fig 3-4). According to the AD-concept (Fig 3-8), polyalkenoic acid is a polymer with a multitude of carboxyl functional groups that act as chemical 'hands' that grab well-spread individual calcium ions along the mineral substrate. This chemical bonding along with micro-mechanical interlocking through shallow hybridization explains the effective self-adhesiveness of glass-ionomers (even without any form of pre-treat-

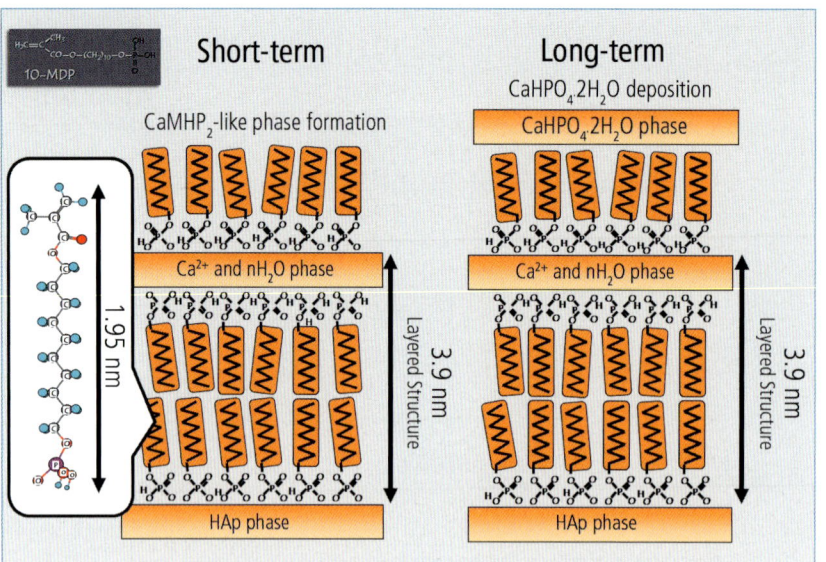

**Fig 3-9** Schematic illustrating the self-assembled nano-layered structure of 10-MDP upon interaction with hydroxyapatite.

ment). The functional monomer 10-MDP bonds through its phosphate groups to hydroxyapatite and forms a regularly layered structure at the hydroxyapatite surface (Fig 3-9).[69] Each layer of this self-assembled nano-layered structure consists of two 10-MDP molecules with their methacrylate groups directed towards each other and their functional hydrogen phosphate groups directed away from one another. In between the layers, calcium salts are deposited.[69]

The adhesive performance of an adhesive material depends on the chemical structure of the functional monomer, and this was recently confirmed when the adhesive performance of four experimental Ivoclar-Vivadent cements was investigated (Fig 3-10).[70] Three cements provided primers that contained derivatives of the phosphonate monomer HAEPA (2-[4-(dihydroxyphosphoryl)-2-oxabutyl]acrylate), of which the carboxyl group was esterified in EAEPA (2,4,6trimethylphenyl 2-[4-(dihydroxyphosphoryl)-2-oxabutyl]acrylate) and MAEPA (ethyl 2-[4-(dihydroxyphosphoryl)-2-oxabutyl]acrylate) with an ethyl and a phenyl group, respectively. The fourth experimental cement provided a primer that contained 10-MDP and served as control. The phosphonate monomers were designed with the aim of good adhesive performance along with high hydrolytic stability.[71] High bond strength of the adhesive cement corresponded to a low dissolution rate of the calcium salt of the respective functional monomer, as measured by AAS. The latter is according to the AD-concept (Fig 3-8) and is suggestive of a high chemical bonding capacity. Consequently, this study showed that improvement of current adhesives is achievable by synthesis of functional monomers tailored to exhibit good chemical bonding potential.

Unfortunately, the bonding of mild self-etch adhesives to enamel (and certainly to unground, aprismatic enamel) remains their weak point.[72-74] Clinical research has obviously revealed that restoration marginal defects at the enamel margins develop rather rapidly, whereas the dentin margins appear to maintain their marginal integrity for much longer.[53] This is somewhat odd if one could expect that the chemical bonding potential to hydroxyapatite must also have its benefit with regard to the bonding effectiveness to enamel which contains even more hydroxyapatite than dentin does. Hence, enamel as a substrate to bond to, apparently requires some degree of micro-mechanical interlocking through some kind of etching process. Therefore, selective etch-

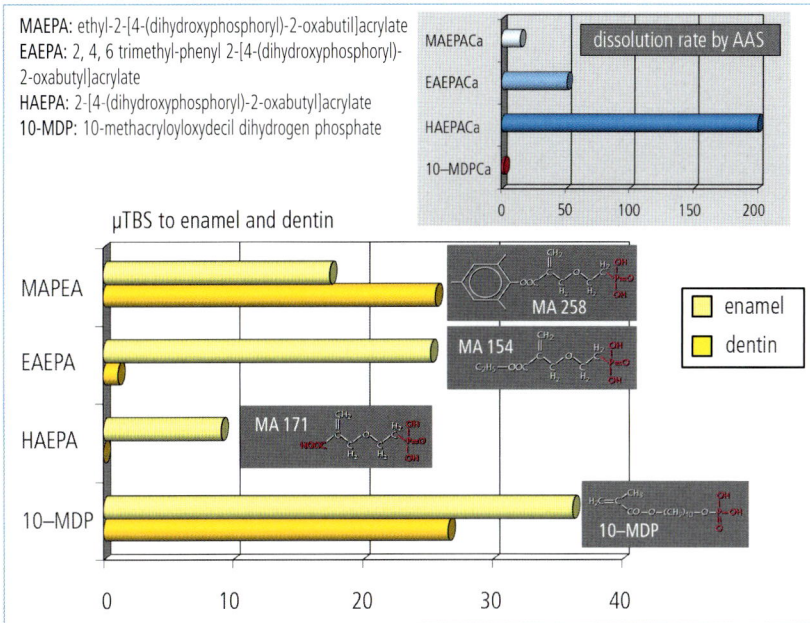

**Fig 3-10** Dissolution rate of the respective calcium salts of three Ivoclar-Vivadent phosphonic-acid monomers as compared to that of the 10-MDP calcium salt, and micro-tensile bond strength to enamel and dentin of the respective luting composites that only differ for the functional monomer added to the self-etching primer.

ing of enamel margins with phosphoric acid, basically turning a two-step self-etch into a three-step adhesive, is a methodology that clinically is frequently applied with much success.[74-76]

# Current Concerns of One-Step Adhesives

Although 'one-step' (self-etch) adhesives are most attractive thanks to their fast and simple application procedure, many concerns have been raised, especially in terms of durability.[6,46] Actually, none of the contemporary all-in-one adhesives can today compete with the classical multi-step systems.[77-79] First, one-step (one-component) adhesives are complex blends of cross-linking and functional monomers, dissolved in water-ethanol or water-acetone.[3,40] Owing to their high hydrophilicity, they remain permeable upon polymerization, permitting movement of water from both the host tooth as well as from the outer oral cavity across the interface.[43,80,81]

HEMA is a water-soluble methacrylate monomer frequently present in dental adhesives in order to increase their wettability and hydrophilicity.[24,82]

Moreover, when incorporated in relatively high concentrations, the miscibility of hydrophobic and hydrophilic components in an adhesive solution is improved, avoiding phase separation (see below), and the possible entrapment of water droplets within the adhesive layer.[83] However, disadvantages have also been related to the presence of HEMA as an adhesive ingredient, especially when it is incorporated in high amounts in so-called 'HEMA-rich' one-step adhesives. Besides the potential allergenic and cytotoxic effects of the uncured monomer,[84,85] HEMA may increase the water sorption of adhesives, adversely influencing the mechanical properties and stability of the adhesive interface.[86] Moreover, such monomer possesses only one polymerizable group, resulting in a polymer with reduced cross-links and, thus, lower mechanical properties.[35,36,86] The high water sorption of HEMA-rich one-step adhesives is due to osmosis (Fig 3-11). Water is actively pulled from the underlying hydrated dentin through the adhesive towards the restorative composite by osmotically induced forces,[43,80,83] potentially produced by calcium and phosphorus ions that are dissolved from the mineralized substrate and are deposited within the oxygen-inhibited layer on the top of the polymerized adhesive.

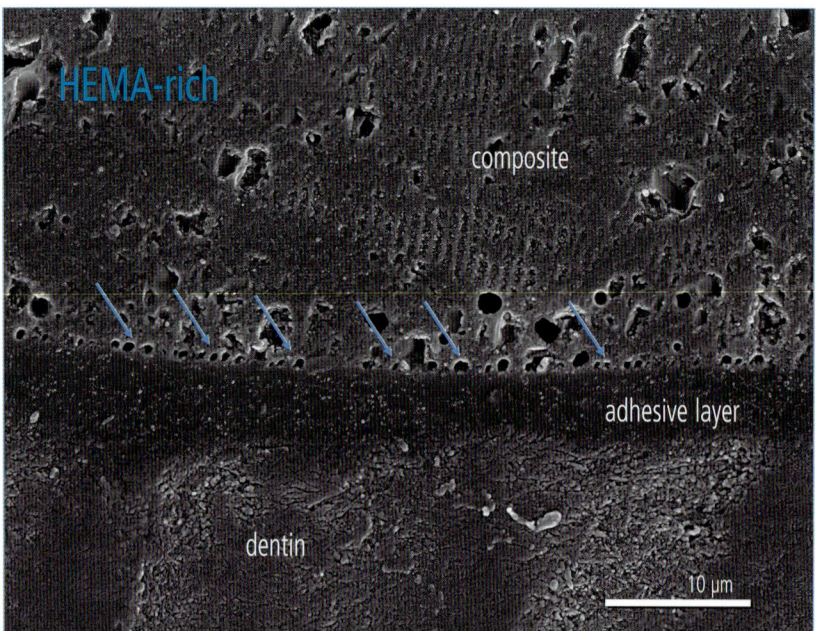

**Fig 3-11** Feg-SEM photomicrograph of the adhesive-dentin interface produced by a HEMA-rich one-step adhesive. Through osmosis, water was abundantly absorbed and resulted in a layer of blisters (arrows) just on top of the adhesive layer in the bottom part of the restorative composite (when light-curing of the latter was postponed for 20 min).

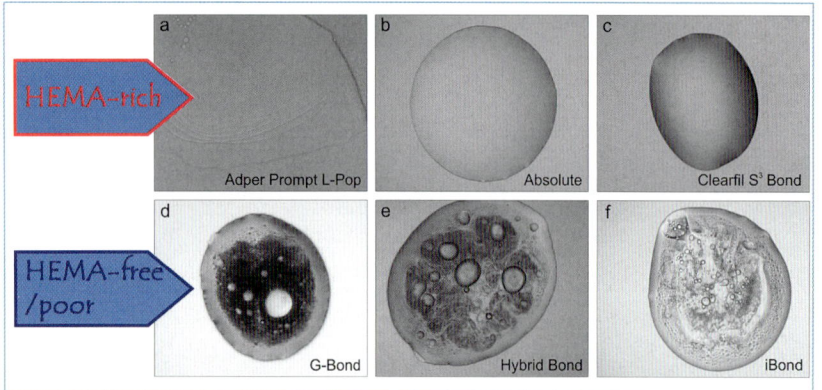

**Fig 3-12** Digital photomicrographs of drops of HEMA-rich and HEMA-free/poor one-step adhesives on a glass plate, showing respectively no and abundant droplet formation due to phase separation.

The above-mentioned drawbacks related to HEMA have led to the introduction of 'HEMA-free' one-step adhesives in an attempt to improve the hydrolysis resistance and, thus, bond durability.[86,87] Indeed, the shallow depth of the hybrid layer produced by these (ultra) mild adhesives should enable resin monomers to interdiffuse relatively fast, decreasing the need for small and, thus, easily diffusing monomers such as HEMA. However, without HEMA the adhesive becomes more sensitive to phase separation (Fig 3-12). Water then separates from the other adhesive ingredients, once the ethanol or acetone solvent starts to evaporate.[87] As a result, these basically water-filled droplets[88] become entrapped in the polymerized adhesive layer, although they can be relatively easily removed by means of strong and prolonged air-blowing prior to light-curing. This adapted application technique is advantageous in removing most water that was provided at the surface by the adhesive, leading to a less water-containing and, thus, theoretically a more stable adhesive–dentin interface.[87] However, how successful this technique can be applied *in vivo*, especially in complex cavity configurations, remains unclear.

Not surprisingly, numerous papers dealing with one-step adhesives have reported on their low resistance to nano-leakage.[6,7,45,46] Their immediate bond strength to enamel and dentin is commonly significantly lower than that of multi-step adhesives.[3] In addition, upon artificial ageing (such as thermo-cycling, mechanical loading in a chewing simulator, simple long-term water storage, exposure to NaOCl, being imposed to high polymerization stress when applied in high C-factor cavities, etc.), their bonding effectiveness has been repeatedly demonstrated to be dramatically reduced.[6,7] In contrast to what is often claimed in commercial advertisements, one-step adhesives are very technique sensitive. For example, air-drying of one-step adhesives has a significant effect on the degree of solvent evaporation and also on the mechanical properties upon setting.[89] Solvents of HEMA-free one-step adhesives should definitely be removed as much as possible by thorough, strong air-drying in order to achieve a strong adhesive layer at the interface. Likewise, the restorative composite should be immediately applied on top of HEMA-rich adhesives in order to avoid abundant osmotic water sorption.

True one-step (one-component) adhesives have generally a shorter shelf life due to in-the-bottle degradation/hydrolysis of the functional monomers.[40,90,91] Therefore, some manufacturers have opted for water-free adhesives (e.g. Absolute 2, Dentsply-Sankin), as this monomer hydrolysis will not take place in a water-free environment. However, in order to activate etching, such a water-free adhesive should obtain its water from the surface, which immediately creates the problem of how wet the surface should be.[92] Of course, shelf life is much less of a problem when water is separated from the functional monomers in two-component one-step adhesives (e.g. Adper Prompt L-Pop, 3M-ESPE; Futurabond NR, VOCO, Cuxhaven, Germany; One-up Bond F plus, Tokuyama; Xeno III, Dentsply).[40,46] More recently synthesized monomers such as amide-linked polymerizable analogs, instead of conventional ester derivatives, and phosphonic-acid monomers (see above) instead of phosphoric-acid monomers (both in AdheSE One, Ivoclar-Vivadent) are more hydrolytically stable, and, thus, prolong the shelf-life.[70,91] Another possibility to improve the adhesive stability is to

increase the pH of the adhesive solution, resulting in the 'ultra-mild' one-step adhesives (e.g. Clearfil S3 Bond, Kuraray). As mentioned above, potential risk of interference on the surface smear with bonding is higher with these relatively high-pH self-etch adhesives (pH ≈ 2.7).[16,20] Therefore, these adhesives could profit from techniques and instruments that produce thinner and less compact smear layers, for example, finishing of the cavity walls with extra-fine diamond burs, or the use of sono- or air-abrasion.[93]

# Durability of Adhesion to Tooth Substrate

Several currently available dental adhesives have been shown to provide reliable short-term bonding effectiveness. However, the durability of adhesion to dental substrate remains a major concern.[6,7,94-96] Actually, current literature has proved that immediate bond strength values do not always correlate with long-term bonding stability.[6,7] In this respect, the current challenge in adhesive dentistry is to create a more stable bonding interface, thereby rendering the restorative treatment more predictable in terms of clinical performance in the long term. The longevity of bonded restorations is, to a large extent, related to the degradation of the adhesive interface, which may occur in a relatively short time, depending on the way the adhesive has been manipulated, the actual adhesive approach and the adhesive composition. In fact, none of the current adhesives or techniques is able to produce an interface that is absolutely resistant to degradation, but many research efforts are currently devoted to improving bonding durability.

The hybrid layer seems to be the most susceptible part of the composite restoration as far as degradation is concerned. Two degradation patterns can be observed within the hybrid layer: loss of resin from interfibrillar spaces and disorganization of unprotected collagen fibrils.[6,7] Such degradation may result from the hydrolysis of resin and/or collagen, thereby weakening the physical properties of the resin-dentin interface. The resin

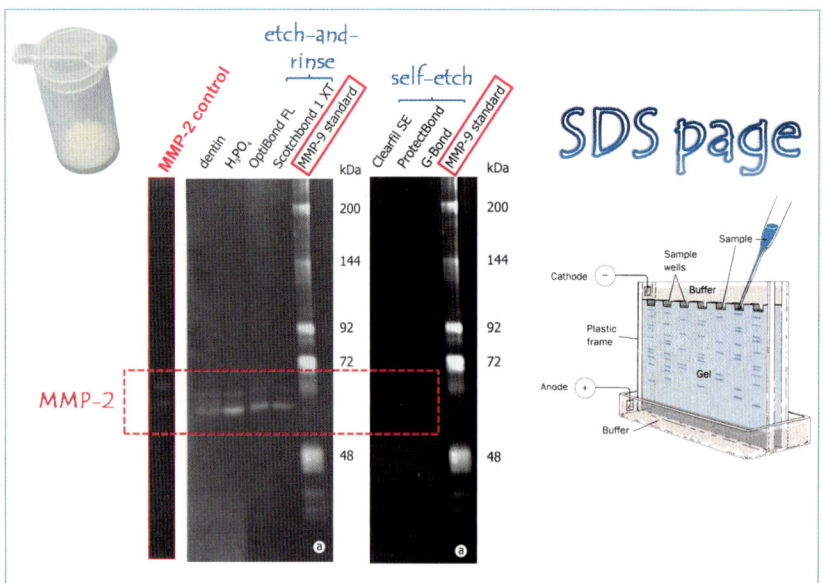

**Fig 3-13** Sodium dodecyl sulfatic polyacrylamide gel electrophoresis (SDS-page) analysis of different etch-and-rinse and self-etch adhesives mixed with dentin powder on their ability to release and activate MMP-2 and MMP-9 enzymes. While etch-and-rinse adhesives that make use of phosphoric-acid etching, released MMP-2, mild self-etch adhesives did not. Release of MMP-9 was not detected with any of the adhesive treatments.

within the hybrid layer is expected to be more prone to hydrolysis than that in the adhesive layer itself. For example, this is the case when the hybrid layer is primarily filled with a poorly cross-linked poly-HEMA matrix, simply due to the higher infiltration potential of this monomer, whereas the adhesive layer contains a higher amount of a strongly cross-linked Bis-GMA/HEMA matrix.

Degradation of collagen within the hybrid layer occurs not only due to activity of collagenases produced *in vivo* by bacteria, but also due to host-derived enzymes that are released and iatrogenically activated by specific adhesive procedures (Fig 3-13).[45,46,97] Such collagenolytic and gelatinolytic activities are triggered by endogenous enzymes, which are naturally present in the mineralized dentin matrix and known as the so-called matrix metalloproteinases (MMPs). During bonding procedures, acid-etching of dentin has been shown to release and activate such MMPs,[97-99] which may in part 'digest' non-resin-enveloped collagen within the hybrid layer.[100] Phosphoric acid (pH ≈ 0.03) probably denatures the MMP activity as rapidly as it exposes more MMP during dentin demineralization, so that the resultant gelatinolytic activity is very low. Actually, pH values near to zero seem to destroy whatever gelatinolytic activity is exposed by acid-etching.[99] On the other hand, mild self-etch adhesives (pH ≥ 2) may activate MMPs far above the non-activity level, but may not be acidic enough to denature them. A simple method to protect the interface against such enzymatic degradation processes is the use of MMP inhibitors, of which one, chlorhexidine, is already commonly used in dentistry and seems effective *in vitro* as well as *in vivo*.[101-103] However, how long this inhibition would be effective remains to be determined. The actual relevance of this enzymatic breakdown of the hybrid layer may be less dramatic clinically than has been suggested in some papers, as the endogenic enzymes gradually decrease with age, commonly disappearing before one reaches the age of 40.[104]

Altogether, different strategies can be followed to render the adhesive interface more resistant against degradation. Improving resin impregnation into demineralized dentin, decreasing the permeability of the bonding interface, optimizing the degree of resin polymerization, avoiding the occurrence of phase separation and inhibiting the activation of endogenous collagenolytic enzymes have been reported as the most important goals to be achieved in search for a more resistant and durable adhesive interface.

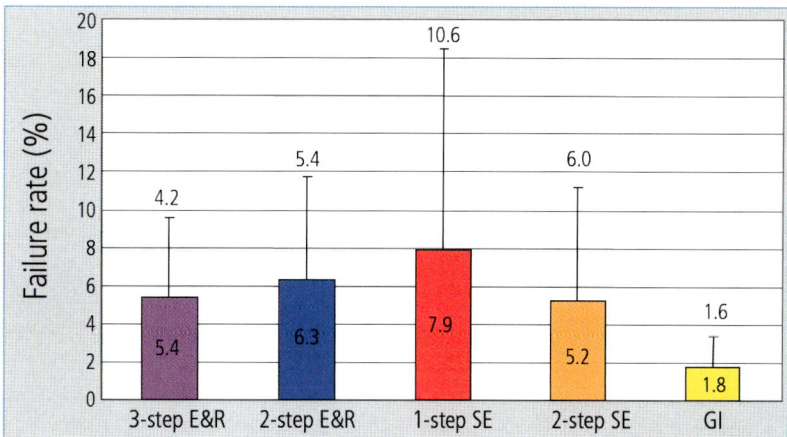

**Fig 3-14** Mean annual failure rates (restoration losses) of the different adhesive approaches when applied in class-V restorations.[5]

# Clinical Performance

Despite the importance of laboratory studies attempting to predict clinical performance of biomaterials, clinical trials remain the ultimate way to collect scientific evidence on the clinical effectiveness of a restorative treatment.[5] The popularity of *in vitro* studies in the field of adhesive dentistry may in part be attributed to the rapid evolution of dental adhesive technology and the resultant high turnover of adhesive systems, which often tempts manufacturers to release a successor product on the market even before its precursor has been clinically evaluated at least in the long term. By carrying out *in vivo* studies, all possible ageing factors occur at the same time, thereby disclosing whether or not an adhesive is truly reliable for routine clinical practice. Retention, marginal integrity and clinical micro-leakage are usually the key parameters recorded to judge the clinical effectiveness of adhesives.

The best clinical performance with regard to retention (the most objective criterion to judge clinical effectiveness) has so far been achieved by glass-ionomers (Fig 3-14).[5] Their low annual failure rates can be attributed to their unique self-adhesiveness, based on the two-fold micro-mechanical and chemical bonding mechanism (see above). Despite their excellent clinical performance in terms of retention, glass-ionomers commonly present with lower esthetic features when compared with resin-based restorative materials. The poorer mechanical properties of glass-ionomers also explains the lower scores achieved in bond strength tests when compared with those of resin-based adhesives, by which a glass-ionomer typically fails cohesively rather than it de-bonds from the tooth surface.

Besides glass-ionomers, three-step etch-and-rinse adhesives exhibit reasonably good clinical effectiveness (Fig 3-14).[5] The clinical durability of three-step etch-and-rinse adhesives confirms their generally superior laboratory results, in which they are considered as gold standard and used as a control to compare the performance of new-generation adhesives.

According to the same standard, mild two-step self-etch adhesives tend to approach three-step etch-and-rinse adhesives in terms of low annual failure rates (Fig 3-14).[5] Their ability to provide a shallow, but uniform hybrid layer, along with their capability to chemically bond to the dentin substrate seems to play an important role to resist long-term hydrolytic degradation. Commonly, the clinical performance of such self-etch adhesives does not vary substantially from one study to another, which is indicative of their rather low technique-sensitivity. Furthermore, another clinically important benefit is, as mentioned previously, that these self-etch adhesives are repeatedly associated with very low levels of postoperative sensitivity.[76]

In general, two-step etch-and-rinse adhesives have performed less favorably compared with the conventional three-step version (Fig 3-14).[5] Laboratory studies have corroborated these results, relating their poorer performance to their higher hydrophilicity and reduced hybridization potential. It is noteworthy that irrespective of the number of application steps, acetone-based etch-and-rinse adhesives have performed less satisfactorily than their water/ethanol-based alternatives. The above-mentioned high technique-sensitivity of acetone-based adhesives must be the reason for their compromised long-term clinical data.

A so far rather inefficient clinical performance has been noted for the newest generation of one-step adhesives. Widely varying retention scores have been recorded, indicating high technique sensitivity despite their user-friendliness (Fig 3-14).[5] Such lower bonding performance must be ascribed to the many concerns advanced earlier.

## Some Directions for Future Development of Adhesive Technology

Design and synthesis of functional monomers is definitely a worthwhile pathway towards new and improved adhesive technology. Many studies on dental adhesive technology are nowadays empirical, basically testing the bond strength of different cocktails of adhesive solutions to enamel and dentin in the laboratory. The adhesive formulation that scores best, commonly makes it rapidly to the market, after which the superior laboratory performance of the product is hopefully confirmed in independent RCTs. Much knowledge on the underlying mechanisms of adhesion to enamel and dentin has been provided by numerous imaging studies of adhesive-tooth interfaces with all sorts of microscopes. In contrast, the actual molecular interactions at the interface have hardly been explored. Many basic questions still remain unanswered, for example why certain functional monomers have better bonding potential than others, and why mild self-etch adhesives with additional chemical bonding do not perform better at enamel. Thus, fundamental for future design and development of dental adhesives is the further unravelling of the molecular interfacial interactions.

## Conclusions

Adhesive technology has undergone great progress in the last decade.

In light of the major drawbacks attributed to all-in-one self-etch adhesives, conventional three-step etch-and-rinse adhesives and two-step self-etch adhesives are still the benchmark for dental adhesion in routine clinical use.

When bonding to enamel, an etch-and-rinse approach is definitely preferred, indicating that simple micro-mechanical interaction appears sufficient to achieve a durable bond to enamel.

When bonding to dentin, a mild self-etch approach is superior, as it additionally chemically interacts with residual hydroxyapatite and this definitely should contribute most to the bond durability.

Altogether, when bonding to both enamel and dentin, selective etching of enamel followed by the application of the self-etch adhesive to both enamel and dentin currently appears the best choice to effectively and durably bond to tooth tissue.

Along with the fast evolution of multi-step adhesives towards one-step adhesives, luting composites so as to adhesively lute indirect ceramic restorations underwent a similar evolution towards simple-to-use and less technique-sensitive one-step luting agents. Hence, these self-adhesive luting composites do not need any kind of pre-treatment of the tooth substrate, thereby bringing the development of self-adhesive composites closer to reality.

# References

1. Black GV. A work in operative dentistry in two volumes, 1917 ed 3. Chicago: Medico-Dental Publishing.

2. Degrange M, Roulet JF. Minimally invasive restorations with bonding, 1997 ed 1. Chicago: Quintessence Publishing.

3. Van Meerbeek B, Yoshida Y, Van Landuyt K, Perdigão J, De Munck J, Lambrechts P, Inoue S, Peumans M (2006). In: Summitt JB, Robbins JW, Hilton TJ, Schwartz RS. Fundamentals of operative dentistry. A contemporary approach. ed 3. Chicago: Quintessence Publishing. 2006;183-260.

4. Manhart J, Chen H, Hamm G, Hickel R. Buonocore Memorial Lecture. Review of the clinical survival of direct and indirect restorations in posterior teeth of the permanent dentition. Oper Dent 2004;29:481-508.

5. Peumans M, Kanumilli P, De Munck J, Van Landuyt K, Lambrechts P, Van Meerbeek B. Clinical effectiveness of contemporary adhesives: a systematic review of current clinical trials. Dent Mater 2005;21:864-881.

6. De Munck J, Van Landuyt K, Peumans M, Poitevin A, Lambrechts P, Braem M, Van Meerbeek B. A critical review of the durability of adhesion to tooth tissue: methods and results. J Dent Res 2005;84:118-132.

7. Breschi L, Mazzoni A, Ruggeri A, Cadenaro M, Di Lenarda R, Dorigo ES. Dental adhesion review: aging and stability of the bonded interface. Dent Mater 2008;24:90-101.

8. Mjör IA, Shen C, Eliasson ST, Richter S. Placement and replacement of restorations in general dental practice in Iceland. Oper Dent 2002;27:117-123.

9. Van Meerbeek B, De Munck J, Yoshida Y, Inoue S, Vargas M, Vijay P, Van Landuyt K, Lambrechts P, Vanherle G (2003). Buonocore memorial lecture: adhesion to enamel and dentin: current status and future challenges. Oper Dent 2003;28:215-235.

10. Buonocore MG. A simple method of increasing the adhesion of acrylic filling materials to enamel surfaces. J Dent Res 1955;34:849-853.

11. Gwinnett AJ, Matsui A. A study of enamel adhesives. The physical relationship between enamel and adhesive. Arch Oral Biol 1967;12:1615-1620.

12. De Munck J, Van Meerbeek B, Yoshida Y, Inoue S, Vargas M, Suzuki K, Lambrechts P, Van Meerbeek B. Four-year water degradation of total-etch adhesives bonded to dentin. J Dent Res 2003;82:136-140.

13. Terkla LG, Brown AC, Hainisch AP, Mitchem JC. Testing sealing properties of restorative materials against moist dentin. J Dent Res 1987;66:1758-1764.

14. Pashley DH, Tao L, Boyd L, King GE, Horner JA. Scanning electron microscopy of the substructure of smear layers in human dentine. Arch Oral Biol 1988;33:265-270.

15. Pashley DH. Smear layer: an overview of structure and function. Proc Finn Dent Soc 1992;88:215-224.

16. Ermis RB, De Munck J, Cardoso MV, Coutinho E, Van Landuyt KL, Poitevin A, Lambrechts P, Van Meerbeek B. Bond strength of self-etch adhesives to dentin prepared with three different diamond burs. Dent Mater 2008;24:978-985.

17. Fusayama T, Nakamura M, Kurosaki N, Iwaku M. Non-pressure adhesion of a new adhesive restorative resin. J Dent Res 1979;58:1364-1370.

18. Heymann HO, Sturdevant JR, Bayne S, Wilder AD, Sluder TB, Brunson WD. Examining tooth flexure effects on cervical restorations: a two-year clinical study. J Am Dent Assoc 1991;122:41-7.

19. Inoue S, Van Meerbeek B, Vargas M, Yoshida Y, Lambrechts P, Vanherle G. Adhesion mechanism of self-etch adhesives. In: Tagami J, Toledano M, Prati C: Advanced adhesive dentistry. Granada international symposium 1999. Cirimido (Como): Grafiche Erredue. 2000;131-148.

20. Cardoso MV, Coutinho E, Ermis RB, Poitevin A, Van Landuyt K, De Munck J, Carvalho RC, Van Meerbeek B. Influence of dentin cavity surface finishing on micro-tensile bond strength of adhesives. Dent Mater 2008;24:492-501.

21. Van Meerbeek B, Inokoshi S, Braem M, Lambrechts P, Vanherle G. Morphological aspects of the resin-dentin interdiffusion zone with different dentin adhesive systems. J Dent Res 1992;71:1530-1540.

22. Van Meerbeek B, Dhem A, Goret-Nicaise M, Braem M, Lambrechts P, Vanherle G. Comparative SEM and TEM examination of the ultrastructure of the resin-dentin interdiffusion zone. J Dent Res 1993;72:495-501.

23. Perdigao J, Lambrechts P, Van Meerbeek B, Braem M, Yildiz E, Yucel T, Vanherle G. The interaction of adhesive systems with human dentin. Am J Dent 1996;9:167-173.

24. Nakabayashi N, Takarada K. Effect of HEMA on bonding to dentin. Dent Mater 1992;8:125-130.

25. Carvalho RM, Mendonca JS, Santiago SL, Silveira RR, Garcia FC, Tay FR, Pashley DH. Effects of HEMA/solvent combinations on bond strength to dentin. J Dent Res 2003;82:597-601.

26. Yoshiyama M, Carvalho R, Sano H, Horner J, Brewer PD, Pashley DH. Interfacial morphology and strength of bonds made to superficial versus deep dentin. Am J Dent 1995;8:297-302.

27. Finger WJ, Balkenhol M. Practitioner variability effects on dentin bonding with an acetone-based one-bottle adhesive. J Adhes Dent 1999;1:311-314.

28. Van Meerbeek B, Van Landuyt K, De Munck J, Hashimoto M, Peumans M, Lambrechts P, Yoshida Y, Inoue S, Suzuki K. Technique-sensitivity of contemporary adhesives. Dent Mater J 2005;24:1-13.

29. Van Meerbeek B, Yoshida Y, Lambrechts P, Vanherle G, Duke ES, Eick JD, Robinson SJ (1998). A TEM study of two water-based adhesive systems bonded to dry and wet dentin. J Dent Res 1998;77:50-59.

30. Kanca III J. Resin bonding to wet substrate. I. Bonding to dentin. Quintessence Int 1992;23:39-41.

31. Tay FR, Gwinnett AJ, Pang KM, Wei SH. Resin permeation into acid-conditioned, moist, and dry dentin: a paradigm using water-free adhesive primers. J Dent Res 1996;75:1034-1044.

32. Wang Y, Spencer P. Hybridization efficiency of the adhesive/dentin interface with wet bonding. J Dent Res 2003;82:141-145.

33. Tay FR, Gwinnett JA, Wei SH. Micromorphological spectrum from overdrying to overwetting acid-conditioned dentin in water-free acetone-based, single-bottle primer/adhesives. Dent Mater 1996;12:236-244.

34. Jacobsen T, Soderholm KJ. Some effects of water on dentin bonding (1995). Dent Mater 1995;11:132 136.

35. Ikeda T, De Munck J, Shirai K, Hikita K, Inoue S, Sano H, Lambrechts P, Van Meerbeek B (2005). Effect of fracture strength of primer-adhesive mixture on bonding effectiveness. Dent Mater 2005;21:413-20.

36. Ikeda T, De Munck J, Shirai K, Hikita K, Inoue S, Sano H, Lambrechts P, Van Meerbeek B (2005). Effect of evaporation of primer components on ultimate tensile strengths of primer-adhesive mixture. Dent Mater 2005;21:1051-8.

37. Gwinnett AJ. Chemically conditioned dentin: a comparison of conventional and environmental scanning electron microscopy findings. Dent Mater 1994;10:150-155.

38. Perdigão J, Lambrechts P, van Meerbeek B, Tomé AR, Vanherle G, Lopes AB. Morphological field emission-SEM study of the effect of six phosphoric acid etching agents on human dentin. Dent Mater 1996;12:262-71.

39. Moszner N, Salz U, Zimmermann J. Chemical aspects of self-etching enamel-dentin adhesives: a systematic review. Dent Mater 2005;21:895-910.

40. Van Landuyt KL, Snauwaert J, De Munck J, Peumans M, Yoshida Y, Poitevin A, Coutinho E, Suzuki K, Lambrechts P, Van Meerbeek B. Systematic review of the chemical composition of contemporary dental adhesives. Biomaterials 2007;28:3757-3785.

41. Sano H, Takatsu T, Ciucchi B, Horner JA, Matthews WG, Pashley DH. Nanoleakage: leakage within the hybrid layer. Oper Dent 1995;20:18-25.

42. Sano H, Shono T, Takatsu T, Hosoda H. Microporous dentin zone beneath resin-impregnated layer. Oper Dent 1994;19:59-64.

43. Tay FR, Pashley DH. Water treeing - a potential mechanism for degradation of dentin adhesives. Am J Dent 2003;16:6-12.

44. Van Meerbeek B. The „myth" of nanoleakage. J Adhes Dent 2007;9:491-2.

45. Pashley D, Tay F. Mechanical stability of resin-dentine bonds. In: Curtis RV, Watson TF. Dental Biomaterials. Imaging, testing and modelling. Cambridge: Woodhead publishing in materials. 2008;112-161.

46. Van Meerbeek B, De Munck J, Van Landuyt KL, Mine A, Lambrechts P, Sarr M, Yoshida Y, Suzuki K (2008). Dental adhesives and adhesive performances. In: Curtis RV, Watson TF. Dental Biomaterials. Imaging, testing and modelling. Cambridge: Woodhead publishing in materials. 2008;81-111.

47. Tay FR, Pashley DH. Have dentin adhesives become too hydrophilic? J Can Dent Assoc 2003;69:726-731.

48. Pashley DH, Tay FR, Carvalho RM, Rueggeberg FA, Agee KA, Carrilho M, Donnelly A, García-Godoy F (2007). From dry bonding to water-wet bonding to ethanol-wet bonding. A review of the interactions between dentin matrix and solvated resins using a macromodel of the hybrid layer. Am J Dent 2007;20:7-20.

49. Tay FR, Pashley DH, Kapur RR, Carrilho MR, Hur YB, Garrett LV, Tay KC (2007). Bonding BisGMA to dentin - a proof of concept for hydrophobic dentin bonding. J Dent Res 2007;86:1034-1039.

50. Becker TD, Agee KA, Joyce AP, Rueggeberg FA, Borke JL, Waller JL, Tay FR, Pashley DH (2007). Infiltration/evaporation-induced shrinkage of demineralized dentin by solvated model adhesives. J Biomed Mater Res B Appl Biomater 2007;80:156-165.

51. Nishitani Y, Yoshiyama M, Donnelly AM, Agee KA, Sword J, Tay FR, Pashley DH (2006). Effects of resin hydrophilicity on dentin bond strength. J Dent Res 2006;85:1016-1021.

52. Van Meerbeek B, Vargas M, Inoue S, Yoshida Y, Perdigão J, Lambrechts P, Vanherle G. Microscopy investigations. Techniques, results, limitations. Am J Dent 2000;13(Spec No):3D-18D.

53. Peumans M, De Munck J, Van Landuyt K, Lambrechts P, Van Meerbeek B. Five-year clinical effectiveness of a two-step self-etching adhesive. J Adhes Dent 2007;9:7-10.

54. Koshiro K, Sidhu SK, Inoue S, Ikeda T, Sano H. New concept of resin-dentin interfacial adhesion: The nanointeraction zone. J Biomed Mater Res Part B: Appl Biomater 2006;77B:401–408.

55. Shirai K, De Munck J, Yoshida Y, Inoue S, Lambrechts P, Suzuki K, Shintani H, Van Meerbeek B. Effect of cavity configuration and aging on the bonding effectiveness of six adhesives to dentin. Dent Mater 2005;21:110-24.

56. De Munck J, Shirai K, Yoshida Y, Inoue S, Van Landuyt K, Lambrechts P, Suzuki K, Shintani H, Van Meerbeek B (2006). Effect of water storage on the bonding effectiveness of 6 adhesives to Class I cavity dentin. Oper Dent 2006;31:456-65.

57. Yoshida Y, Nagakane K, Fukuda R, Nakayama Y, Okazaki M, Shintani H, Inoue S, Tagawa Y, Suzuki K De Munck J, Van Meerbeek B. Comparative study on adhesive performance of functional monomers. J Dent Res 2004;83:454-458.

58. Yoshida Y, Van Meerbeek B, Nakayama Y, Snauwaert J, Hellemans L, Lambrechts P, Vanherle G, Wakasa K (2000). Evidence of chemical bonding at biomaterial-hard tissue interfaces. J Dent Res 2000;79:709-714.

59. Fukuda R, Yoshida Y, Nakayama Y, Okazaki M, Inoue S, Sano H, Suzuki K, Shintani H, Van Meerbeek B (2003). Bonding efficacy of polyalkenoic acids to hydroxyapatite, enamel and dentin. Biomaterials 2003;24:1861-7.

60. Yiu CK, Tay FR, King NM, Pashley DH, Sidhu SK, Neo JC, Toledano M, Wong SL (2004). Interaction of glass-ionomer cements with moist dentin. J Dent Res 2004;83:283-9.

61. Tay FR, Sidhu SK, Watson TF, Pashley DH. Water-dependent interfacial transition zone in resin-modified glass-ionomer cement/dentin interfaces. J Dent Res 2004;83:644-9.

62. Coutinho E, Van Landuyt K, De Munck J, Poitevin A, Yoshida Y, Inoue S, Peumans M, Suzuki K, Lambrechts P, Van Meerbeek B (2006). Development of a self-etch adhesive for resin-modified glass ionomers. J Dent Res 2006;85:349-53.

63. Coutinho E, Yoshida Y, Inoue S, Fukuda R, Snauwaert J, Nakayama Y, De Munck J, Lambrechts P, Suzuki K, Van Meerbeek B. Gel phase formation at resin-modified glass-ionomer/tooth interfaces. J Dent Res 2007;86:656-61.

64. Inoue S, Koshiro K, Yoshida Y, De Munck J, Nagakane K, Suzuki K, Sano H, Van Meerbeek B (2005). Hydrolytic stability of self-etch adhesives bonded to dentin. J Dent Res 2005;84:1160-4.

65. Yoshida Y, Van Meerbeek B, Nakayama Y, Yoshioka M, Snauwaert J, Abe Y, Lambrechts P, Vanherle G, Okazaki M (2001). Adhesion to and decalcification of hydroxyapatite by carboxylic acids. J Dent Res 2001;80:1565-9.

66. Yoshioka M, Yoshida Y, Inoue S, Lambrechts P, Vanherle G, Nomura Y. Okazaki M, Shintani H, Van Meerbeek B (2002). Adhesion/decalcification mechanisms of acid interactions with human hard tissues. J Biomed Mater Res 2002;59:56-62.

67. Sano H, Yoshikawa T, Pereira PN, Kanemura N, Morigami M, Tagami J, Pashley DH (1999). Long-term durability of dentin bonds made with a self-etching primer, in vivo. J Dent Res 1999;78:906-911

68. Salz U, Mücke A, Zimmermann J, Tay FR, Pashley DH (2006). pKa value and buffering capacity of acidic monomers commonly used in self-etching primers. J Adhes Dent 8:143-50.

69. Fukegawa D, Hayakawa S, Yoshida Y, Suzuki K, Osaka A, Van Meerbeek B. Chemical interaction of phosphoric acid ester with hydroxyapatite. J Dent Res 2006;85:941-4.

70. Van Landuyt KL, Yoshida Y, Hirata I, Snauwaert J, De Munck J, Okazaki M, Suzuki K, Lambrechts P, Van Meerbeek B (2008). Influence of the chemical structure of functional monomers on their adhesive performance. J Dent Res 2008;87:757-761.

71. Moszner N, Salz U, Zimmermann J. Chemical aspects of self-etching enamel-dentin adhesives: a systematic review. Dent Mater 2005;21:895-910.

72. Pashley DH, Tay FR. Aggressiveness of contemporary self-etching adhesives. Part II: etching effects on unground enamel. Dent Mater 2001;17:430-444.

73. Perdigão J, Geraldeli S. Bonding characteristics of self-etching adhesives to intact versus prepared enamel. J Esthet Restor Dent 2003;15:32-41.

74. Van Landuyt KL, Kanumilli P, De Munck J, Peumans M, Lambrechts P, Van Meerbeek B (2006). Bond strength of a mild self-etch adhesive with and without prior acid-etching. J Dent 2006;34:77-85.

75. Lührs AK, Guhr S, Schilke R, Borchers L, Geurtsen W, Günay H. Shear bond strength of self-etch adhesives to enamel with additional phosphoric acid etching. Oper Dent 2008;33:155-62.

76. Perdigão J. New developments in dental adhesion. Dent Clin North Am 2007;51:333-57.

77. Bouillaguet S, Gysi P, Wataha JC, Ciucchi B, Cattani M, Godin C, Meyer JM (2001). Bond strength of composite to dentin using conventional, one-step, and self-etching adhesive systems. J Dent 2001;29:55-61.

78. Inoue S, Vargas MA, Abe Y, Yoshida Y, Lambrechts P, Vanherle G, Sano H, Van Meerbeek B (2001). Microtensile bond strength of eleven contemporary adhesives to dentin. J Adhes Dent 2001;3:237-245.

79. Inoue S, Vargas MA, Abe Y, Yoshida Y, Lambrechts P, Vanherle G, Sano H, Van Meerbeek B (2003). Microtensile bond strength of eleven contemporary adhesives to enamel. Am J Dent 2003;16:329-334.

80. Tay FR, Pashley DH, Suh BI, Carvalho RM, Itthagarun A. Single-step adhesives are permeable membranes. J Dent 2002;30:371-382.

81. Tay FR, Pashley DH, Yoshiyama M. Two modes of nanoleakage expression in single-step adhesives. J Dent Res 2002;81:472-476.

82. Toledano M, Osorio R, Moreira MA, Cabrerizo-Vilchez MA, Gea P, Tay FR, Pashley DH (2004). Effect of the hydration status of the smear layer on the wettability and bond strength of a self-etching primer to dentin. Am J Dent 2004;17:310-314.

83. Van Landuyt KL, Snauwaert J, De Munck J, Coutinho E, Poitevin A, Yoshida Y, Suzuki K, Lambrechts P, Van Meerbeek B (2007). Origin of interfacial droplets with one-step adhesives. J Dent Res 2007;86:739-44.

84. Goossens A. Contact allergic reactions on the eyes and eyelids. Bull Soc Belge Ophtalmol 2004;292:11-17.

85. Paranjpe A, Bordador LC, Wang MY, Hume WR, Jewett A. Resin monomer 2-hydroxyethyl methacrylate (HEMA) is a potent inducer of apoptotic cell death in human and mouse cells. J Dent Res 2005;84:172-177.

86. Van Landuyt KL, Snauwaert J, Peumans M, De Munck J, Lambrechts P, Van Meerbeek B. The role of HEMA in one-step self-etch adhesives. Dent Mater in press. Dent Mater Apr 21 2008. [Epub ahead of print].

87. Van Landuyt KL, De Munck J, Snauwaert J, Coutinho E, Poitevin A, Yoshida Y, Inoue S, Peumans M, Suzuki K, Lambrechts P, Van Meerbeek B (2005). Monomer-solvent phase separation in one-step self-etch adhesives. J Dent Res 2005;84:183-188.

88. Gaintantzopoulou M, Rahiotis C, Eliades G. Molecular characterization of one-step self-etching adhesives placed on dentin and inert substrate. J Adhes Dent 2008;10:83-93.

89. Ikeda T, De Munck J, Shirai K, Hikita K, Inoue S, Sano H, Lambrechts P, Van Meerbeek B (2008). Effect of air-drying and solvent evaporation on the strength of HEMA-rich versus HEMA-free one-step adhesives. Dent Mater Apr 16. 2008 [Epub ahead of print].

90. Nishiyama N, Tay FR, Fujita K, Pashley DH, Ikemura K, Hiraishi N, King NM (2006). Hydrolysis of functional monomers in a single-bottle self-etching primer—correlation of 13C NMR and TEM findings. J Dent Res 2006;85:422-6.

91. Salz U, Zimmermann J, Zeuner F, Moszner N. Hydrolytic stability of self-etching adhesive systems. J Adhes Dent 2005;7:107-16.

92. Van Landuyt KL, Mine A, De Munck J, Countinho E, Peumans M, Jaecques S, Lambrechts P, Van Meerbeek B (2008). Technique sensitivity of water-free one-step adhesives. Dent Mater Apr 2. 2008 [Epub ahead of print].

93. Van Meerbeek B, De Munck J, Mattar D, Van Landuyt K, Lambrechts P. Microtensile bond strengths of an etch & rinse and self-etch adhesive to enamel and dentin as a function of surface treatment. Oper Dent 2003;28:647-660.

94. Hashimoto M, Ohno H, Sano H, Kaga M, Oguchi H. In vitro degradation of resin-dentin bonds analyzed by microtensile bond test, scanning and transmission electron microscopy. Biomaterials 2003;24:3795-3803.

95. Koshiro K, Inoue S, Sano H, De Munck J, Van Meerbeek B. In vivo degradation of resin-dentin bonds produced by a self-etch and an etch-and-rinse adhesive. Eur J Oral Sci 2005;113:341-348.

96. Tay FR, Pashley DH, Suh BI, Hiraishi N, Yiu CK. Water treeing in simplified dentin adhesives - déjà vu? Oper Dent 2005;30:561-579.

97. Pashley DH, Tay FR, Yiu C, Hashimoto M, Breschi L, Carvalho RM, Ito S (2004). Collagen degradation by host-derived enzymes during aging. J Dent Res 2004;83:216-221.

98. Tay FR, Pashley DH, Loushine RJ, Weller RN, Monticelli F, Osorio R. Self-etching adhesives increase collagenolytic activity in radicular dentin. J Endod 2006;32:862-868.

99. Nishitani Y, Yoshiyama M, Wadgaonkar B, Breschi L, Mannello F, Mazzoni A, Carvalho RM, Tjäderhane L, Tay FR, Pashley DH (2006). Activation of gelatinolytic/collagenolytic activity in dentin by self-etching adhesives. Eur J Oral Sci 2006;114:160-166.

100. Armstrong SR, Vargas MA, Chung I, Pashley DH, Campbell JA, Laffoon JE, Qian F (2004). Resin-dentin interfacial ultrastructure and microtensile dentin bond strength after five-year water storage. Oper Dent 2004;29:705-712.

101. Gendron R, Grenier D, Sorsa T, Mayrand D. Inhibition of the activities of matrix metalloproteinases 2, 8, and 9 by chlorhexidine. Clin Diagn Lab Immunol 1999;6:437-439.

102. Carrilho MR, Carvalho RM, de Goes MF, di Hipólito V, Geraldeli S, Tay FR, Pashley DH, Tjäderhane L. Chlorhexidine preserves dentin bond in vitro. J Dent Res 2007;86:90-94.

103. Carrilho MR, Geraldeli S, Tay F, de Goes MF, Carvalho RM, Tjäderhane L, Reis AF, Hebling J, Mazzoni A, Breschi L, Pashley D (2007). In vivo preservation of the hybrid layer by chlorhexidine. J Dent Res 2007;86:529-33.

104. Martin-De Las Heras S, Valenzuela A, Overall CM. The matrix metalloproteinase gelatinase A in human dentine. Arch Oral Biol 2000;45:757-765.

# Anterior Restorations – Direct Composites, Veneers or Crowns?

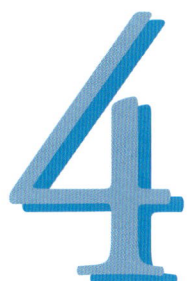

Mutlu Özcan

## Introduction

Being able to eat, swallow and digest food is one of the prerequisites for human life. Chewing in humans starts primarily with the incision of food by the anterior teeth. These teeth not only provide guidance of the mandible (anterior guidance), but also supply lip support. Many of the sounds made during speech are pronounced utilizing the anterior teeth. Some letters require the lips and/or tongue to make contact with anterior teeth for proper pronunciation of the sounds. For example, the fricative consonant sounds of the English language *s, z, x, d, n, l, j, t, th, ch* and *sh* are achieved with tongue-to-tooth contact, and the fricative f and v are achieved through lip-to-tooth contact. In languages other than English, the sounds produced utilizing the anterior teeth may be even more frequent. Thus missing anterior teeth in an individual will affect the way in which these sounds are enunciated. Since during talking or smiling anterior teeth become the most exposed, their role in esthetics is also dominant. Although the perception and definition of esthetics varies between cultures, with its objective and subjective components that are debatable, esthetics is still considered an integral part of oral function in many cultures.

Unfortunately, there is no known method for regenerating large amounts of tooth structures or periodontal tissues. Regrettably, because of either the lack of education in oral hygiene, not practicing preventive measures timely, or simply as a consequence of neglect on the part of the patient or trauma due to various reasons, the form and function of dental tissues must still be restored, repaired, or replaced with artificial materials by the dentist. It has been proven difficult to imitate dental tissues, because of their unique structure. Both structurally and biomechanically, the dental tissues demonstrate a unique combination. Hardness and elastic modulus, for example, vary in different places of the tooth showing anisotropic features. Tooth material, in short, is a perfectly designed, intelligent composite material that can resist the chewing forces without damaging its own durability. Fortunately, the dental profession has profited from remarkable technologies from other disciplines of science, which allow the substitution of missing dental tissues or teeth. However, we are still faced with the challenge of imitating the tooth tissues mechanically, physically, biologically or optically, if not completely.

Some 50 years ago, clinicians had to drill extensively not only the infected but also the sound dental tissues for mechanical retention of the restorative materials.

One of the greatest innovations of recent times is the discovery of enamel and dentin etching with phosphoric acid, with which it has become possible to adhere synthetic resins to the tooth tissues.[1,2] This led to new treatment possibilities in orthodontics and minimally invasive interventions. Dominant factors in decision making for the particular restoration type are usually related to the amount of leftover tissue after caries removal or the size of the remaining tissues after trauma. Being able to master the existing technology, the availability of the technology on site, and the demands of the individual also play roles in choosing one therapy model over another when restoring anterior teeth. Furthermore, today people even without pathological problems wish to improve the look of their teeth, with particular emphasis on their anterior teeth, mainly concentrating on improvements in color and form.

At the moment, operative treatment concepts could be categorized as non-invasive (reversible), minimally invasive (partially reversible) and (more) invasive strategies (irreversible) using various materials. Dentistry, perhaps, has the unique distinction of using the widest variety of materials, ranging from polymers, metals and metal alloys, to resin-based composites (hereon: composites) and ceramics. Tremendous industrial investments are being made at a rapid pace to improve the quality of composites and ceramics, including in dentistry. These developments in the polymer and ceramic fields have largely eliminated the use of metals and reduced the possible corrosion products in the mouth. Clinicians should be aware of the latest developments, but also realize the disadvantages before selection of the most appropriate material for the right indication. Concentrating only on the material properties is also insufficient. This should be accompanied by the best application method, which sometimes requires a long learning curve. In addition, it is at times frustrating that once experience is gained, new technologies or materials become available that necessitate further education. As the esthetic aspect of dental care becomes increasingly important to patients, the dental practitioner should be aware of the applications and limitations of the var-

ious tooth-colored restorative materials or systems, and keep a balance between the ethical and financial aspects of the applications.

Several techniques are available for the direct or indirect restoration of anterior teeth. Unfortunately, there is some confusion as to which approach is appropriate for each situation and the most durable result, let alone which material to select for the production of the restoration. The purpose of this chapter, based on the available scientific information, is to provide a checklist of esthetic and restorative systems for the maintenance or restoration of anterior teeth, and to cover the important factors and options to consider before choosing a specific treatment.

# Tooth-Colored Restorative Materials: Where Are We Now?

## Composites: Developments and Drawbacks

Developments in the field of adhesive technologies, using the appropriate conditioning methods for the corresponding substrate material (be it either the tooth or the artificial materials), have made it possible to adhere metallic, polymeric or ceramic materials to one another for direct and indirect applications.[3] The fundamental principle of adhesion to tooth substrate is based upon an exchange process by which inorganic tooth material is exchanged for synthetic resins.[4] The hybrid layer then involves infiltration and subsequent in-situ polymerization of resin within the microporosities created by etching, which is a prerequisite for achieving good adhesion of polymeric materials to the tooth.[5] Despite the fact that newer generations of dentin-bonding systems produce better hybrid layers, recently degradation of the hybrid layer has been the topic of interest of in-vitro studies.[6,7] While efforts are being made to improve the durability of adhesive systems for bonding to either to the dental tissues or to the restorative materials, bonded interfaces are prone to changes over time when they are exposed to aggressive conditions, affecting the longevity of the restorations.

There is also considerable development in the composite arena. Despite the rich history for developmental changes of dental composites, polymeric materials still have certain inherent limitations such as polymerization shrinkage, wear, low degree of conversion, and surface luster-related problems. These problems, translated to the clinical situation, become more visible or noticeable in the anterior region. It is claimed that modern polymeric materials are highly filled with glass particles, eliminating the shortcomings of wear and discoloration. The potential use of nanofillers has been adopted from other technologies in dentistry.[8] Generally, increased filler content leads to greater stiffness, higher elastic modulus, improved fracture resistance and wear characteristics. Most fillers in composites are in fact not in the nano-range. This is also related to the fact that with nanofillers, one cannot reach high filler loads because of their large surface area.[9] Some manufacturers claim that certain types of nanofillers may allow for better color match and maintenance as well as radiopacification systems. The classic radiopaque filler is ytterbium fluoride, which is not in the nano-scale by itself, namely 150–200 nm. They are also used as clusters, ca. 10 µm. The common x-ray contrast agent is Ba glass, ca. 0.5–5 µm.[10] Therefore terminology should not be misunderstood and the expectations for the longevity of composite materials should not be based on this information.

Another inherent problem in dental composites is polymerization shrinkage. Polymerization shrinkage in composites is inconsistent. Actual polymerization shrinkages of about 1.5 to 3.5% are common in current composite materials. With adjustments in filler levels or monomer combinations, it is hoped that new composites can control this level by utilizing ring-opening reactions typical to epoxy systems to compensate for the double-bond reaction shrinkage.[11] These particular systems are not entirely trouble-free and not widely stud-

ied. Polymerization shrinkage also affects the matrix and filler interfaces. Incomplete or non-uniform silane bonding to the filler particles prevents appropriate coupling, and local shrinkage may result in either separation or porosity along the filler interfaces. Hydrolytic degradation of the silanes, coupled with the effect of shrinkage reduces the quality of internal interfaces with filler particles. Clinically this may be observed as surface porosity.

There is also continuous development in the field of indirect composites, which are usually classified according to the size of their inorganic particles; hybrid ones contain particles greater than 1.0 µm, micro-hybrid ones have particles smaller than 1.0 µm and micro-particle indirect resin composites have particles smaller than 0.4 µm.[12] They do not require high levels of technical skill from clinicians, occlusal anatomy and proximal contacts could be established by laboratory technicians, and they can be repaired when needed.[13] Indirect composites are said to allow for a higher degree of conversion since polymerization is carried out in the laboratories or at chairside in special photopolymerization units. Unfortunately, dental technicians and some clinicians have to invest not only in the material itself, but also in the polymerization devices. Polymerization modes of such devices also show variations that affect the mechanical and chemical properties of indirect resin composites.

Owing to their chameleon affect and favorable physical properties (i.e. elastic modulus), natural tissues could be mimicked with composite materials. They also offer repair possibilities using different surface conditioning methods. If the above-mentioned shortcomings could be managed, it is certain that their indication would be substantially improved.

## Ceramics: Developments and Drawbacks
With their noteworthy advantages of biocompatibility and mimicry of natural enamel properties, ceramics have played a significant role in dentistry. The latest developments in the arena of all-ceramics eliminated

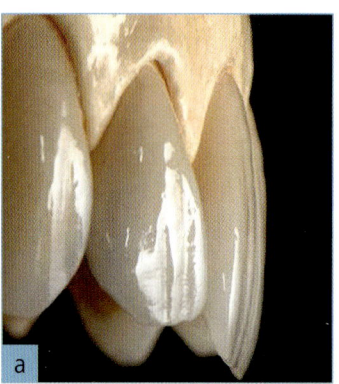
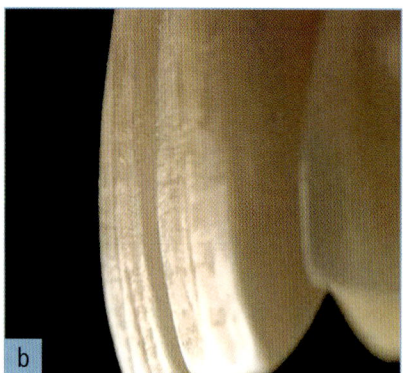
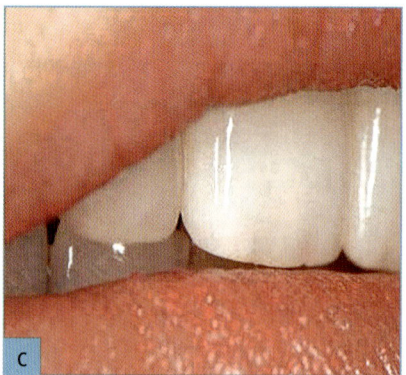

**Fig 4-1a–c** **(a)** Empress Esthetic laminates on the plaster model manufactured for anterior teeth. **(b and c)** *In situ* after cementation – note the excellent surface properties.

the use of metals to a great extent. A wide range of all-ceramic materials has been introduced (feldspathic ceramic, leucite-reinforced, alumina-reinforced, high-density alumina, high-density zirconia, glass-infiltrated alumina ceramics, etc.). In particular, with the silica-based ceramics, frequently used to veneer metal frameworks or high-strength ceramic core materials for all-ceramic restorations, excellent esthetic results can be achieved (Fig 4-1a-c). This made them the material of choice for ceramic laminate veneers and inlays/onlays. In spite of the inherent brittleness and limited flexural strength of silica-based ceramics, with adhesive cementation to the tooth tissues, their fracture resistance has increased. Leucite-reinforced feldspathic porcelain (i.e. IPS Empress, Ivoclar Vivadent) full-coverage fixed dental prostheses (FDP) for both anterior and posterior teeth could be indicated if resin bonding techniques are properly applied. A lithium-disilicate glass-ceramic core veneered with a sintered glass-ceramic (i.e. e.max Press, Ivoclar Vivadent) offers further strength that allows for the fabrication of short-span FDPs. Adhesion of resin cements to such glassy matrix ceramics using hydrofluoric acid and silanization is no problem. Although much progress has been achieved since the introduction of these ceramics in the dental profession, there is still porosity that leads to cracks. With more robust oxide-based ceramic systems, it is hoped these problems will be solved. However, new approaches have introduced different problems. With ceramic materials, clinicians are mainly challenged with cracking problems, high costs, adhesion, and esthetic characterization of some ceramic systems. Today we also know that veneered frameworks are not as strong as the framework ceramic.[14] There is certainly a need for more research. Rapid prototyping, stereolithography, and other printing techniques are being studied for new ceramic systems but they are not yet fully incorporated in dental practice.

In any case, in ceramic restorations, more tooth tissue needs to be sacrificed to achieve a sufficient thickness to overcome the brittleness and chipping problems, especially when compared with gold restorations or direct resin composite layering. Ceramic materials also require complex manufacturing processes and more technical investment. Antagonistic wear is also potentially a greater problem than for composites or alloys.

# Maintenance and Prevention

Since the primary functions of anterior teeth are fulfilling chewing and speaking abilities, and as no current restorative materials can fully replace dental tissues, patients should not be persuaded to undergo invasive therapies of any kind in the first instance. Maintenance of the vitality of the tooth and prevention practices should be initially considered. Non-caries-related rehabilitation, usually using purely esthetic incentives, may be solved with a non-surgical approach. If the chief concern of the patient is esthetic improvement, such as minor color or form corrections, then non-invasive treatment possibilities with their consequences should be communicated and eventually applied if required.

## Non-Invasive Procedures

### Bleaching

Demand for tooth whitening has existed for more than 125 years.[15] During this time, significant efforts have been directed towards understanding the nature of tooth discoloration and devising methods to improve dental esthetics. In today's society, discolored teeth are a potential cause of psychological problems such as lack of self-esteem and confidence. Since teeth are clearly visible during everyday activities such as talking and laughing, today's society dictates that it is the norm for people to have straight, white teeth. Therefore the demand for tooth whitening in dental practice has increased exponentially over the last decade. A common approach to achieving this goal is by bleaching using peroxides. Once the etiology of tooth discoloration is identified, and when administered correctly, vital tooth whitening (as opposed to restorative measures) is by all accounts one of the safest, most conservative, least expensive, and most effective esthetic procedures. Several methods exist to bleach the vital or non-vital teeth. Many changes have occurred in this process during the last 30 years. They are classified mainly as dentist-supervised night-guard bleaching, in-office or power bleaching, and over the counter bleaching products. The U.S. Food and Drug Administration (FDA) classified these products as 'new drugs'. Discolored teeth from aging, chromogenic foods and drinks, smoking, or brown fluorosis-stained teeth, single dark teeth, and tetracycline-stained teeth can be effectively bleached. The chromatic stability of non-vital discol-

ored teeth that have undergone endodontic treatment allows safe correction of the discoloration, preserving the dental tissues with no internal or external root resorption.[16]

The potential side effects related to bleaching are generally reported as sensitivity due to elevation in the intrapulpal temperature.[17] Until long-term safety data become available, the dental practitioner should still approach the use of in-home bleaches with caution, and bleaching should be performed under supervision. Generally, vital tooth bleaching has been found to be effective. However, although not frequent, color relapse may occur after some years.[18] Bleaching agents may also affect some dental materials.[19] It must be communicated to the patient that any existing restorations may look more yellow or prominent after tooth bleaching.

### Orthodontics

Another non-invasive method for diastema closure, correcting anterior crowding or labiolingual aversions in the maxilla or mandible, is orthodontics. Although there is a significant trend to solve these problems with direct resin composite applications, the treatment option of orthodontics should be communicated to the patient as the primary treatment approach (Fig 4-2 a-c). Crown lengths, incisal edge contours and axial inclinations of all maxillary and mandibular incisors, midline corrections, crown torque (canines), smile line (rest position and full smile), right-left symmetry of crown shapes and sizes, and gingival margin levels could be corrected with orthodontic therapy. Decisions to start orthodontic treatment in order to improve esthetics should usually not be taken before a child has reached sufficient maturity for these decisions, normally after the age of 12 years. Special consideration needs to be given to subjects with craniofacial syndromes or disabilities in order to develop effective treatment methods to promote as normal growth and occlusal development as possible. The relapse problem should also be taken into consideration since the use of retainers is to be life-long.[20]

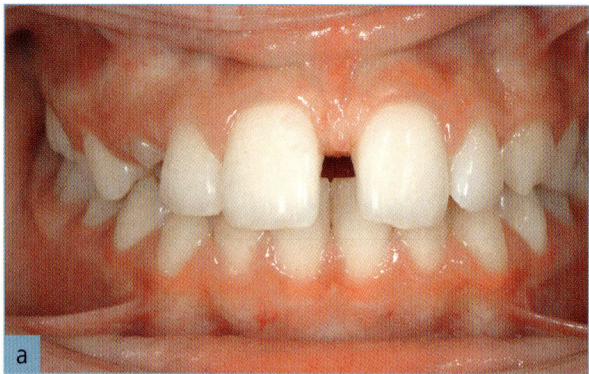

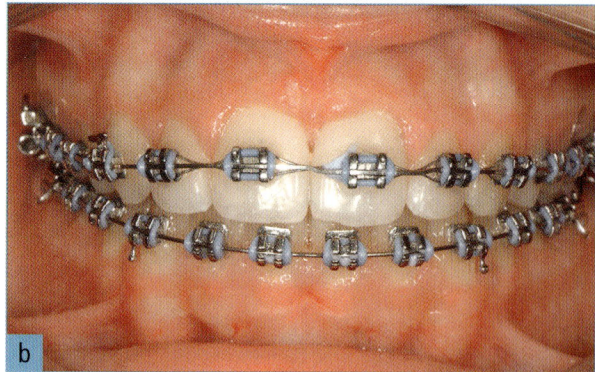

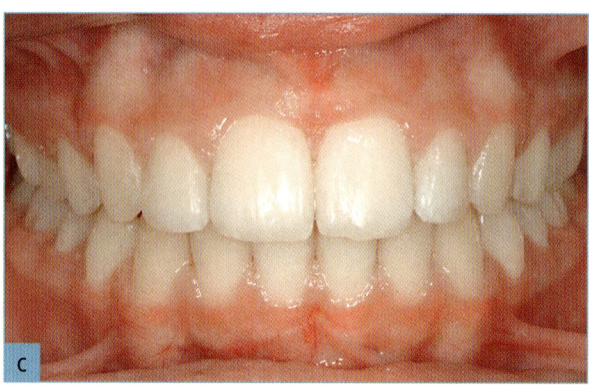

**Fig 4-2a–c** (a) Intraoral photo of a patient concerned with the anterior diastema. (b) Orthodontic treatment with fixed appliances. (c) Diastema closure after orthodontic treatment. (*Courtesy of D. Lie Sam Foek*)

## Minimally Invasive Procedures

### Trauma-related Fracture

Epidemiological studies show that approximately 11.6% to 33% of all boys and 3.6% to 19.3% of all girls suffer dental trauma of varying severity before the age of 12 years.[21] The male-to-female ratio ranges from 1.3 to 2.3:1. The number, type and severity of dental injuries differ according to the age of the patient and the cause of the accident. Coronal fractures of the anterior teeth are a common form of dental trauma, and affect mainly children and adolescents. The majority of fractures and displacements result from accident, collision, sporting activities, domestic violence, automobile accidents, and assaults in developmentally disabled individuals. Most of the time, these result in coronal fractures that are easily recognizable by both the patients and/or their parents. The maxillary central

incisors are the most frequently injured teeth because of their position, followed by mandibular central incisors. The intrusive luxation or avulsion of anterior teeth in children can have a psychological impact on both the parents and the child, especially if the injury affects the permanent dentition. Patients with these types of injuries present themselves years after a traumatic accident with a single discolored tooth caused by pulp calcification and subsequent discoloration. It is also widely accepted that moderate injuries often go unnoticed.

Several factors influence the management of coronal tooth fractures, including extent of fracture (biological width violation, endodontic involvement, alveolar bone fracture), pattern of fracture and restorability of fractured tooth (associated root fracture), secondary trauma injuries (soft tissue status), presence/absence of fractured tooth fragment and its condition for use (fit between fragment and the remaining tooth structure),

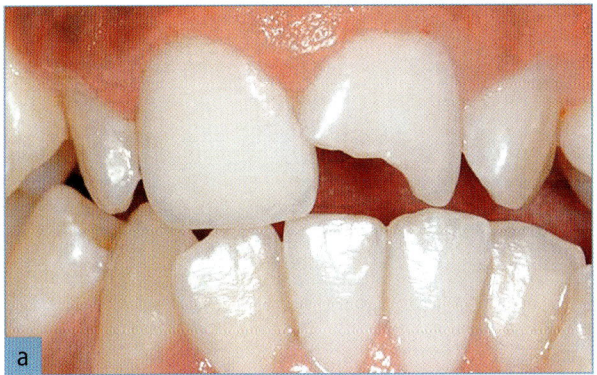
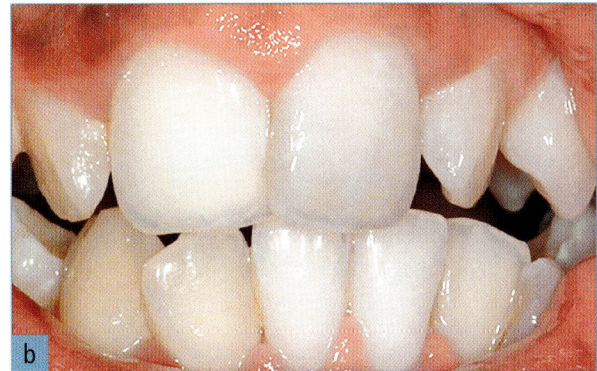
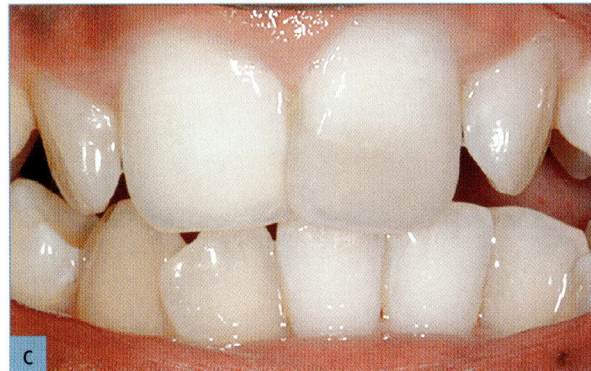

Fig 4-3a–c  (a) Coronal fracture of 21 after trauma.
(b) Direct build-up with resin composite using layering technique, situation immediately after finishing and polishing, and
(c) after 4 years.

occlusion, esthetics, finances, and prognosis.[22] Coronal fractures must be approached in a systematic way to achieve a successful restoration with no invasion. One of the options for managing coronal tooth fractures, especially when there is no or minimal violation of the biological width, is the reattachment of the dental fragment when it is available. Reattachment of fractured tooth fragments can provide good and long-lasting esthetics because the tooth's original anatomic form, color, and surface texture are maintained. It also restores function, provides a positive psychological response, and is a relatively simple procedure. Clinical trials and long-term follow-up have reported that reattachment using modern adhesive systems may achieve functional and esthetic success.[23] It has been shown that a simple reattachment with no further preparation of the fragment or tooth was able to restore only 37.1% of the intact tooth's fracture resistance, whereas a buccal chamfer recovered 60.6% of that fracture resistance.[24] On the other hand, bonding with an overcontour and placement of an internal groove nearly restored the intact tooth fracture strength, recovering 97.2% and 90.5% respectively. In cases of complicated fractures, when endodontic therapy is required, the space provided by the pulp chamber can be used as an inner reinforcement, thus avoiding further preparation of the fractured tooth. In some cases several anterior teeth may be involved and all fragments could be available. In this case, making a template that considers the interocclusal relation, all fragments could be bonded.[25] This approach should be preferred to extensive overlays or full coverage crowns. The technique is reasonably simple. However, the professionals have to keep in mind that a dry and clean working field and the proper use of bonding protocol and materials is the key for achieving success. In case the fragment is not available, a layering technique could be practiced using a silicone template with composite materials (Fig 4-3 a-c). Fabrication of a mouth guard may enhance clinical success, especially in younger patients.

### Incisal or Labial Tooth Surface Loss

Tooth surface loss can be caused by attrition, erosion, abrasion, and abfraction. The frequent clinical finding is that they often act in combination. The problems frequently encountered are the lack of interocclusal space owing to dento-alveolar compensation, and problems related to the diminutive nature of these teeth.[26] One other reason is bruxism, which is usually classified into two categories: centric (vertical loading during waking hours) and eccentric (grinding into lateral excursion while sleeping). There is still discussion on the etiology of bruxism and the controversial role that teeth play in the process. Today's restorative dentist faces an apparent increase in patients exhibiting tooth wear that may result in shortened teeth, making crowning these teeth problematic. In addition, it is evident that patients are becoming more aware of the importance of a pleasing smile. Adopting a conventional prosthodontic approach with FDPs to manage the worn mandibular anterior dentition is not without complication in such patients. Optimal preparation design for a crown will significantly weaken the residual tooth tissue and often compromise the integrity of the pulp. In such situations, the placement of direct composite restorations at an increased occlusal height can be considered as the most conservative approach with no or minimal tooth preparation. This approach is inexpensive, easy to repair, and can provide an acceptable esthetic result. Although the evidence for its use as a medium-term restorative material is increasing, there has been limited research regarding the technique specifically for the worn mandibular anterior dentition. The existing reports showed mild staining (19%) in patients who smoke tobacco products compared with non-smokers, but none of the patients were concerned about this.[27] It was advised that smokers should preoperatively be informed of the likelihood of composite staining and the potential need for fre-

quent maintenance and/or restoration replacement. If restoration staining is likely to be a significant cosmetic issue, then a move towards alternative restorations, such as the use of ceramics, may be required. When marginal adaptation was evaluated, 46% of the restorations had no catch on the labial aspect. The remainder (54%) had evidence of a catch requiring monitoring. There was no evidence of wear of the natural tooth substance by the composite restorations. The improvement in bleeding on probing was explained on the grounds that many patients report difficulty and soreness whilst brushing their teeth when they are short and worn. A lower survival rate of the mandibular restorations was attributed to the fact that mandibular teeth have a smaller bonding area and the restorations are likely to experience greater shear and tensile forces in protrusive guidance. Among the very few clinical studies, one study evaluated the use of indirect palatal veneers placed at an increased vertical dimension of occlusion in patients with advanced localized anterior tooth wear.[28] A total of 75 indirect Artglass palatal veneers were cemented on 12 patients. Follow-up at 2 years showed minor failures in 13.3% of cases. These were repaired with direct composites or polishing only. Hemmings et al.[29], on the other hand, reported from a prospective study bulk failure of only 7 out of 104 (7%) direct composite restorations placed on the anterior dentition at 30 months.

Composite restorations are not the same as conventional extra-coronal restorations, but they serve as a simple and time-efficient method of managing the worn anterior dentition. Marginal breakdown and staining seem to be the more common forms of deterioration of these types of restorations, and bulk failure and fracture were uncommon. Since these patients present a continuous risk of abrading their teeth, reparability of composite materials also makes this material more forgiving.

Tooth surface loss in anatomical disorders, enamel hypoplasia or amelogenesis imperfecta may also affect esthetics. Further breakdown of such structures could also be restored using direct layering techniques with

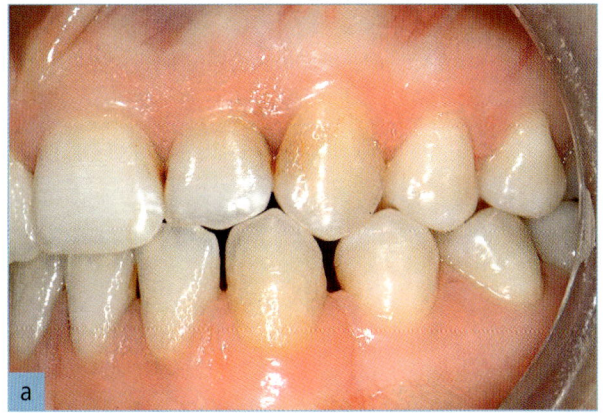
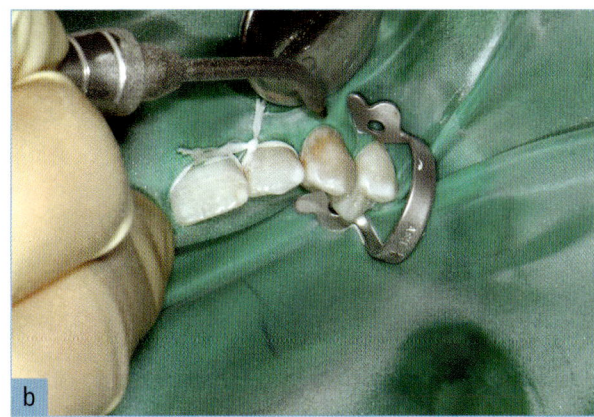
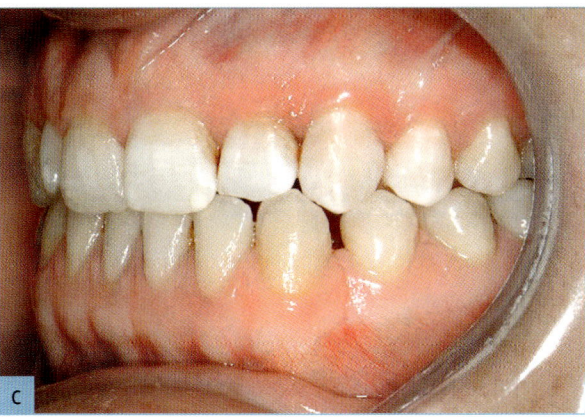
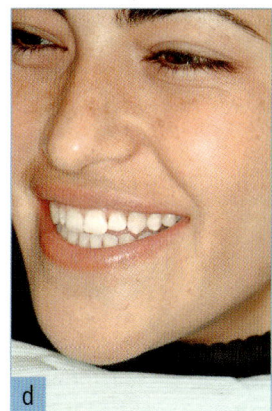

Fig 4-4a–d  (a) Fluorosis presenting itself with porous surface on 23. (b) After rubber-dam placement, removal of the enamel using air-abrasion. (c) Situation of directly build-up resin composite after 6 years. (d) Patient pleased with the result.

reliable adhesion with 100% retention up to 4 years (Fig 4-4a-d).[30] Hypersensitivity and color change, in some cases, were the reported problems with the used composite.

## Non-Caries or Caries-Dominated Situations

### *Direct Applications*

Depending on the size of the cavity (Class III, IV, V) after caries removal or in non-caries lesion treatments, restoration of the missing tissues could be realized with direct application of composite materials. This approach would serve as the most conservative and surely the most convenient and cost-effective method that could be accomplished in one session. With the dramatic developments and modifications of adhesive systems, much effort has been given during the last two

decades on their better performance and at the same time simplification. Although adhesives and composites have become easier to use compared with earlier generations of these materials, their use is still technique-sensitive (Fig 4-5). Three-step etch-and-rinse, two-step and one-step self-etching adhesive systems are at present frequently used adhesive systems.

Dental literature contains overwhelming information on the in-vitro performance of adhesive systems. A critical review on the studies evaluating the hydrolytic stability of adhesive systems in Class III, IV and V composite restorations bonded to enamel and dentin primarily looked at the percentages of 'continuous margins' as well as ultra-structural evaluations.[31] After only 18 months of water storage, significant differences were observed among the materials. Marginal adaptation either in enamel, dentin, or both of all the materials

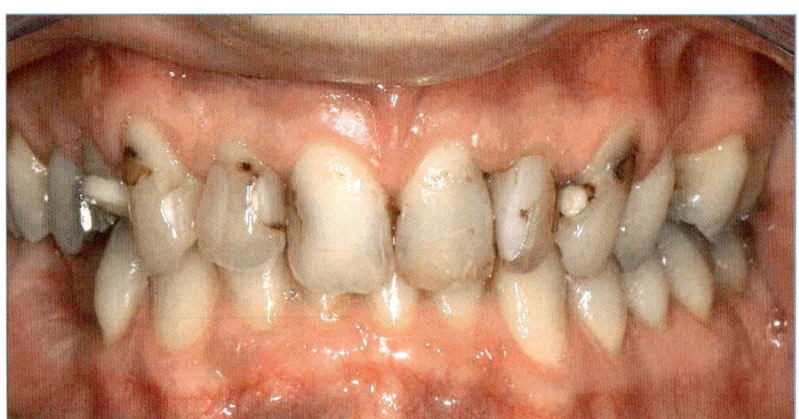

**Fig 4-5** Poor anterior composite restorations 3 years after placement, caused by improper handling of the adhesive systems.

tested so far was affected by water storage. None of the restorative systems tested exhibited hydrolytically stable marginal adaptation with 100% continuous margins with respect to the total marginal length. On the other hand, clinical examinations are usually performed based on modified Ryge or United States Public Health Service (USPHS) criteria concentrating on the marginal integrity, anatomical form, secondary caries, color, marginal discoloration, and surface roughness. The American Dental Association (ADA) recommends 90% retention after 18 months, and many studies have taken this statement as a guideline for assessing their success rate. Unfortunately, high-quality long-term clinical studies are very few. One such clinically controlled split-mouth study on the quality after 2 years of Class III, IV and V restorations using hybrid or microfilled composites, rated the quality of these restorations after 12 and 24 months. At the end of the observation period all evaluation criteria, except color, were assessed as level A, with the hybrid composite being superior to the microfilled composites.[32] This study still indicated problems related to the surface properties of the composites.

Five-year clinical effectiveness of a two-step self-etching adhesive in Class V restorations, in a prospective randomized controlled clinical study showed the clinical performance of a 'mild' two-step self-etching adhesive with and without selective acid-etching of the enamel cavity margins with 40% phosphoric acid prior to placement of the composite in 100 cavities.[33] Only one restoration in the group where enamel was not selectively etched prior to the application of self-etching adhesive was lost at the 5-year recall. Marginal integrity deteriorated over time in both groups. The number of restorations with defect-free margins was significantly lower in the non-etched group. This latter group presented significantly more frequent small marginal defects. Superficial marginal discoloration increased in both groups, but was more pronounced in the non-etch group and was related to the higher frequency of small marginal defects. The results of this study indicated that additional etching of the enamel cavity margins resulted in an improved marginal adaptation on the enamel side; however, this was not critical for the overall clinical performance of the restorations.

Clinical evaluation of an anterior hybrid composite based on USPHS criteria over 8 years in a single-centre clinical trial on Class III, IV and V restorations, reviewed independently by two clinicians, showed low incidence of secondary caries.[34] Life table analysis demonstrated 73% survival, with no scores below Bravo at 8 years. Although the particular material was no longer available, the authors suggested that these results might be applicable to currently available similar materials.

Clinical long-term retention of etch-and-rinse and self-etch adhesive systems in non-carious cervical lesions in a 13-year evaluation comparing seven adhesive systems in a total of 337 non-carious cervical lesions, with Class V restorations of three three-step etch-and-rinse, one two-step etch-and-rinse and three self-etch adhesive systems placed showed the following. Over the 13 years of the study, 275 restorations were evaluated.[35] The cumulative loss rate at 13 years was 60.3%, with significantly different failures rates for the different systems, varying between 26.3 and 94.7%. Three materials fulfilled the ADA 18-month full acceptance criteria. Three systems showed by 18 months or earlier catastrophic debonding rates. The annual failure rate for the three-step etch-and-rinse systems ranged between 2% and 7.3%. For the two-step etch-and-rinse systems, it was between 3.2% and 6.5%. A continuous degradation of the resin-dentin bond was observed for all bonding systems during the follow-up. A wide variation of dentin bonding effectiveness was seen between the systems independent from adhesion strategy.

An extensive literature research was conducted on the clinical effectiveness of contemporary adhesives for restoring cervical non-carious Class V lesions.[36] Restoration retention as a function of time was recorded in order to find out if adhesives with a simplified application procedure were clinically as effective as conventional three-step adhesives. Literature published from January 1998 to May 2004 was reviewed for university-centered clinical trials. Restoration retention rates per adhesive reported were included and depicted as a function of time for each of the five adhesive classes (three- and two-step etch-and-rinse adhesives, two- and one-step self-etch adhesives, and glass-ionomers). The guidelines from the ADA for dentin and enamel adhesive materials were used as a reference. The results revealed glass-ionomers as the most effectively and durably bonded material to tooth tissues. Three-step etch-and-rinse adhesives and two-step self-etch adhesives showed a clinically reliable clinical performance. The clinical effectiveness of two-step etch-and-rinse adhesives was less favorable, while an inefficient clinical performance was noted for the one-step self-etch adhesives. Although there is a tendency towards adhesives with simplified application procedures, simplification so far appears to induce loss of effectiveness. Similar findings were obtained in a 13-year clinical study presented recently.[37]

## Moderately Invasive Procedures

### Indirect Applications

More moderate invasive restorations of discolored or damaged anterior teeth could be achieved with the application of laminate veneers made of either ceramics or particulate filler composites (PFC). Compared with full coverage FDPs, laminates (veneers) could be considered minimally invasive, but compared with direct applications, laminates could be considered moderately invasive irreversible procedures. To date, little information is available in the literature on the survival rates of indirect composite laminate materials.[38] Furthermore, the Cochrane Collaboration concluded that there was no evidence as to whether indirect laminates are better than the direct ones.[39] Direct composite laminate veneers are less expensive than those of indirect options and they could be accomplished in one session. However, they still suffer from a limited longevity since they are susceptible to discoloration, wear and marginal fractures, thereby reducing the esthetic result in the long term. Indirect techniques in the form of laminates are usually attained when veneering multiple anterior teeth.

### Composite Laminates

The new PFCs are characterized by a filler/matrix ratio that is significantly greater (up to 92%) than that of the preceding generation of resin composite materials, with improved wear resistance, physical properties, and color stability. However clinical information is limited on the performance of this material. A clinical trial of a composite laminate veneer system for masking discoloration or hypoplasia on 320 anterior teeth could follow 273 restorations in 68 patients over a 2-year period.[40] The technique produced an acceptable improvement in the esthetics of the patients in the trial. However, 52% of veneers on lateral incisors and 79% on central incisors and canines showed some evidence of chipping after 2 years. Also, 75% of the veneers showed some marginal staining after 2 years. The veneer restorations had a deleterious affect upon the gingival health of the teeth on which they were placed.

Clinical and scanning electron microscopic (SEM) assessments of ceramic and PFC veneers showed good esthetic quality, surface finish and good anatomic form after 1 year, but later depicted changes in color, surface appearance, marginal adaptation, increased marginal discoloration, and tissue response. Inability to achieve a good finish with high gloss was a major drawback for the PFC tested. In return, ceramic laminates exhibited better esthetics, marginal adaptation, finish qualities, and tissue response.[41] The SEM results showed good to excellent marginal fit at baseline in PFC and ceramic veneers, but loss of luting resin at the margins in both materials after 12 months, leading to visible gaps in a number of veneer restorations.

In another clinical trial, 180 veneers made of either direct composite, indirect composite or ceramic showed that veneers on vital teeth showed a significantly better survival rate than on non-vital teeth, with ceramic veneers showing the best overall survival.[42] Unfortunately this is the only study where these restoration options were compared with one another.

*Ceramic Laminates*
The idea of ceramic laminates dates back to 1938, when Charles Pincus described a technique where laminates were retained by a denture adhesive during cinematic filming.[43] After the hydrofluoric acid-etching and silanization of ceramic veneers prior to cementation with adhesive resins was introduced,[44] ceramic veneers started to be frequently prescribed as esthetic restorations for the anterior teeth. The treatment of discolored, fractured, worn, or congenitally malformed teeth, esthetic reshaping of anterior teeth, and also elimination of discolorations could be achieved using ceramic laminates. A substantially reduced preparation or no tooth preparation is required compared with conventional complete crown preparations. The long-term

clinical success of ceramic laminates depends on careful case selection and diagnostic approach, as well as appropriate adhesive bonding procedures. Moreover, inherent properties of the ceramic material, such as its strength, optical properties, color, wear resistance, and durability of the adhesion in the tooth–luting-cement–ceramic complex are important factors for their durability. Excellent adhesion to the enamel, coupled with the compatible adhesion of the adhesive resin to the ceramic increased their reliability. Restoration of one anterior tooth with an indirect ceramic laminate is difficult at best. The blending of the ceramic color with the color of the cement and the underlying tooth structure color requires significant artistic ability of the dental technician. Although ceramic veneers are excellent restorations for multiple anterior teeth, the difficulty of matching the color of one veneered tooth to the adjacent teeth still remains difficult.

On the clinicians' side, although it does not require outstanding skills, and early concepts suggested minimal or no tooth preparation, current beliefs support removal of the aprismatic top surface of unprepared enamel. The advised preparation depth varies between 0.3 and 1 mm. Preparation completely in enamel is most desirable for reliable adhesion. With incisal preparation, the dental technician has more control of the esthetic characteristics, and overlapping was not found to add to the adhesion. Although the results of the newest generation of dentin adhesive systems are very promising, the adhesion quality of resin cements to enamel is still superior compared with that of dentin. Thickness of the ceramic, preparation, temporization, adhesion, material choice, etching duration, ultrasonic cleaning, and silanization modes all play significant roles in the success, and they have been widely studied.[45] Ceramic laminates are mainly fabricated from conventional low-fusing feldspathic porcelain using the platinum foil and the refractory die technique, pressed reinforced ceramic techniques that are widely employed today.

An early meta-analysis on laminates reported that all-ceramics had a better survival rate of 92%, compared with resin veneers, 74%.[38] In another review, 10-year results were presented as 90%, and when preparations are made in enamel the survival rate is even longer.[46] Recent results show a success rate of 96% at 5 to 6 years and 91% at 12 to 13 years.[47] When the laminates were made on canines overlapping the incisal edge and compared to full laminates extended to the palatal cingulum area, after 5 years overlapped ones showed 97.5% and full laminates 100% success rate.[48] When laminates are used for establishing canine guidance, a 76% success rate was noted in this high-loading area. A review of clinical trials between 1990 and 2000 confirmed the strong bond between a laminate and the underlying tooth tissues, as most short- and medium-term clinical studies reported a very low annual failure rate (0 to 5%) because of loss of bonding.[45] Somewhat higher failure rates were noted by Christensen and Christensen[49], with 13% failure after 3 years. Although Strassler and Weiner[50] found 7% failure after 7 to 10 years, Walls[51] observed a higher number of fractures and/or debonding (14%) after 5 years of clinical functioning. Unfavorable occlusion and articulation seemed to be a determining factor for the high failure rate when the restorations were placed for esthetic and functional reconstruction of fractured and worn anterior teeth in patients with a history of bruxism. The large exposed dentine surfaces to be bonded in these fractured and worn teeth were thought to have contributed to the high failure rate. Higher failure rates were noted when laminates were partly bonded to underlying composite restorations.[45] Marginal opening or loss of the marginal seal, and luting cement wear, especially in case of larger gaps compared with smaller ones, indicated that it is desirable to maximize the close adaptation of the laminate, especially at the gingival margins. Clinically this poorer fit, especially at the gingivo-proximal corners of the laminates, made finishing of the luted laminates difficult. Finishing the margins corrects the inherent marginal defects but results in removal of the glaze from the ceramic. This will cause increased plaque retention and gingival reaction. Regarding the marginal adaptation of the veneers after several years of clinical functioning,

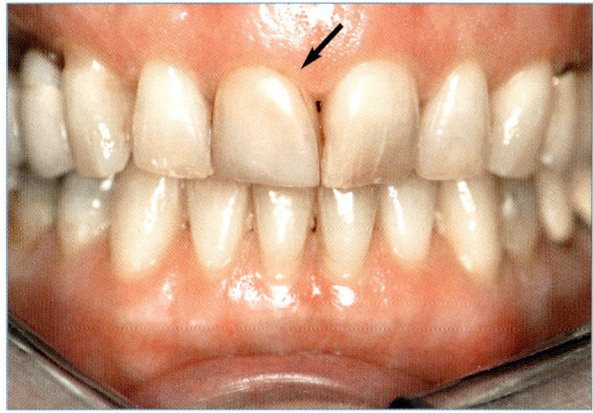

**Fig 4-6**  Discoloration at the margins of a ceramic laminate (arrow) after 10 years due to either poor fit or degradation of the adhesive systems.

most studies reported excellent marginal adaptation, ranging between 65% and 98%. Microleakage was more frequently observed when dentin was exposed during tooth preparation, even in the case of third generation dentin adhesive systems (Fig 4-6). In the reviewed studies, for the clinical studies that had complete intra-enamel preparations, microleakage was reported less frequently.

While Kourkata et al.[52] described a significantly lower bacterial plaque vitality immediately after placement, Peumans et al.[53] observed a slight increase in plaque retention at the cervical margins of 5-year old ceramic laminates. This slight increase was explained by the increased surface roughness at the cervical border of the restoration caused by removal of the glaze of the ceramic during finishing with microfine finishing diamonds. Concerning the gingival response, only a few clinical studies reported a slight gingival inflammation at the restored teeth, especially in patients with moderate or bad oral hygiene. According to Pippin et al.,[54] the location of the cervical extension of the restoration towards the gingival margin plays an important role in the reaction of the gingival tissues, that is gingival reaction increase as the extension was located closer to or below the gingival margin. However, the gingival reaction to ceramic laminates was less than for metal-ceramic restorations at similar locations. The periodontal response to ceramic laminates varied, pointing to patient-related factors. In the study of Carlsson et al.,[55] for example, 30% of the cases presented bleeding on probing.

While a private practice report on the survival of the 83 anterior ceramic laminates was 98.8% at 5 years[56] and 94.4% in 182 veneers at 12 years,[57] in another study marginal imperfections were noted at 1 year.[58] When laminates were used for management of fractured and worn anterior teeth, a 5-year follow-up showed a tendency for marginal staining after 3 to 4 years in service, although without significant alteration in the periodontal or gingival status of the teeth. On the other hand, clinical evaluation of 546 tetracycline-stained teeth restored with ceramic laminates showed less than 1% debonding in the first 6 months of application, and 99% of them presented excellent marginal adaptations, stable color, and no evident staining according to Ryge criteria after 2.5 years.[59]

In a prospective 10-year clinical trial, ceramic laminates on 87 maxillary anterior teeth in 25 patients made by one single operator were evaluated.[60] All patients were recalled at 5 years, leading to observation of 93% of the restorations at 10 years. Clinical performance was assessed in terms of esthetics, marginal integrity, retention, clinical microleakage, caries, fracture, vitality, and patient satisfaction. Failures were recorded either as 'clinically unacceptable but repairable' or as 'clinically unacceptable with replacement needed'. Esthetic results were maintained after 10 years and none of the veneers were lost. The percentage of restorations that remained 'clinically acceptable' (without need for intervention) significantly decreased from an average of 92% at 5 years to 64% at 10 years. Ceramic fractures (11%) and large marginal defects (20%) were the main reasons for failure. Marginal defects were especially noticed at locations where the veneer ended in an existing composite filling. At such vulnerable locations, severe marginal discoloration (19%) and caries recurrence (10%) were frequently observed. Most of the restorations that presented one or more 'clinically unacceptable' problems

(28%) were repairable. Only 4% of the restorations needed to be replaced at the 10-year recall. Occlusion, preparation design, presence of composite fillings, and the adhesive used to bond veneers to tooth substrate were considered as covariables that contribute to the clinical outcome of these restorations in the long term.

A practice-based study within the general dental services in England and Wales evaluated the 10-year outcome of ceramic laminates, looking at the history of intervention on that tooth.[61] Data for over 80,000 adult patients were analyzed, of whom 46% were male and 54% female. Information from a total of 2562 ceramic laminates in 1177 patients was obtained from the data over a period of 11 years. Factors that were found to influence the survival included patient gender, patient age, changing dentist, patient's treatment need, patient charge-paying status and geographical area. While clinician factors do not appear to play a part, a variety of patient factors have been found to influence the re-intervention. Overall, only 53% of the laminates survived without re-intervention at 10 years.

## Invasive Procedures

### Single Tooth Full-coverage FDPs: Metal-ceramic Versus All-ceramic

Single-unit metal-ceramic FDPs have played a major role in dentistry for the restoration of both the anterior and the posterior teeth in the last 50 years. The metal-ceramic FDP system is still selected most frequently because of its strength and versatility. Unfortunately, achieving an exact color match between metal-ceramic restorations and adjacent natural teeth can be extremely difficult because of the metal component. In particular, single anterior FDPs seldom match adjacent teeth. Among other alloys, high-noble metal, with its gold-like color, covered with fired ceramic and including a ceramic facial margin, provides one of the best possibilities to match adjacent natural teeth. Efforts were made to eliminate the metal component in FDPs since grayish colour is usually evident in the cervical third (Fig

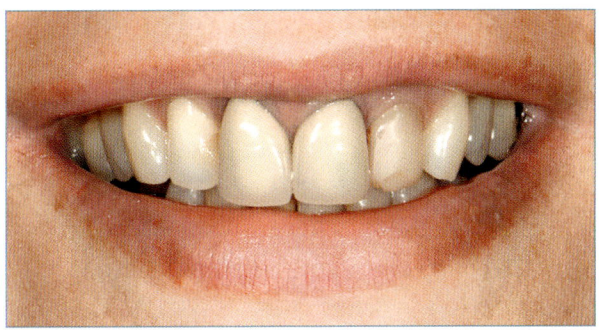

**Fig 4-7** Metal ceramic single unit FPDs on 11 and 21 with greyish cervical margins and lack of adequate translucency.

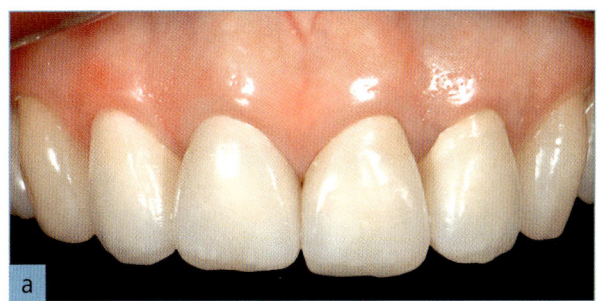

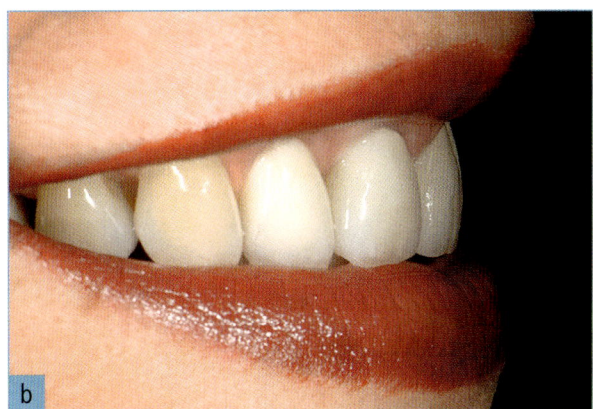

**Fig 4-8a–b** Pressed-ceramic FDPs on 22,21,11,12 indicating that an adequate aesthetic result could be achieved with this material when technical and artistic skills of the dental technician exist.

4-7). Several all-ceramic options are currently available to address the challenge of restoring a single tooth, especially in the maxillary anterior region. In fact, porcelain jacket crowns were introduced more than five decades ago.[62] The porcelain available then was high fusing and not resistant to fracture. Later, alumina oxides were added to their composition. This innovation in metal-free ceramics provided stronger and more durable restorations, but it still restricts adequate translucency in teeth where minimal tooth reduction is allowed.

When a qualified ceramist is engaged, pressed ceramics provide outstanding results for single anterior FDPs compared with almost all other restorative options with suitable marginal fit, minimal abrasion and conservative tooth preparation (Fig 4-8a-b). However, they are not as strong as the reinforced ceramics and patients should be cautioned to practice care in

chewing hard substances to prevent premature failures. In case bruxism signs are evident (Fig 4-9), all ceramic FDPs should not be inserted unless bruxism is eliminated. All-ceramic FDPs can also be achieved using milled aluminous or zirconia copings. Slightly deeper tooth preparation is needed, but the presence of the relatively opaque internal ceramic core still may provide an impediment to matching some tooth colors. With the slip castings method, the initial coping is infiltrated with glass and covered with fired ceramic. The relatively opaque internal core blocks the color of discolored tooth preparations, such as tetracycline-stained teeth.

If moderate tooth structure is lost or moderate staining is present, glassy matrix ceramics are preferably indicated for anterior restorations. In those instances in which heavy staining is present, a foil or core system should be considered to completely block out the back-

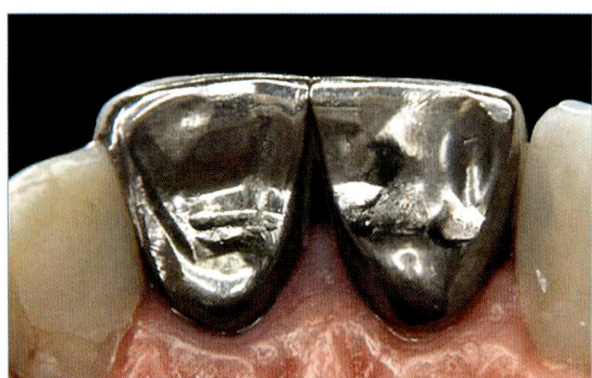

**Fig 4-9** Wear facettes on the metal-ceramic FDPs on 11 and 21. Before replacing them with all-ceramics, patient history with such traces may help to choose the right material.

ground colors.[63] If the occlusal forces become more of a factor, selection of a restorative system will depend more on strength than esthetic demands. When most of the color is on the surface of the teeth, or when there is a high translucency to the teeth, pressed ceramics can provide very good esthetic results. Intrinsic shading is also possible using adhesive cements. When greater strength is required and metal must be eliminated from the restoration because of other reasons, selection of an oxide ceramic could be a better option. These stronger core materials will render improved flexural and compressive strengths, but esthetic outcomes in terms of light transmission and achieving translucency may not be as good as with pressed ceramics.

Burke and Lucarotti,[64] in a meta-analysis, reported an annual clinical failure rate for both metal-ceramics and all-ceramic systems of approximately 3%. Patient selection and technique sensitivity may be more critical with all-ceramics versus metal-ceramic FDPs. Usually, studies on all-ceramic crowns have exclusion criteria for patients with severe parafunction, moderate gingival inflammation, high caries rates, and poor oral hygiene – eventually increasing their success rate. Furthermore, the coping design and luting system seem to be critical to maximize long-term success. A coping design allowing for optimal ceramic thicknesses, a thin and uniform cement layer, and reduction of the mismatch in thermal

expansion of the veneering and core ceramics may decrease combined stresses for all-ceramic FDPs. Ongoing concerns regarding wear of the opposing enamel with all-ceramic restorations have been substantiated in the review of literature. The abrasive potential of ceramic is dependent on fracture toughness, the presence of porosities, crystal size, and surface finish, but there is little understanding of wear patterns, wear occurrence, and amount of wear for a particular individual.

A recent systematic review assessed the 5-year survival rates of all-ceramic single-unit FDPs, compared it with the survival rates of metal-ceramic single-unit FDPs, and described the incidence of biological and technical complications.[65] Prospective and retrospective cohort studies were evaluated with a mean follow-up time of at least 3 years. Thirty-four studies met the inclusion criteria. In meta-analysis, the 5-year survival of all-ceramic FDPs in general was estimated at 93.3%, and 95.6% for metal-ceramic. From the selected studies that met the inclusion criteria, when anterior single FDPs were extracted, the total number of restorations reached 2048. The results showed the highest 5-year survival rate of 96.4% for densely sintered alumina (Procera) FDPs, followed by reinforced glass-ceramic FDPs (Empress) and In-Ceram with survival rates of 95.9% and 96.7%, respectively. All-ceramic FDPs, when used for anterior teeth, showed survival rates at 5 years comparable to those seen for metal-ceramic crowns. When used for posterior teeth, the survival rates at 5 years of densely sintered alumina (94.9%) and reinforced glass-ceramic (93.7%) were similar to those obtained for metal-ceramic single-unit FDPs.

These figures are different when these materials are used for multiple-unit FDPs. Another systematic review assessed the 5-year survival rates and incidences of complications of multiple-unit all-ceramic FDPs and compared them with those of metal-ceramic FDPs.[66] Prospective and retrospective cohort studies on all-ceramic and metal-ceramic reconstructions with a mean follow-up time of at least 3 years resulted in 39 articles, of which nine studies met the inclusion criteria for all-ceramics. The 5-year survival of metal-ceramic FDPs was significantly higher, with 94.4%, than the survival of all-ceramic FDPs, being 88.6%. The frequencies of framework and veneering material fractures were significantly higher for all-ceramic FDPs (6.5% and 13.6%) compared with those of metal-ceramic FDPs (1.6% and 2.9%). Other technical complications such as loss of retention, biological complications like caries and loss of pulp vitality were similar for the two types of reconstructions over the 5-year observation period. When zirconia was used as framework material, the reasons for failure were primarily biological and technical complications other than framework fracture. Extensive laboratory testing to date has confirmed the strength and marginal fit of zirconia ceramic, but 5- to 10-year clinical studies are lacking on the success rate and primary mode of failure. Nevertheless, the application of zirconia-based ceramics for anterior reconstructions would be less favorable due to esthetic reasons.

# Discussion and Concluding Remarks

Advances in material science and technology have given practicing dentists the ability to mimic nature when restoring missing dental tissues. Depending on the society and cultural or subjective priorities, the perception of health and beauty varies. Today's clinicians are not only treating disease-related dental problems, but also trying to find solutions for fulfilling the esthetic demands of the patients. The growing number of patients who are dissatisfied with the color or form of their anterior teeth, or who have worn anterior dentitions from several causes, is also striking. Interestingly, these patients do not complain about their function, but are concerned with their dentition when it starts to impair their smile. For esthetic reasons, some patients are today more willing than their clinicians to sacrifice their dental tissues, without considering the longevity of their restorations.

The term 'longevity' has also changed in meaning over the years, with changes in measurement tools, definition of quality, and expectations. Yesterday's 'success' is not comparable with success in today's terms. In particular, with concerns regarding esthetics or mimicking nature and the steady development of materials that present similar optical properties to dental tissues, together with increased life expectancy, clinicians have started to be more critical of the final outcome and longevity, be it restoration with a direct composite, ceramic laminate, or single-unit ceramic FDPs with and without metal substructure. The term 'longevity' today comprises not only biological and mechanical aspects, but also optical aspects of any restoration, at the same time applying the least invasive method. Clinicians meet the challenge of choosing the most suitable and long-lasting treatment approach from a growing plethora of dental materials. Material technologies also need to be blended with traditional functional concepts in order to be successful. In fact, with any of the materials or restorative approaches the function of tearing, incising, chewing or speaking could be accomplished, but the major concern is now to keep the vitality and biological integrity, simultaneously mimicking the neighboring teeth. For many years, the most predictable and durable esthetic correction of anterior teeth has been achieved by preparing the teeth and restoring them with full-coverage metal-ceramic FDPs. This approach was surely less invasive compared with extraction, and certainly more esthetically pleasing than their gold counterparts. Generally speaking, dentistry has become a lot more conservative and less invasive than it used to be. Hence, in today's sense metal-ceramic FDPs are being questioned undoubtedly because of the need for substantial removal of large amounts of sound tooth substance and the possible adverse effects for the adjacent pulp and periodontal tissues.

Since polymeric, ceramic, or metallic materials belong to different families, and preparation techniques may vary from non-invasive to minimal, moderate to more invasive styles, from the ethical point of view it is almost impossible to conduct clinical trials comparing different treatment modalities or materials in the same mouth. Consequently, dental literature with particular emphasis on individual clinical trials or meta-analysis is taken as the highest level of evidence. In the absence of evidence, however, common sense dictates that the least invasive and the most cost-effective treatment modality should be practiced. Against all the recent developments, no material to date is flawless. Survival rates of restorative materials inevitably decrease over the years.

For these reasons, to answer the question 'Direct composites, veneers or crowns?' for anterior restorations, based on today's knowledge, biological, mechanical and optical aspects need to be considered using the most biocompatible material as a result of their functioning in the aggressive oral environment. Anterior function and esthetics could also be achieved without utilizing any material or by practicing no invasion. For aligning healthy teeth with composite or ceramic laminates, claiming that they are less invasive than metal-ceramics or claiming that metal-ceramics are more durable are not valid arguments. Moreover none of these are conservative procedures when we have options such as bleaching, orthodontics, direct bonding or layering.

When non-invasive methods are evaluated, depending on the dietary habits etc, informed consent should be given to the patients that color relapse may occur after some years following bleaching and that lingual retainers are needed to avoid orthodontic relapse. When a fragment is reattached to a broken anterior tooth using adhesive systems or a direct layering technique, preventive measures should be advised to high-risk patients. After any kind of therapy, repair and maintenance should be practiced using the most conservative approach.

Regarding direct applications, it can be said that composite materials are cost-effective, less invasive, patient-pleasing options compared with other available materials. They are also well studied compared with many other restorative materials. However, long-term data is available for only a few composite materials. This is partly because of the increasing number of composites and adhesives being introduced to the dental mar-

ket. Since their introduction, only a few remain as benchmark materials. Until long-term information is obtained from in-vitro or in-vivo studies, many direct composites either disappear from the market or an improved version is introduced. There are countless case reports in dental journals with appealing results or cases related to application techniques, but long-term results are rarely mentioned. Evidence, on the other hand, clearly shows that retention of direct composite fillings is not a problem at all for restoration of defects using either total-etch systems or self-etch adhesives after removal of caries. Even though they are inferior in terms of esthetics, clinical studies show that glass ionomers seem to work better in the restoration of non-carious lesions. From the mechanical point of view, considering the excellent retention rate, it can be stated that adhesion to enamel and dentin is not a problem anymore. Perhaps aiming for higher bond strengths is not necessary in material development. Current problems for direct composite applications are related to the hydrolytic instability of adhesives and shrinkage-related problems that show themselves clinically with significant deterioration in marginal adaptation and cavosurface marginal discoloration after only few years. The majority of the clinical studies report outcome measures as successful, fulfilling the less-than-10% failure in 18 months recommendation by the ADA. In fact, ADA specifications for resin composites and adhesives could be seen as too tolerant considering the lifetime of other restorations, and recently it has been amended.

For direct composites, technique sensitivity is often brought as an argument. However when carefully considered, all kinds of restorative materials, and even dentistry per se, are technique-sensitive. Nonetheless, as mentioned above for the disadvantages of composites and ceramics, inherent problems regarding the loss of surface luster underscore with composites compared with ceramics. This may require repolishing or refinishing or relayering, with which survival rate can be prolonged.[67] However, in none of the studies are the surface-related problems compared with the natural teeth, which may also necessitate plaque or calculus removal.

Whether the surface defect is a patient-related problem, an inherent problem of the composite or a lack of meticulous work on the part of the clinician remains to be identified. According to the reviewed literature, it is a common finding after several years of clinical function, so the maintenance of the surface characteristics of composites even after finishing and polishing requires technological improvement in the future. Also, considering the outcome measures of clinical studies, critical clinical analysis of dentin bonding agents must continue. In particular, for patients with a history of parafunction, or unknown diagnosis, composite materials still serve as more forgiving options for repair as they are more predictable than other materials.

Generally, operator factors are suspected to be the most important and materials factors may be very minor or smaller, especially when long-term survival rates are considered even with more inferior composites and adhesives.[68] The question of how to improve operator diligence then remains to be answered. Considering the increasing demand for postgraduate education courses, perhaps during undergraduate education a deeper understanding of the fundamental layering, contouring, and polishing principles, and meticulous application of adhesives with sufficient practice should be taught more in depth. Only then could better outcomes with direct composite restorations be achieved. For direct composites, it is the responsibility of the clinician to outperform both the artistic and the technical aspects of the profession, without doubt in a less invasive way than with indirect laminates.

When multiple single-unit anterior restorations are in question, clinicians prefer to delegate the work to the dental technician. Two materials are then in question, either indirect composites or ceramics. Very limited evidence is available with indirect composites, but gradual improvements are being made. Although perhaps not as important during tooth preparation, during cementation operator diligence is still required with these laminates for isolation, etching the tooth and the ceramic, placement, bonding, polymerization, finishing and polishing the margins etc. In addition, for final color, the

ceramic, adhesive cement and the underlying tooth structure play a role. Therefore clinicians may need to spend more time optimizing all these aspects before final cementation is performed. There are often more than two sessions required and close cooperation with the technician is compulsory. When these conditions do not exist, added to the higher costs, direct composite application could be preferable.

According to the majority of studies, it is clear that from the mechanical point of view, retention of laminates is not a problem. Clinical studies rarely report debonding, indicating that the adhesion of the luting cement not only to dental tissues but also to the hydrofluoric etched and silanized ceramic is very reliable. Therefore the choice of full coverage FDPs over laminates because of mechanical retention reasons cannot be justified. The esthetic outcome resulting from the lack of metal surely outweighs their choice over metal-ceramics.

From the reviewed literature, it is clear that the ceramic laminates are not problem-free. Even though the retentive quality is ideal, especially when the margins are located in the enamel, marginal deteriorations are frequently reported. This finding is consistent with the findings obtained from direct composites. Unfortunately, the real indication of ceramic laminates is usually in dentin after extensive caries removal or for replacement of multiple discolored pre-existing composites, or teeth with a history of several restoration cycles. In these occasions, the substrates are dentin, composite, or a combination. In the cervical area, intra-enamel preparations are not usually possible. These factors may be associated with marginal quality problems in the future, but studies do not usually report the substrate material or marginal qualities. The wear of the luting cement and marginal degradation observations indicate the need for excellent fit of the ceramic laminates. Hence, precision is still required when using ceramic laminates.

Experience over 25 years with ceramic laminates showed mismatch in color between the natural dentition and the more color-persistent ceramic laminates.[69] Over the years, the natural teeth may change color, and

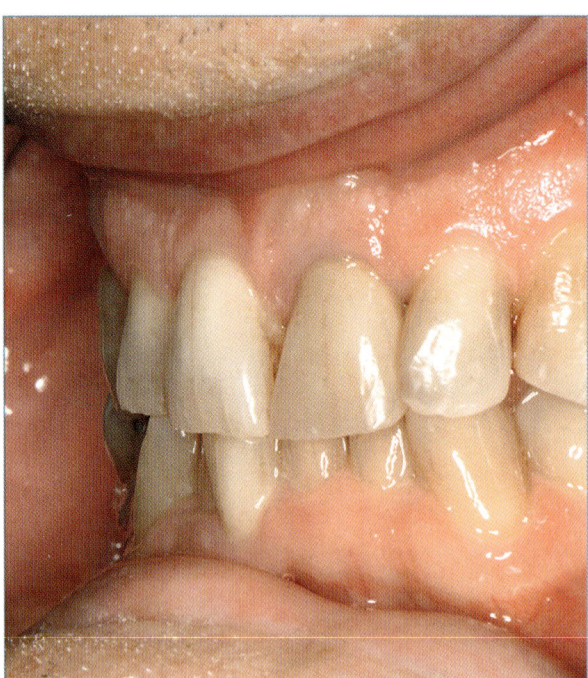

**Fig. 4-10** Twenty-year-old metal-ceramic FDP on 21.

Although we have the longest record of using metal-ceramic FDPs (Fig 4-10), when a decision needs to be made between a laminate and a full-coverage FDP for anterior restoration, the information derived from the literature should be evaluated with caution. Metal-ceramic FDPs have been used in dentistry for more than 50 years. Much has been learnt from failures and many developments have been made in metals, ceramics, and their processing techniques. From the mechanical point of view, when the fit is ideal, and there is enough coronal length and close to parallel convergence, retention of FDPs is not a problem. Specific biological and technical complications such as caries, loss of vitality, and periodontal disease recurrence as well as loss of retention, loss of vitality, and tooth and material fractures are considered problems. These factors are not consistently evaluated in all clinical trials but such problems seem not to pose much danger for single-unit FDPs.

In case of replacement of an aged FDP, if a decision has to be made between a metal-ceramic or all-ceramic restoration, elimination of metal and eventually better optical properties may favor the indication of the latter. The available information shows that incidence of loss of abutment vitality in all-ceramics and metals-ceramics is identical, with 2.1% up to 5 years.[65] Loss of retention, chipping and marginal discoloration occurred less frequently. Unfortunately, observation times reported for metal-ceramics are twice as long as for all-ceramic single-unit FDPs, indicating the need for longer observations. Even though the observation period is still considerably shorter, clinical performance of all-ceramic single-unit anterior FDP applications could be considered similar to metal-ceramics. Elimination of the metal and the good optical properties are advantages over metal-ceramics, but since adhesive cementation is compulsory (especially for glass ceramics), more careful work is required using all-ceramics compared with metal-ceramics. Considering that metal-ceramics are applied worldwide, the number of follow-up studies is dramatically lower than for all-ceramics. Interestingly, a systematic review of studies reported between 1966 and

the ceramics may not follow this trend. Although durations of studies are not similar, the likelihood of this mismatch occurring is reduced when direct composites are used.

If ceramic laminates are to be chosen over direct composites, two recent reports should be evaluated with caution.[59,60] In a university setting, with fewer time constraints, 28% of ceramic laminates needed repair after 10 years, indicating that refinishing, repolishing or repair of chipping and fracture using composites was necessary. On the other hand, practice-based evidence that 53% of laminates survived without re-intervention at 10 years indicates that the situation is different in the practice. There is a clear need for long-term data. Meticulous work could have been lacking at the practices with a heavy workload, or the clinicians and dental technicians had not mastered the techniques adequately, which again emphasizes the need for implementation of these systems in undergraduate education. These two studies specify the need for optimization of the materials and the application techniques.

2006 provided only 39 articles that could fulfill the inclusion criteria.[66] Perhaps metal-ceramics should be revisited, with longer observation durations in better-controlled trials.

When a decision has to be made between a ceramic laminate and an all-ceramic FDP for anterior reconstructions, based on the survival rate reports a full-coverage FDP may seem to be superior to using ceramic laminates. It should also be noted that fewer clinical data are available for laminates compared with single-unit FDPs. When evaluating the success rate of direct or indirect laminates, the modified USPHS criteria are usually used. This kind of evaluation and scoring criteria unfortunately does not exist for full-coverage restorations.[70] For example, marginal deteriorations are frequently reported with direct composites and indirect composite or ceramic laminates according to the defined criteria of USPHS, adding to the failure rate of such restorations. However, such changes at the crown margins are usually hidden at the cervical area of the FDPs and they do not become visible unless caries is noted or the restoration detaches. The so-called 'technical failures' or definition of quality is not similar for direct or indirect laminates and full coverage restorations. Also, pulp vitality is often not considered as one of the evaluation criteria for direct composites or ceramic laminates, whereas it is more commonly recorded for FDPs. This can be partially attributed to the fact that much emphasis is given to the esthetic outcome and therefore biological factors are overseen. This indicates the necessity for standardized or comparable evaluation criteria for outcome measures for direct and indirect restorations.

When biological factors are considered, one factor is important for all types of extensive restorations – the preservation of the cementoenamel junction in order to avoid periodontal problems. This has been reported for ceramic laminates and single-unit FDPs.

In terms of esthetics in the anterior region, mastering the artistic skill to imitate the neighboring teeth is still challenging for both the clinician and dental technician, as slight variation can be observed. Perhaps with the development of computer-generated restorations this problem may be solved.

With all the advances in adhesive technologies, classic prosthetic dentistry is shifting towards more operative and reparative dentistry. This has strongly influenced current concepts, with the goal of less invasive interventions that conserve the healthy tooth structure. It should be emphasized that today's clinicians should be able to master both composite and ceramic materials, since depending on the size or location of the restorations, material choice may differ. When selecting composite or ceramic materials, common sense surely dictates that the least invasive option and the corresponding material to achieve this should be of preference. However, we have to accept the fact that the oral environment is harsh. Long exposure to oral conditions changes material properties such as porosity, water sorption, corrosion, and degradation, diminishing their lifetime. Generally, teeth surrounded by healthy periodontal tissues yield a very high longevity, with up to 99.5% survival over 50 years.[71] If periodontally compromised, but treated and maintained regularly, the survival of such teeth is still very high, at 92% to 93%. It should be noted that all materials have a certain lifetime, and none of the available restorative materials yet surpass the lifetime of a natural tooth. Until technologies are able to preserve the dental hard and soft tissues completely, or regeneration of new tissues is achieved, clinicians are destined to use dental materials. In addition, patient-related factors will continue to dominate when choosing one restoration type over another, or the most suitable restorative materials for an individual. In a sense, this reflects the art of dentistry.

# References

1.  Buonocore MG. A simple method of increasing the adhesion of acrylic filling materials to enamel surfaces. J Dent Res 1955;34:849–853.
2.  Fusayama T, Nakamura M, Kurosaki N, Iwaku M. Non-pressure adhesion of a new adhesive restorative resin. J Dent Res 1979;58:1364–1370.
3.  Özcan M, Pfeiffer P, Nergiz I. A brief history and current status of metal- and ceramic-surface-conditioning concepts for resin bonding in dentistry. Quintessence Int 1998;29:713–724.

4. Van Meerbeek B, De Munck J, Yoshida Y, Inoue S, Vargas M, Vijay P, et al. Buonocore memorial lecture. Adhesion to enamel and dentin: current status and future challenges. Oper Dent 2003;28:215–235.

5. Nakabayashi N, Nakamura M, Yasuda N. Hybrid layer as a dentin-bonding mechanism. J Esthet Dent 1991;3:133–138.

6. Spencer P, Wang Y, Bohaty B. Interfacial chemistry of moisture-aged class II composite restorations. J Biomed Mater Res B Appl Biomater 2006;77:234–240.

7. Breschi L, Mazzoni A, Ruggeri A, Cadenaro M, Di Lenarda R, De Stefano Dorigo E. Dental adhesion review: aging and stability of the bonded interface. Dent Mater 2008;24:90–101.

8. Kaehler T. Nanotechnology: Basic concepts and definitions. Clin Chem 1994;40:1797–1799.

9. Moszner N, Salz U. Recent developments of new components for dental adhesives and composites. Macromol Mater Eng 2007;292:245–271.

10. Bayne SC. Dental biomaterials: where are we and where are we going? J Dent Educ 2005;69:571–585.

11. Eick JD, Byerly TJ, Chappell RP, Chen GR, Bowles CQ, Chappelow CC. Properties of expanding SOC/epoxy copolymers for dental use in dental composites. Dent Mater 1993;9:123–127.

12. Touati B, Aidan N. Second generation laboratory composite resins for indirect restorations. J Esthet Dent 1997;9:108–118.

13. Özcan M, Alander P, Vallittu PK, Huysmans MC, Kalk W. Effect of three surface conditioning methods to improve bond strength of particulate filler resin composites. J Mater Sci Mater Med 2005;16:21–27.

14. Kohorst P, Dittmer MP, Borchers L, Stiesch-Scholz M. Influence of cyclic fatigue in water on the load-bearing capacity of dental bridges made of zirconia. Acta Biomater 2008;4:1440–1447.

15. Tredwin CJ, Naik S, Lewis NJ, Scully C. Hydrogen peroxide tooth-whitening (bleaching) products: Review of adverse effects and safety issues. Brit Dent J 2006;200:371–376.

16. Amato M, Scaravilli MS, Farella M, Scully C. Bleaching teeth treated endodontically: long-term evaluation of a case series. J Endod 2006;32:376–378.

17. Sulieman M, Addy M, Rees JS. Surface and intra-pulpal temperature rises during tooth bleaching: an in vitro study. Br Dent J 2005;199:37–40.

18. Karpinia KA, Magnusson I, Barker ML, Gerlach RW. Placebo-controlled clinical trial of a 19% sodium percarbonate whitening film: initial and sustained whitening. Am J Dent 2003;16:12B–16B.

19. Rosentritt M, Lang R, Plein T, Behr M, Handel G. Discoloration of restorative materials after bleaching application. Quintessence Int 2005;36:33–39.

20. Zachrisson BU. Facial esthetics: guide to tooth positioning and maxillary incisor display. World J Orthod 2007;8:308–314.

21. Hamilton FA, Hill FJ, Holloway PJ. An investigation of dento-alveolar trauma and its treatment in an adolescent population. Part 1: the prevalence and incidence of injuries and the extent and adequacy of treatment received. Br Dent J 1997;182:91–95.

22. Olsburgh S, Jacoby T, Krejci I. Crown fractures in the permanent dentition: pulpal and restorative considerations. Dent Traumatol 2002;18:103–115.

23. Andreasen FM, Norén JG, Andreasen JO, Engelhardtsen S, Lindh-Strömberg U. Long-term survival of fragment bonding in the treatment of fractured crowns: a multicenter clinical study. Quintessence Int 1995;26:669–681.

24. Reis A, Loguercio AD, Kraul A, Matson E. Reattachment of fractured teeth: a review of literature regarding techniques and materials. Oper Dent 2004;29:226–233.

25. Macedo GV, Diaz PI, De O Fernandes CA, Ritter AV. Reattachment of anterior teeth fragments: a conservative approach. J Esthet Restor Dent 2008;20:5–18; discussion 19–20.

26. Berry DC, Poole DFG. Attrition: possible mechanisms of compensation. J Oral Rehabil 1976;3:201–206.

27. Poyser NJ, Briggs PF, Chana HS, Kelleher MG, Porter RW, Patel MM. The evaluation of direct composite restorations for the worn mandibular anterior dentition-clinical performance and patient satisfaction. J Oral Rehabil 2007;34:361–376.

28. Gow AM, Hemmings KW. The treatment of localized anterior tooth wear with indirect Artglass restorations at an increased occlusal vertical dimension. Results after two years. Eur J Prosthodont Restor Dent 2002;10:101–105.

29. Hemmings KW, Darbar UR, Vaughan S. Tooth wear treated with direct composite restorations at an increased vertical dimension: results at 30 months. J Prosthet Dent 2000;83:287–293.

30. Lygidakis NA, Chaliasou A, Siounas G. Evaluation of composite restorations in hypomineralised permanent molars: a four year clinical study. Eur J Paediatr Dent 2003;4:143–148.

31. De Munck J, Van Landuyt K, Peumans M, Poitevin A, Lambrechts P, Braem M, et al. A critical review of the durability of adhesion to tooth tissue: methods and results. J Dent Res 2005;84:118–132.

32. Geitel B, Kwiatkowski R, Zimmer S, Barthel CR, Roulet JF, Jahn KR. Clinically controlled study on the quality of class III, IV and V composite restorations after two years. J Adhes Dent 2004;6:247–253.

33. Peumans M, De Munck J, Van Landuyt K, Lambrechts P, Van Meerbeek B. Five-year clinical effectiveness of a two-step self-etching adhesive. J Adhes Dent 2007;9:7–10.

34. Millar BJ, Robinson PB, Inglis AT. Clinical evaluation of an anterior hybrid composite resin over 8 years. Br Dent J 1997;182:26–30.

35. van Dijken JW, Sunnegårdh-Grönberg K, Lindberg A. Clinical long-term retention of etch-and-rinse and self-etch adhesive systems in non-carious cervical lesions. A 13 years evaluation. Dent Mater 2007;23:1101–1107.

36. Peumans M, Kanumilli P, De Munck J, Van Landuyt K, Lambrechts P, Van Meerbeek B. Clinical effectiveness of contemporary adhesives: a systematic review of current clinical trials. Dent Mater 2005;21:864–881.

37. van Dijken JW, van Dijken JW. Retention of a resin-modified glass ionomer adhesive in non-carious cervical lesions. A 6-year follow-up. J Dent 2005;33:541–547.

38. Kreulen CM, Creugers NH, Meijering AC. Meta-analysis of anterior veneer restorations in clinical studies. J Dent 1998;26:345–353.

39. Wakiaga J, Brunton P, Silikas N, Glenny AM. Direct versus indirect veneer restorations for intrinsic dental stains. Cochrane Database Syst Rev 2004;4: CD004347.

40. Walls AW, Murray JJ, McCabe JF. Composite laminate veneers: a clinical study. J Oral Rehabil 1988;15:439–454.

41. Chen JH, Shi CX, Wang M, Zhao SJ, Wang H. Clinical evaluation of 546 tetracycline-stained teeth treated with Cerinate laminate veneers. Zhonghua Kou Qiang Yi Xue Za Zhi 2003;38:199–202.

42. Meijering AC, Creugers NHJ, Roeters FJ, Mulder J. Survival of three types of veneer restorations in a clinical trial: a 2.5-year interim evaluation. J Dent 1998;26:563–568.

43. Pincus CR. Building mouth personality. J South Calif Dent Assoc 1938;14:125–129.
44. Simonsen RJ, Calamia JR. Tensile bond strength of etched porcelain. J Dent Res 1983;62:297(Abstract 1154).
45. Peumans M, van Meerbeek B, Lambrechts P, Vanherle G. Porcelain veneers: a review of the literature. J Dent 2000;28:163–177.
46. Kerschbaum T. Long-term survival of dental restorations. A review. Quintessenz 2004;55:1113–1126.
47. Layton D, Walton T. An up to 16-year prospective study of 304 porcelain veneers. Int J Prosthodont 2007;20:389–396.
48. Schaffer H, Kulmer S. Functional reconstruction of abraded canines by resin-bonded all-ceramic guiding elements. Int J Prosthodont 1990;3:538–544.
49. Christensen GJ, Christensen RP. Clinical observations of porcelain veneers: a three year report. J Esthet Dent 1991;3:174–179.
50. Strassler HE, Weiner S. Seven to ten year clinical evaluation of etched porcelain veneers. J Dent Res 1995;74:176(Abstract 1316).
51. Walls AWG. The use of adhesively retained all-porcelain veneers during the management of fractured and worn anterior teeth. Part II: clinical results after 5-years follow-up. Br Dent J 1995;178:337–339.
52. Kourkata S, Walsh TF, Davis LG. The effect of porcelain laminate veneers on gingival health and bacterial plaque characteristics. J Clin Periodontol 1994;21:638–640.
53. Peumans M, Van Meerbeek B, Lambrechts P, Vuylsteke-Wauters M, Vanherle G. Five-year clinical performance of porcelain veneers. Quintessence Int 1998;29:211–221.
54. Pippin DJ, Mixson JM, Sodan-Els P. Clinical evaluation of restored maxillary incisors: veneers vs. PFM crowns. J Am Dent Assoc 1995;126:1523–1529.
55. Karlsson S, Landahl I, Stegersjö G, Milleding P. A clinical evaluation of ceramic laminate veneers. Int J Prosthodont 1992;5:447–451.
56. Fradeani M. Six-year follow-up with Empress veneers. Int J Periodontics Restorative Dent 1998;18:216–225.
57. Fradeani M, Redemagni M, Corrado M. Porcelain laminate veneers: 6- to 12-year clinical evaluation-a retrospective study. Int J Periodontics Restorative Dent 2005;25:9–17.
58. Coyne BM, Wilson NH. Indirect laminate veneers: a review. J Ir Dent Assoc 1988;34:98–102.
59. Chen JH, Shi CX, Wang M, Zhao SJ, Wang H. Clinical evaluation of 546 tetracycline-stained teeth treated with porcelain laminate veneers. J Dent 2005;33:3–8.
60. Peumans M, De Munck J, Fieuws S, Lambrechts P, Vanherle G, Van Meerbeek B. A prospective ten-year clinical trial of porcelain veneers. J Adhes Dent 2004;6:65–76.
61. Burke FJ, Lucarotti PS. Ten-year outcome of porcelain laminate veneers placed within the general dental services in England and Wales. J Dent 2008. [Epub ahead of print].
62. McLean JW. A higher strength porcelain for crown and bridge work. Br Dent J 1965;119:268–272.
63. Wassell RW, Walls AW, Steele JG. Crowns and extra-coronal restorations: materials selection. Br Dent J 2002;192:199–202, 205–211.
64. Burke FJ, Lucarotti PS. Ten-year outcome of crowns placed within the General Dental Services in England and Wales. J Dent 2008. [Epub ahead of print]
65. Pjetursson BE, Sailer I, Zwahlen M, Hämmerle CH. A systematic review of the survival and complication rates of all-ceramic and metal-ceramic reconstructions after an observation period of at least 3 years. Part I: Single crowns. Clin Oral Implants Res 2007;18(Suppl 3):73–85.
66. Sailer I, Pjetursson BE, Zwahlen M, Hämmerle CH. A systematic review of the survival and complication rates of all-ceramic and metal-ceramic reconstructions after an observation period of at least 3 years. Part II: Fixed dental prostheses. Clin Oral Implants Res 2007;18(Suppl 3):86–96.
67. Moncada G, Fernández E, Martín J, Arancibia C, Mjör IA, Gordan VV. Increasing the longevity of restorations by minimal intervention: a two-year clinical trial. Oper Dent 2008;33:258–264.
68. Pallesen U, Qvist V. Composite resin fillings and inlays. An 11-year evaluation. Clin Oral Investig 2003;7:71–79.
69. Calamia JR, Calamia CS. Porcelain laminate veneers: reasons for 25 years of success. Dent Clin North Am 2007;51:399–417.
70. Hickel R, Roulet JF, Bayne S, Heintze SD, Mjör IA, Peters M, et al. Recommendations for conducting controlled clinical studies of dental restorative materials. Science Committee Project 2/98-FDI World Dental Federation study design (Part I) and criteria for evaluation (Part II) of direct and indirect restorations including onlays and partial crowns. J Adhes Dent 2007;9(Suppl 1):121–147.
71. Holm-Pedersen P, Lang NP, Müller F. What are the longevities of teeth and oral implants? Clin Oral Implants Res 2007;18(Suppl 3):15–19.

# Posterior Composite Restorations – Direct or Indirect Technique

Roberto Spreafico and Jean-François Roulet

## Introduction

When composites were introduced in the late 1960s, it was believed that they could be used also for posterior restorations, based on their good mechanical properties. However, extensive clinical studies with this first generation of composites showed very poor wear behavior (Fig 5-1).[1,2] Furthermore, in early times, composites were applied without adhesive techniques. The inherent polymerization shrinkage led to marginal gaps. These gaps, coupled with poor oral hygiene, led to a higher recurrent caries rate than with amalgam. This formed the basis for the poor reputation of composites, especially for application in the posterior area.[3] Since then, there have been substantial technological improvements in composites. Modern resin composites are optimized for wear resistance, smooth surface, and low polymerization shrinkage (Figs 5-2 to 5-4). Furthermore, self-curing was replaced by light curing;[4] reliable adhesives were introduced (reviewed by Eick et al.,[5] Perdigão et al.[6] and Lopes et al.[7]), and a layering technique was introduced to control shrinkage.[8] The knowledge of the c-factor,[9] which describes the effect of cavity configuration on bonding of composite, has led to more sophisticated layering techniques that reduce the stress at the interface and increase the positive effect on margin quality.

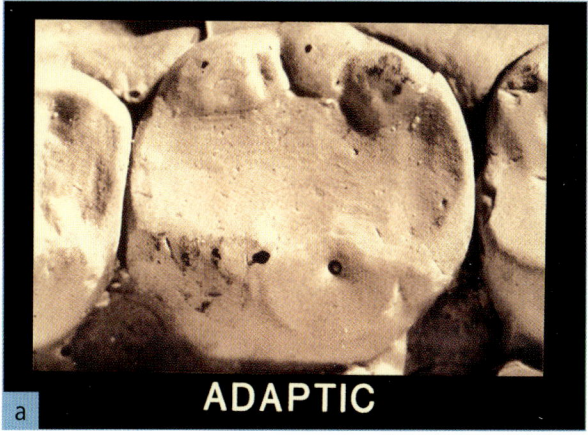

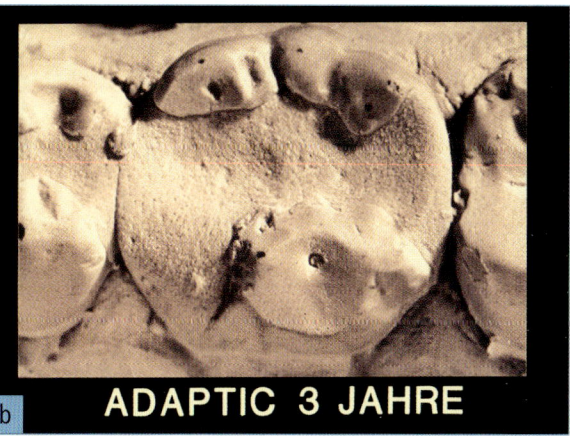

Fig 5-1a–b  Replica of posterior composite restoration. (a) Baseline. (b) Same restoration after 3 years. Note the heavy substance loss owing to wear. *(From Mettler et al. 1978, 1986)*

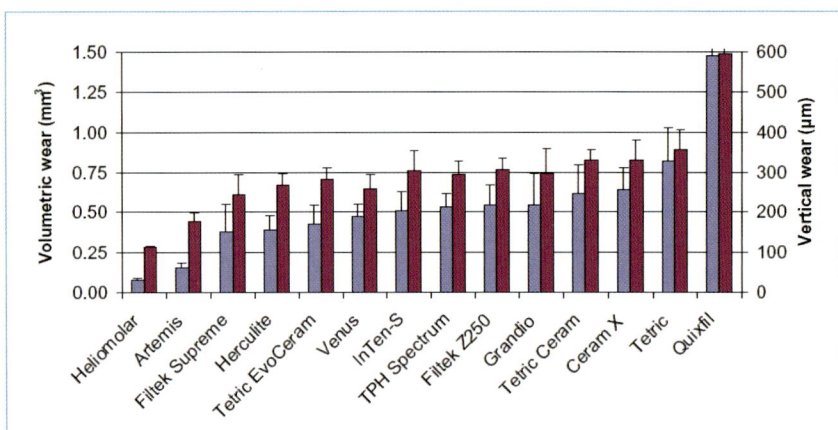

**Fig 5-2** *In vitro* wear of different composites measured with Willitec wear simulation. *(courtesy of Ivoclar Vivadent)*

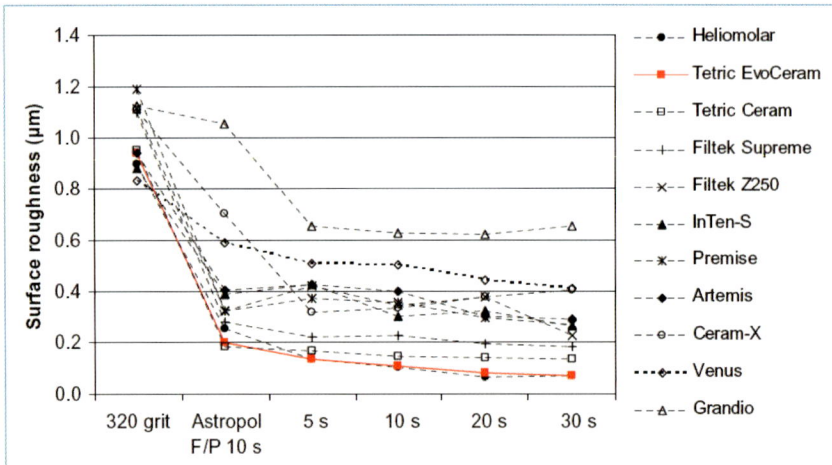

**Fig 5-3** Surface roughness of different composites. *(courtesy of Ivoclar Vivadent)*

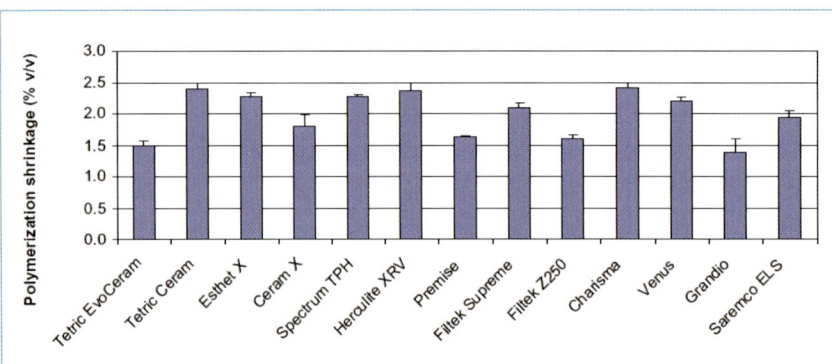

**Fig 5-4** Polymerization shrinkage of different composites (measured with mercury dilatometer). *(courtesy of Ivoclar Vivadent)*

In the early 1980s, it was believed that the wear resistance of a composite could be improved by optimizing its polymerization. This led to the idea of indirect application of composite in the form of composite inlays.[10] However clinical examinations showed that heat curing did not improve wear resistance over auto-

or light-cured composites.[11,12] However, the margin quality of the restorations was definitely improved and seemed to remain stable over time.[11,12]

Parallel to the experiments with composite inlays, also in the 1980s, castable and later pressable ceramics were introduced into the market. In the Dental School of the Free University in Berlin, early experiments were performed to test if the castable ceramic would be suitable for the manufacture of ceramic inlays. *In vitro* studies elucidated the correct treatment of interfaces and the luting technology for adhesive cementation.[13] An *in vitro* study also proved the clinical applicability of these techniques.[14] Other researchers have shown that it is also possible to produce ceramic inlays by layering and sintering ceramics on refractory dyes.[15–17] In 1985, the Cerec technology was introduced by Mörmann and Brandestini.[18] At this time, the only restorations possible with this system were inlays. Because of the innovative character of this technology, a multitude of scientific investigations were undertaken with ceramic inlays during the late 1980s. It was clearly shown that good margin integrity would remain intact over the years with the exception of wear of the luting composite.[19]

# Direct Posterior Restorations

As described above, modern composites with excellent physical and mechanical properties allow a high standard of filling therapy. Such restorations are virtually invisible because the optical properties of the composites mimic those of dentin and enamel. This creates a chameleon effect, in that the restorations are optically integrated into the tooth.

Figure 5-5 demonstrates the steps to produce such a restoration. After the appropriate cavity preparation (Fig 5-5b), the desired bonding system is applied. Note the slight bevel on the lateral and occlusal finishing lines. Cervical enamel is best for an excellent cervical margin quality. The wedge has a double function: first, to protect the rubber dam/gingiva and the neighboring tooth from being damaged during cavity preparation and, second, to separate both teeth slightly in order to obtain a tight contact point later on. The first step is to recreate the correct proximal relation to the neighbor-

ing tooth. This is best achieved with a sectional, precontoured matrix band. Then the first composite increment ('enamel') is carefully adapted to the matrix band and cured (Fig. 5-5c). With this technique, the maximum advantage of the configuration is exploited, since only a small proportion of the whole increment is bonded to the tooth (cervical, buccal, and oral). Both large surfaces are allowed to freely shrink during light-curing. With this procedure, the difficult class II situation is converted into an easy class I situation. Then, the dentin is covered with a thin layer of flowable composite (Fig 5-5d). In the authors' experience, this reliably avoids post-operative sensitivity after placing composite restorations. The next step is to build up the 'dentin' core. It is important to create the occlusal anatomy at this step. The central grove must be correctly placed and the dentin should also follow the intended inclination of the cusps. The dentist must take care to leave enough space for the final layer of the 'enamel' composite (Fig 5-5e). Using a rather stiff composite, with good thixotropic behavior, the dentist can sculpture the final occlusal anatomy in great detail before curing the composite. This reduces the final contouring polishing to a minimum (Fig 5-5f). After rehydratation of the enamel, excellent optical integration can be observed (Fig 5-5g).

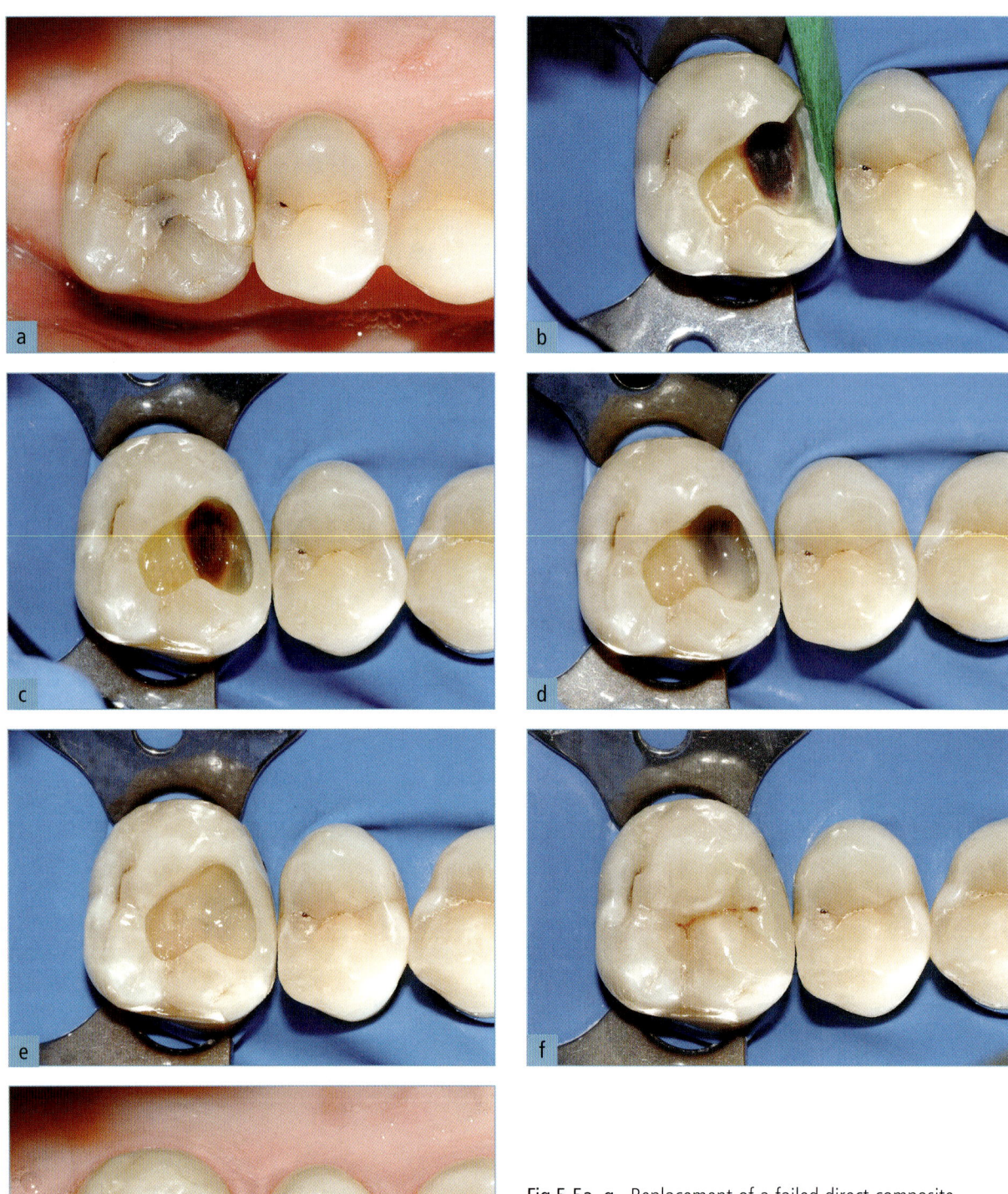

**Fig 5-5a–g** Replacement of a failed direct composite restoration. **(a)** Preoperative view. **(b)** The cavity is prepared and the size is appropriate to receive a direct restoration. **(c)** The class II cavity is transformed into a class I cavity using a small amount of an 'enamel' mass. **(d)** A thin layer (< 0.5 mm) of flowable composite is layered covering the dentin. **(e)** A 'dentin' mass is applied leaving sufficient space for the last enamel layer. **(f)** The restoration completed. **(g)** The same restoration some weeks later.

In the next case presentation, a whole quadrant is restored with proximal composite restorations (Fig 5-6). The methodology is similar to that used in Fig 5-5. Note that the characterization or structuring of the fissures should be carried out on top of the 'dentin' layer, or in other words under the 'enamel' layer. Minute amounts of intensely stained composite (e.g. Tetric color) should be used. Seen from the front, it is not apparent that this quadrant has been restored with composite restorations (Fig 5-6h). Notice also the excellent stability of the restoration over the years (Fig 5-6j).

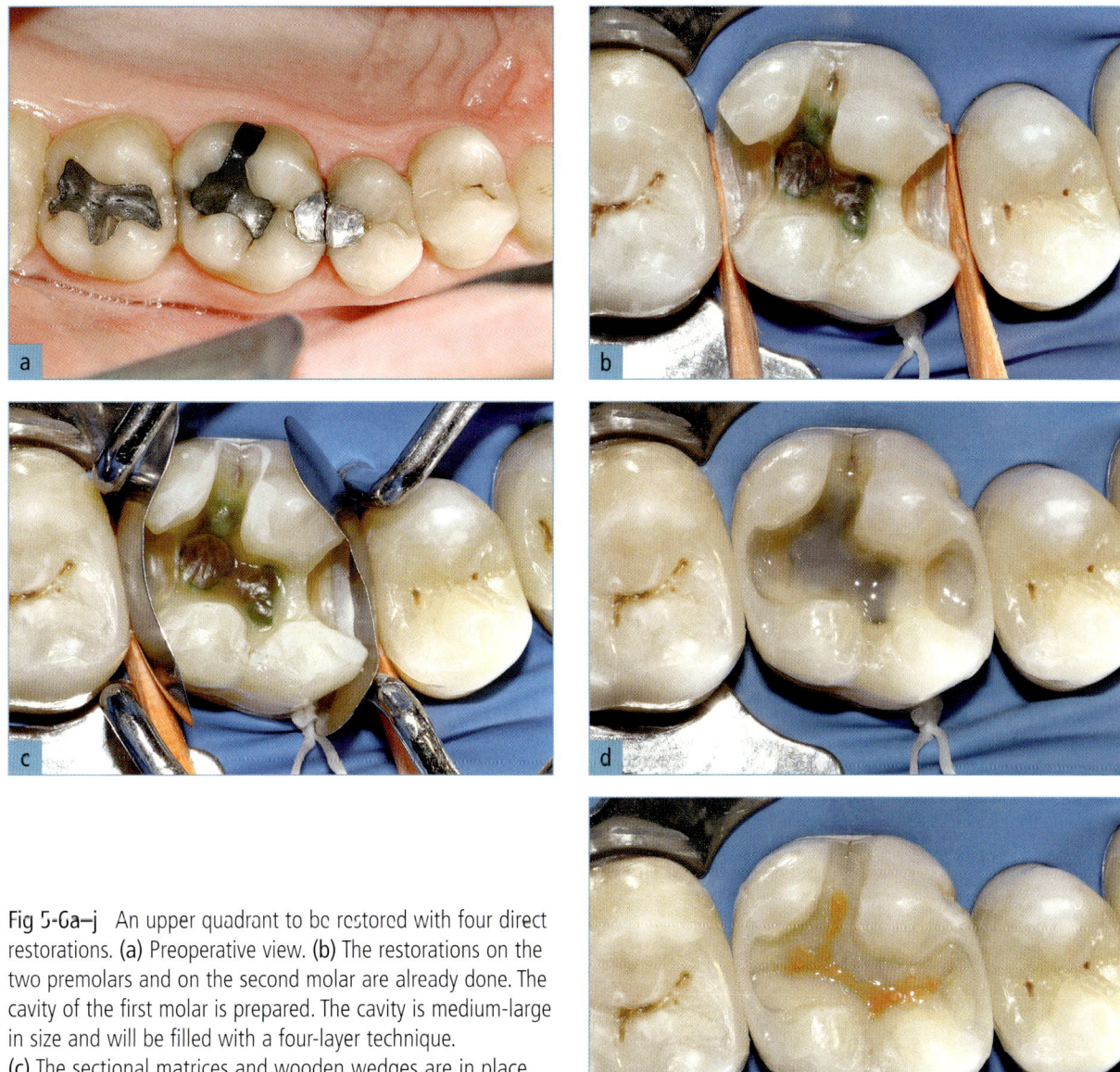

**Fig 5-6a–j** An upper quadrant to be restored with four direct restorations. **(a)** Preoperative view. **(b)** The restorations on the two premolars and on the second molar are already done. The cavity of the first molar is prepared. The cavity is medium-large in size and will be filled with a four-layer technique.
**(c)** The sectional matrices and wooden wedges are in place.
**(d)** The class II cavity is transformed in a class I cavity and then the flowable material is applied. **(e)** The third layer (dentin) is characterized with some liquid stain.

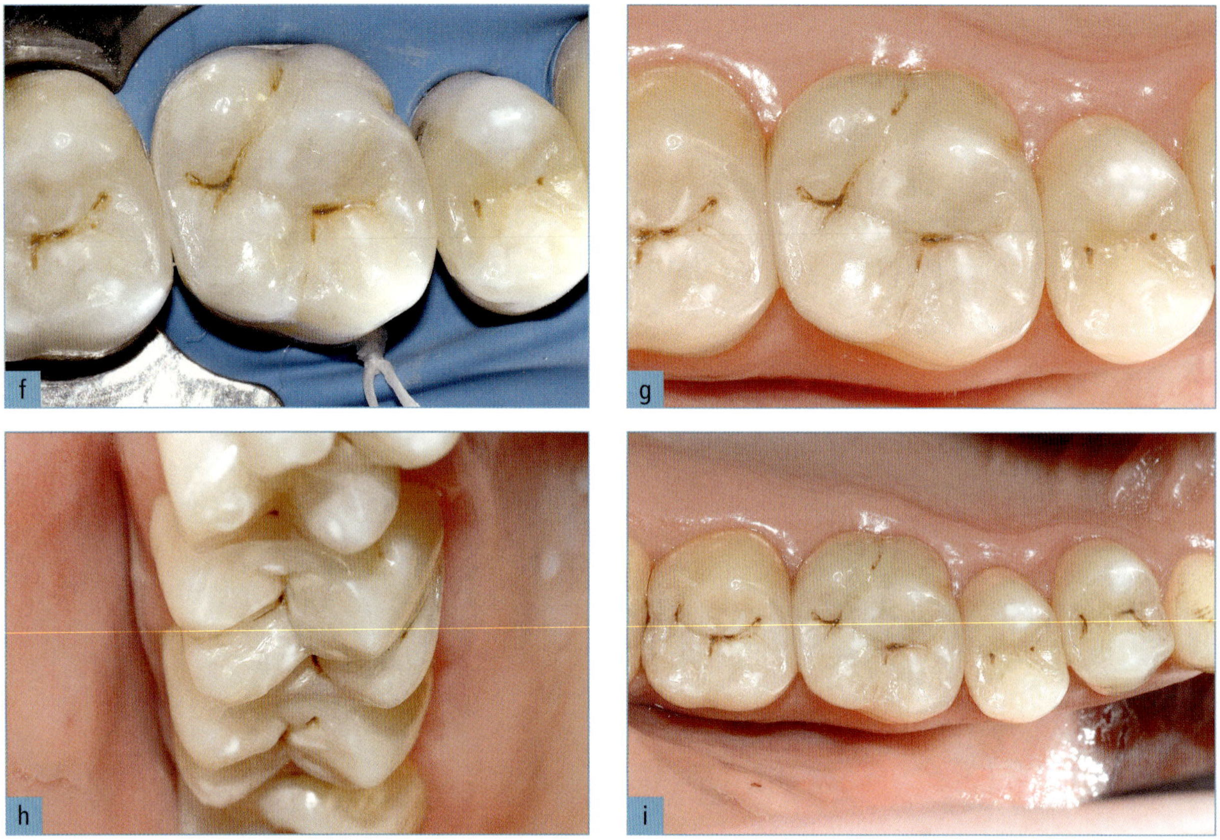

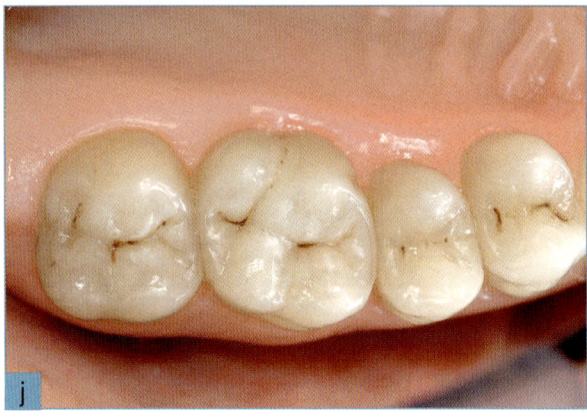

Fig 5-6a–j  An upper quadrant to be restored with four direct restorations. **(f)** The last layer of enamel is modeled and the restoration is finished and polished. **(g)** The same restoration after the occlusal adjustments. **(h)** The front view of the quadrant. **(i)** The quadrant some months later. **(j)** The same quadrant after 6 years.

# Indirect Posterior Restorations

Tooth-colored indirect posterior restorations can be made in different ways.

## Composite or Ceramic Inlays/Onlays

If it is decided to follow a composite route, there are three options.

♦ *Direct composite inlay.* With this technique, an inlay cavity without any undercuts is insulated with a separating liquid. Then the inlay is built up in the cavity using an incremental technique. Because of the insulation, the inlay can be removed from the cavity and its margins finished outside the oral cavity. The inlay can also be heat cured and then seated with adhesive techniques.

♦ *Indirect composite inlay.* This technique is identical to the traditional way of making gold inlays. A stone model, based on an impression, is used by the dental technician to build up the inlay with light-cured composite in an incremental technique. The advantage is that there is an articulated model of the opposing teeth, so the occlusal relationship can be carefully

built up and checked in the articulator. Additional heat curing is optional. Luting is as described below.

♦ *Chairside composite inlay.* In principle, this is placed in the same way as in the indirect technique; however all steps are optimized for speed. The model is made out of a extremely fast-working silicone material (e.g. Mach 1 by Parkell). The dentist can start the build up of the inlay a few minutes after pouring the silicone into the insulated impression. However, there is no antagonist, so the occlusal morphology is extrapolated from the remaining cusps. The advantage of this technique is that the dentist has the best articulator at his/her disposal: the patient.

For the luting process, the tooth interface is treated with an adhesive system. The inlay inner surface is roughened with a diamond burr and lined with an unfilled resin for good wetting. Then it can be cemented with either a dual cured composite-based luting agent (e.g. Variolink) or with the same composite material as used for the inlay. The latter is the authors' preferred method. Using an ultrasonic insertion technique facilitates the seating of the inlay still further.[20]

Figure 5-7 shows a molar with extensive destruction that was reconstructed with an indirect composite onlay.

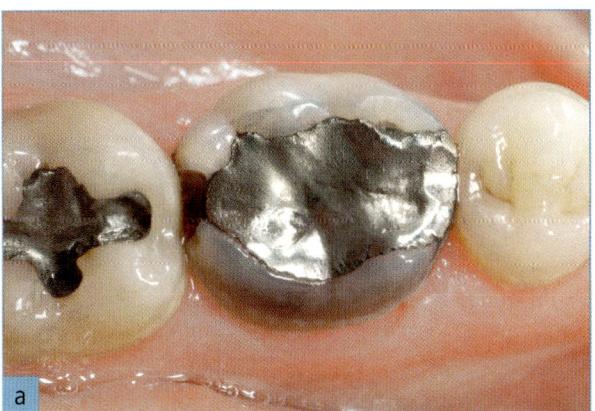 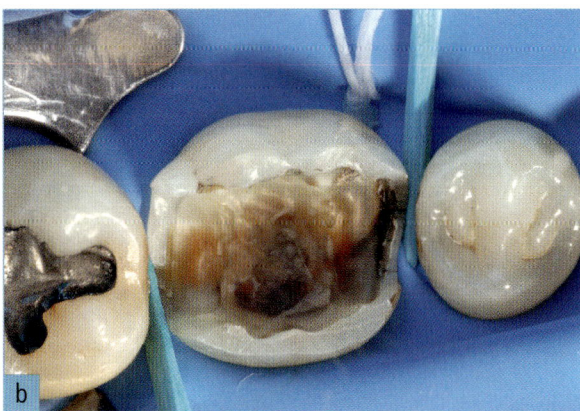

**Fig 5-7a–f**  Restoration of a molar with an indirect composite inlay. **(a)** Preoperative view. **(b)** Since the buccal and lingual walls are very thin, they have to be cut down.

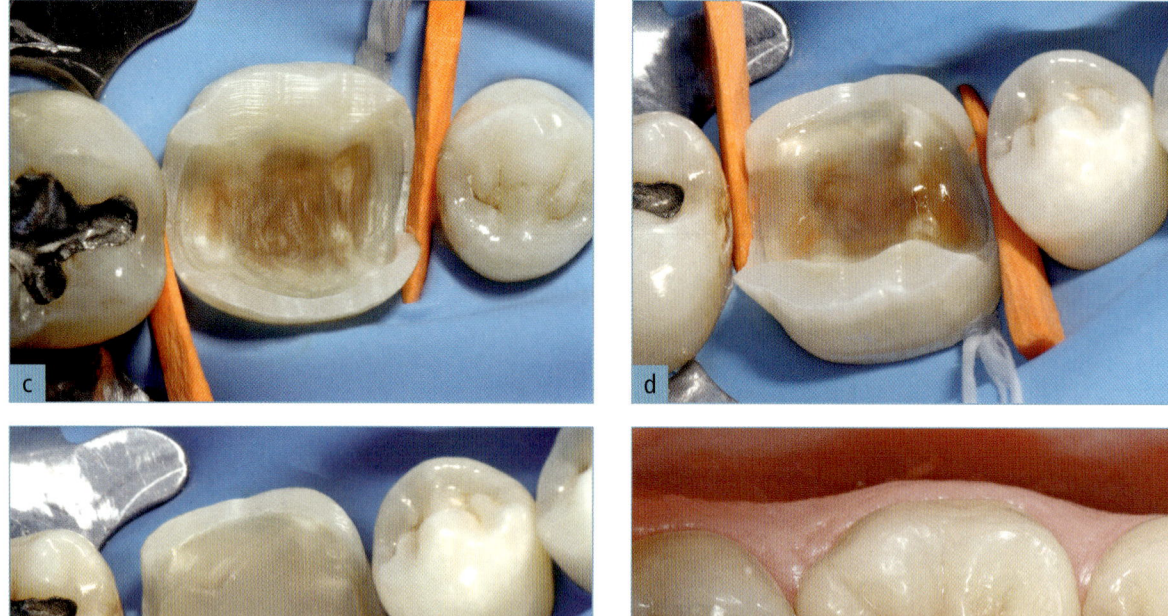

**Fig 5-7a–f** Restoration of a molar with an indirect composite inlay. **(c)** The tooth is prepared for a composite overlay. **(d)** The dentin is hybridized. **(e)** A composite resin build up is placed. It allows for an ideal cavity preparation for an inlay. Now the tooth is ready for the impression. **(f)** The same tooth 2 weeks later with an indirect composite onlay *in situ*.

*Ceramic Inlays*

There are also various options for the manufacture of ceramic inlays.

- *Conventional feldspar ceramic* fired on a refractory dye. As mentioned in the introducion, a conventional feldspar ceramic can be layered on a refractory dye to produce an inlay.
- *Pressable ceramic*. The most common way to produce ceramic inlays is to use a pressable ceramic (e.g. Empress). This has the advantage that the lost wax technique is used, which allows a 1:1 transfer from the wax object to the ceramic inlay.
- *Computer-aided design and manufacture* (CAD/CAM). The third possibility is to use a CAD/CAM device to produce ceramic inlays. Cerec is the system

with the longest experience and, in our view, with the highest degree of sophistication. After taking an optical impression of the teeth with a powdered covering to create the required non-reflective surface, the actual configuration of the area is known and the system can even account for the occlusal relationship and function.

For cementing ceramic inlays, the inlay's inner surface must be roughened by etching with hydrofluoric acid and silanated for good wetting with the resinous luting cement. The luting materials are the same as those used for composite inlays.

Figure 5-8 shows a reconstruction with Cerec inlays made with Empress CAD (Ivoclar Vivadent).

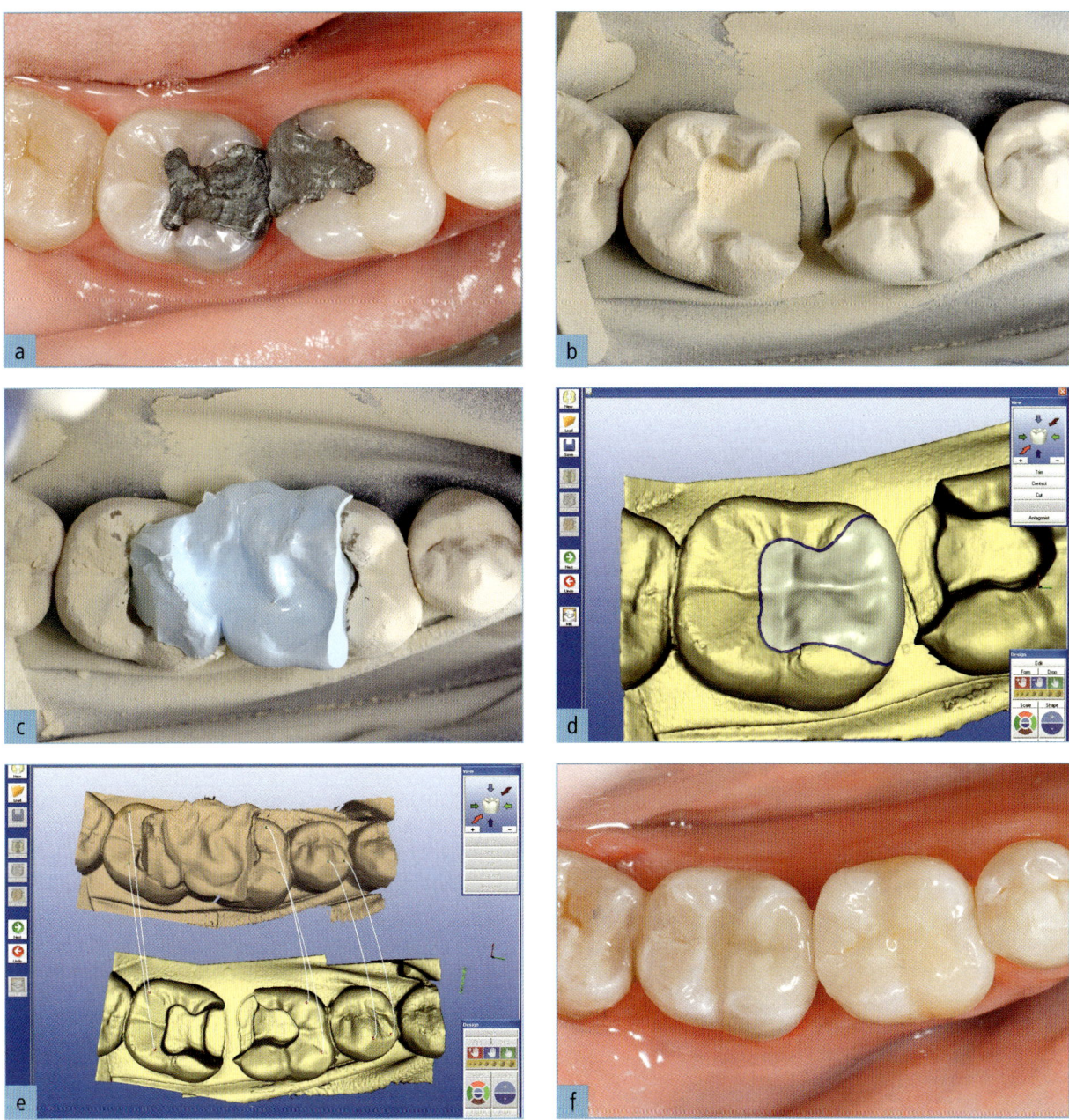

**Fig 5-8a–f**  Two insufficient amalgam restorations to be replaced. **(a)** Preoperative view. **(b)** The cavities are prepared with a rubber dam *in situ*. The whole area is powdered to create a non-reflective surface and to prepare the teeth for the optical impression. **(c)** Registration of the antagonistic relation with a silicone suitable for optical impressions. **(d)** Construction of the inlay on the virtual model. **(e)** Virtual working models to create the occlusal relationship and function. **(f)** Adhesively luted inlays. *(Courtesy of Dr. A Peschke)*

## Comparison of the Techniques

Opinions on how to approach restorations and the use of composites has changed in recent years. When composites first became available, most dentists were not in favor of their application in the posterior segments, and in the 1990s the indirect technique was considered to allow the best marginal adaptation in any clinical situation for medium and large cavities.[21–23] More recently, it has been demonstrated that indirect restorations perform better, particularly for large cavities.[24] *In vivo* studies have demonstrated that there is not a significant difference in the performance of luted restorations and direct restorations.[25–27] However, von Dijken[26] has re-ported that composite inlays and onlays performed better than direct composite restorations in patients with high caries activity (high risk) and when the enamel in the cervical box was reduced or completely absent.

In our own study,[28] we could show that there is no difference in terms of longevity and marginal adaptation between direct restorations and inlays in medium-sized cavities.

The advantages and disadvantages of the different options to restore posterior teeth are summarized in Table 5-1. The luting procedures are very demanding from a clinical point of view and require a certain clinical experience.

**Table 5-1** Advantages and disadvantages of the different posterior restoration options.

| Restoration type | Advantages | Disadvantages |
|---|---|---|
| Direct composite restorations | Less invasive<br>Single visit<br>Less expensive<br>Excellent longevity data | Shrinkage stress control<br>Anatomic issues: proximal contact, occlusal anatomy |
| Indirect composite restorations | Better shrinkage stress control<br>Optimal anatomical outcomes<br>Less expensive (when compared with ceramic inlays and onlays) | The indirect technique is more invasive (path insertion)<br>Two visits required (indirect technique)<br>Clinical skill required (chairside technique) |
| Ceramic inlays/onlays | Durable high esthetics<br>Optimal anatomical outcomes<br>Excellent longevity data | The indirect technique is more invasive (path insertion )<br>Very expensive<br>Two visits required |

### Longevity

Basically, the restoration that yields the best longevity should be the preferred one. Most studies of longevity, however, focus on the material, despite the fact that the dentist has a much larger influence on the outcome. An example illustrates this: In a study of Pallesen,[29] composite direct restorations were observed for 20 years. Therefore, on today's standards, the materials used (Miradapt, P-10, P-30) were technologically quite old.

Despite this, she reported an excellent longevity, with an annual failure rate of 1.6% after 10 years and 1.3% after 20 years!

Mannhard and colleagues have looked at the longevity of posterior restorations.[30,31] In the summary to their review,[30] it can be seen that direct composite restorations behave as well as amalgam. Statistically, there was almost no difference between the different restoration types analyzed (Table 5-2).

**Table 5-2** Longevity of posterior restorations in terms of percentage annual failure rate. *(From Manhart et al. 2004 and Manhart 2006)*[30,31]

| Restoration type | All studies | | | | Longitudinal studies, class II, 1990–2003 | | | |
|---|---|---|---|---|---|---|---|---|
| | Range | Mean (SD) | LSD test | Median | Range | Mean (SD) | LSD test | Median |
| Amalgam | 0–7.4 | 3.0 (1.9) | C | 2.6 | 0–7.4 | 2.6 (2.0) | B | 2.0 |
| Direct composite | 0–9.0 | 2.2 (2.0) | ABC | 1.8 | 0–7.0 | 2.2 (1.9) | AB | 1.7 |
| Composite inlay/onlay | 0–10.0 | 2.9 (2.6) | BC | 2.3 | 0–10 | 2.9 (2.6) | B | 2.3 |
| Ceramic inlay/onlay | 0–7.5 | 1.9 (1.8) | AB | 1.3 | 0–7.5 | 1.9 (1.9) | AB | 1.3 |
| CAD/CAM inlay/onlay | 0–5.6 | 1.7 (1.6) | A | 1.2 | 0–5.6 | 1.7 (1.4) | AB | 1.2 |
| Gold inlay/onlay | 0–5.9 | 1.4 (1.4) | A | 1.0 | 0–4.0 | 0.9 (1.1) | A | 0.9 |
| LSD, Fisher's least significant difference; CAD/CAM, computer-aided design and manufacture. | | | | | | | | |

# Conclusions

Based on the facts discussed above, it can be concluded that it is not the material that dictates the indication (direct filling versus inlay/only) but rather the ability of the dentist to reconstruct the damaged tooth flawlessly. Basically, the less destruction there is of the tooth, the easier it is to reconstruct directly in the mouth. In other words, as long as there is sufficient left from the occlusal surface that the dentist can orient him/herself for the reconstruction, a good result should be obtained.

# Recommendations

♦ Direct restorations are indicated to restore small and medium-sized cavities.
♦ Indirect restorations are indicated to restore large class I and II cavities.
♦ When one or all the cusps are missing, indirect restorations perform better especially for anatomic reasons (proximal contact and occlusal anatomy).

♦ Multiple large restorations can more easily be performed in the dental laboratory and in these cases it seems that there is a time advantage for the dentist.
♦ There is no scientific evidence to prefer ceramic over composite or vice versa for the inlay/onlay material.

# References

1. Phillips RW, Avery DR, Mehra R, Swartz ML, McCune RJ. Observations on a composite resin for class II restorations: three year report. J Prosthet Dent 1973;30:891–897.
2. Mettler P, Friedrich U, Roulet J-F. Studie über die Abrasion von Amalgam und Komposits im Seitenzahnbereich. Schweiz Mschr Zahnheilk 1987;88:324–344.
3. Lutz F, Mörmann W, Kreici I. Seithenzahnkomposite: Ja, Nein oder Jein? Dtsch Zahnärztl Z 1985;40:892–896.
4. Dart EC, Nemcek J. Photopolymerizable composition. Br Patent B 408 265 (Oct 1 1975).
5. Eick JD, Gwinnett AJ, Pashley DH, Robinson SJ. Current concepts on adhesion to dentin. Crit Rev Oral Biol Med 1997;8:306–335.
6. Perdigão J, Frankenberger R, Rosa BT, Breschi L. New trends in dentin/enamel adhesion. Am J Dent 2000;13(Spec No):25D–30D.
7. Lopes GC, Baratieri LN, de Andrada MA, Vieira LC. Dental adhesion: present state of the art and future perspectives. Quintessence Int 2002;33:213–224.
8. Spreafico R, Roulet JF. Composite Layering. In: Roulet J-F, Vanherle G (eds). Adhesive Technology for Restorative Dentistry. London: Quintessence, 2005, pp. 11–26.

9. Feilzer AJ, Gee AJd, Davidson CL. Setting stress in composite resin in relation to configuration of the restoration. J Dent Res 1987;66:1636–1639.

10. Mörmann WH. Kompositeinlay: Forschungsmodell mit Praxispotential? Quintessenz 1982;33:1891–1901.

11. Mörmann W, Ameye C, Lutz F. Kompositeinlays: Marginale Adaptation, Randdichtigkeit, Porosität und okklusaler Verschleiss. Dt Zahnärztl Z 1982;37:438—441.

12. Roulet J-F. Degradation of Dental Polymers. Basel: Karger, 1986.

13. Geppert W, Roulet J-F. In virto marginal integrity of mod-Dicor inlays luted with adhesive techniques. J Dent Res 1986;65:731.

14. Herder S. In vivo Untersuchung der marginalen Adaptation adhäsiv befestigter Glaskeramikinlays. Berlin:Zahnmed Diss, 1988.

15. Mönkmeyer U. Die Herstellung ästhetisch wirkender Inlays: Vorstellung von vier Keramiksystemen. Quintessenz Zahntech 1987;13:993–997.

16. Theisen E. Anfertigung keramischer Inlays im Labor mit Duucera-Lay (I). Quintessenz Zahntech 1988;14:675–686.

17. Theisen E. keramischer Inlays im Labor mit Duucera-Lay (II). Quintessenz Zahntech 1988;14:799–812.

18. Mörmann W,H, Brandestini M, Ferru A, Lutz F, Kreici I. Marginale Adaptation von adhäsiven Porzellaninlays in vitro. Schweiz Mschr Zahnmed 1985;95:1118–1129.

19. Kanzler R, Roulet J.-F. Margin quality and longevity in vivo of sintered ceramic inlays luted with adhesive techniques. In: Mörmann W (ed.) CEREC 10 Year Anniversary Symposium: CAD/CIM in Aesthetic Dentistry, , 1986, pp. 537–552.

20. Noack MJ, Roulet, J.-F, Bergmann P. A new method to lute tooth colored inlays with highly filled composite resins. International Association of Dental Research DMG Microfilm, Publ. No. 1528.1991.

21. Haller B, Klaiber B. Kompositinlays als zahnfarbene Seitenzahnrestaurationen. Zahnarztl Mitt 1989;79:920–925.

22. Milleding P. Microleakage of indirect composite inlays. An in vitro comparison with the direct technique. Acta Odontol Scand 1992;50:295–301.

23. Shortall AC, Baylis RL, Baylis MA, Grundy JR. Marginal seal comparisons between resin-bonded Class II porcelain inlays, posterior composite restorations, and direct composite resin inlays. Int J Prosthodont 1989;2:217–223.

24. Iida K, Inokoshi S, Kurosaki N. Interfacial gaps following ceramic inlay cementation vs direct composites. Oper Dent 2003;28:445–452.

25. Pallesen U, Qvist V. Composite resin fillings and inlays. An 11-year evaluation. Clin Oral Invest 2003;7:71–79.

26. van Dijken JW. Direct resin composite inlays/onlays: an 11 year follow-up. J Dent 2000;28:299–306.

27. Wassell RW, Walls AW, McCabe JF. Direct composite inlays versus conventional composite restorations: 5-year follow-up. J Dent 2000;28:375–382.

28. Spreafico RC, Krejci I, Dietschi D. Clinical performance and marginal adaptation of class II direct and semidirect composite restorations over 3.5 years in vivo. J Dent 2005;33:499–507.

29. Pallesen U. Clinical evaluation of three posterior composite resins: 20 year report. In: Joint Meeting of the Continental European and Scandinavian Divisions of the International Association of Dental Research, Amsterdam 2005, abstract 0145.

30. Manhart J, Chen HY, Hamm G, Hickel R. Review of the clinical survival of direct and indirect restorations in posterior teeth of the permanent dentition. Oper Dent 2004;29:481–508.

31. Mannhart J. Charakterisierung direkter zahnärztlicher Füllungsmaterialien für den Seitenzahnbereich: Alternativen zu Amalgam? Die Quintessenz 2006;57:465–481.

# Treatment Goal for the Anterior Segment – Functional Reconstruction or Smile Design?

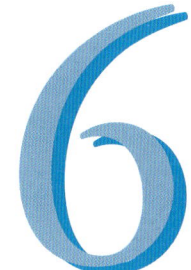

Alessandro Devigus

## Introduction

In today's dentistry, the term smile design is often mis-used and related to cosmetic changes made to the dentition without following any functional guidelines.[1] When planning treatment for esthetic reasons, smile design cannot be isolated from a comprehensive approach to patient care. Achieving a successful, healthy, and functional result requires an understanding of the interrelationship among all the supporting oral structures and occlusion.[2]

Many authors have described the base criteria that are required for an esthetic appearance.[3-5] The criteria for an esthetic appearance of the gingiva are well known. Health and morphology are the most important issues on this checklist. The objective characteristics of natural teeth can also be classified (Fig 6-1).

A treatment starts with a comprehensive dental examination, including a patient interview to find out what the patient's desires are, dental radiographs, photographic records, and a thorough clinical examination of all oral tissues (Fig 6-2).[6]

One of the most important components of a healthy mouth is proper occlusion. The importance of a balanced occlusion without any interference is still valid in individuals with full-mouth or extended rehabilita-tions.[7,8] In the anterior region where at first sight only small corrections are required, the role of occlusion is often overlooked or neglected and this may be the cause of clinical failures. The large number of articles discussing the reconstruction in the anterior segment can be summarized as stating that dental esthetics (form) follows proper occlusion (function).[9,10]

There are few restorative procedures that do not involve occlusal surfaces. Many articles on smile design do not consider the natural irregularities that contribute to the individuality and beauty of a person's smile. Most beautiful and natural smiles are not necessarily symmetric, uniform in color, or perfect by scientific standards.

## Case Presentation

### First Appointment

A 24-year-old woman presented with the chief complaint of chipping at the central incisors, which she felt gave her an unpleasant smile (Fig 6-3). During the first appointment with the patient, in addition to taking a history and comprehensive clinical examination, photographs, radiographs, and alginate impressions were taken. The patient was caries free and had no periodontal problems (probing depth all < 2 mm).

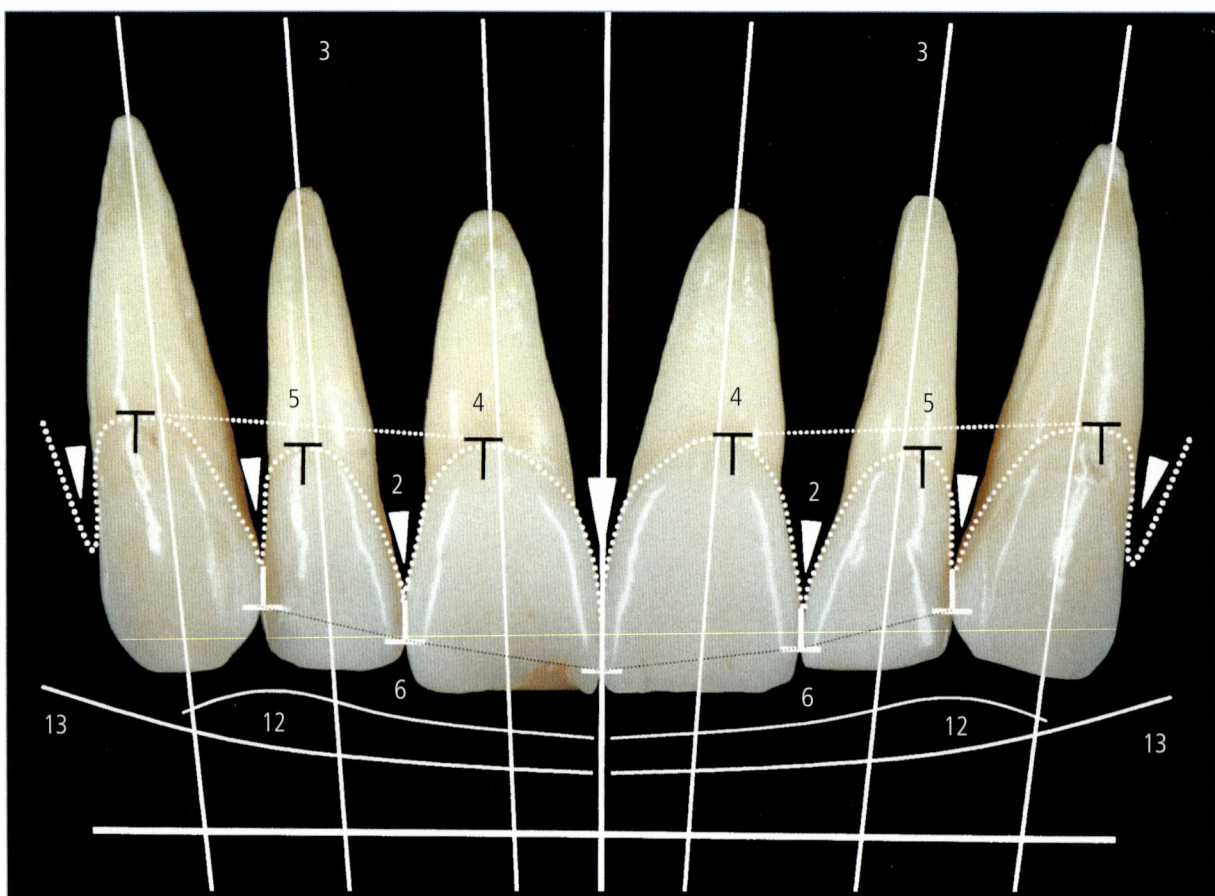

**Fig 6-1** The Esthetic Checklist. *(From Magne and Belser 2002[4])*

### Fundamental objective criteria

| | |
|---|---|
| 1. Gingival health | 2. Interdental closure |
| 3. Tooth axis | 4. Zenith of the gingival contour |
| 5. Balance of the gingival levels | 6. Level of the interdental contact |
| 7. Relative tooth dimensions | 8. Basic features of tooth form |
| 9. Tooth characterization | 10. Surface texture |
| 11. Color | 12. Incisal edge configuration |
| 13. Lower lip line | 14. Smile symmetry |

### Subjective criteria (esthetic integration)

Variations in tooth form
Tooth arrangement and positioning
Relative crown length
Negative space

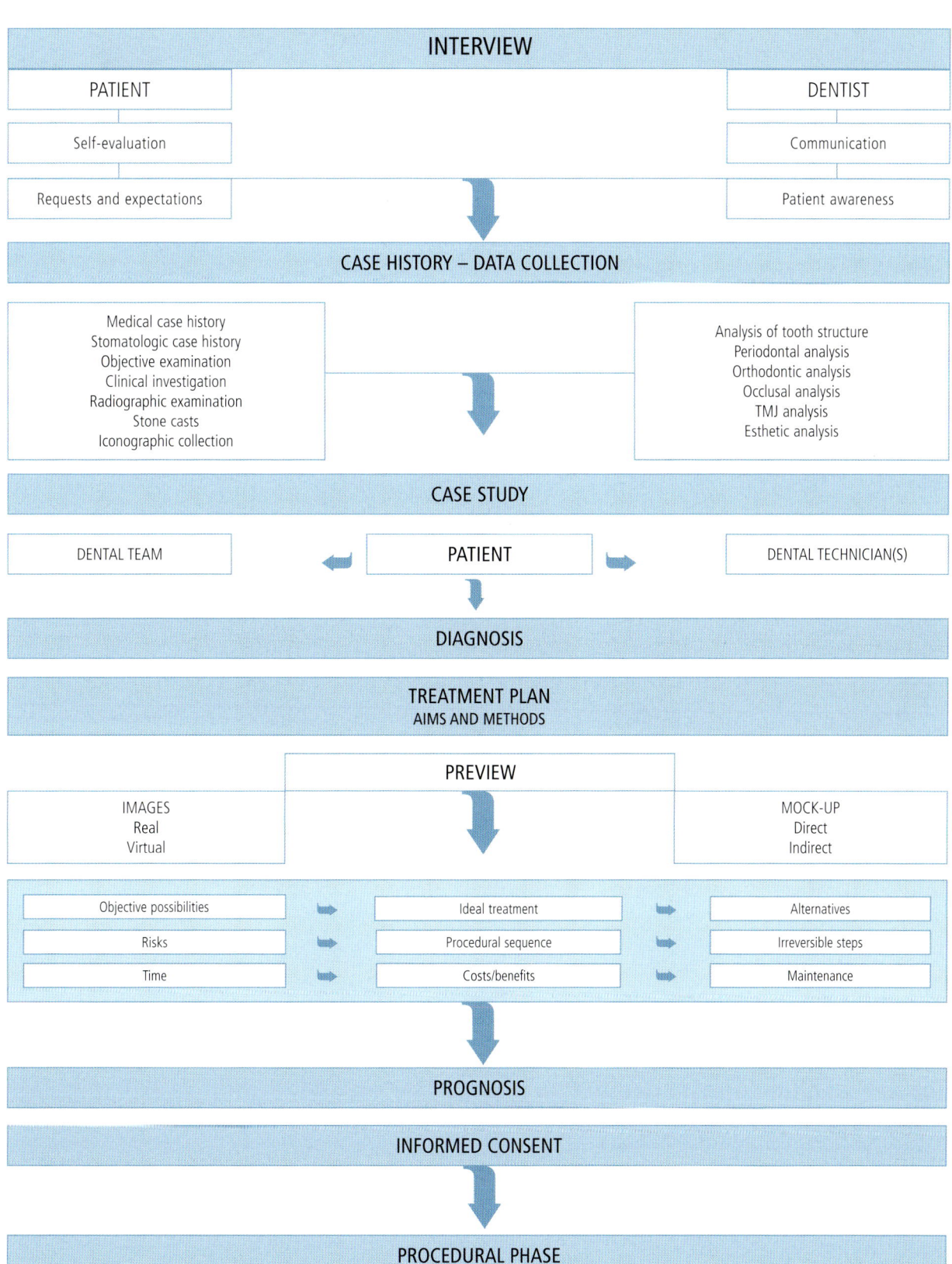

**Fig 6-2** Schematic representation of the phases that must precede the clinical procedures. *(From Fradeani 2004[6])*

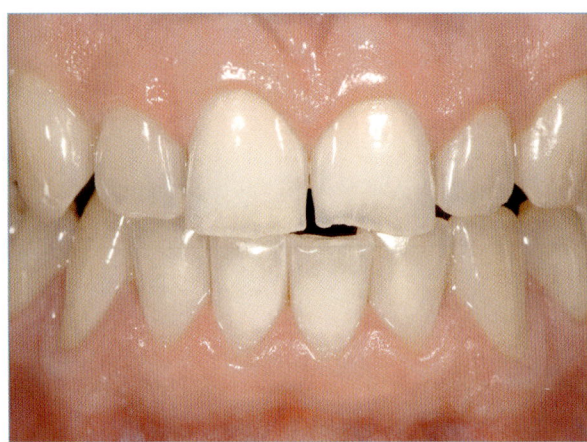

**Fig 6-3** At presentation: the central incisors show signs of wear.

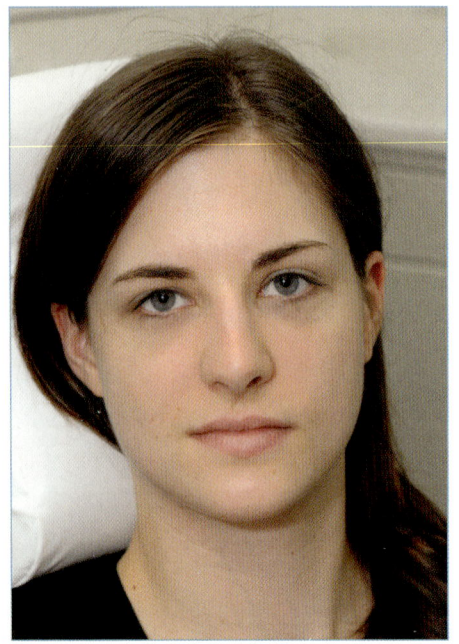

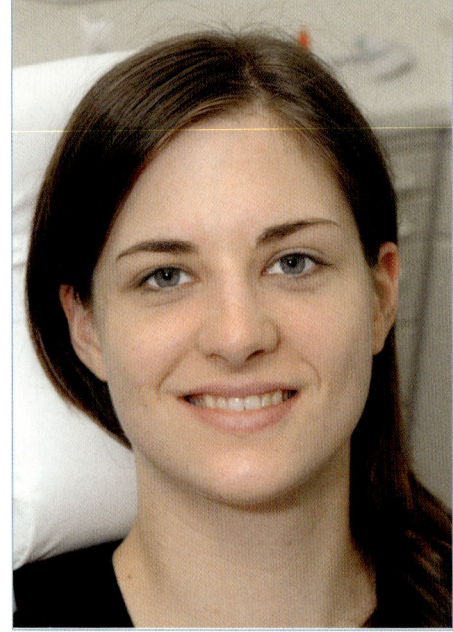

**Fig 6-4** The smile analysis includes a series of photographs of the patient. It is important to start with a portrait and then get closer to end up with details of the teeth involved.

**Fig 6-5** The patient is asked to smile or, if not possible, to show her teeth. This image shows the impact of the teeth on the overall facial appearance.

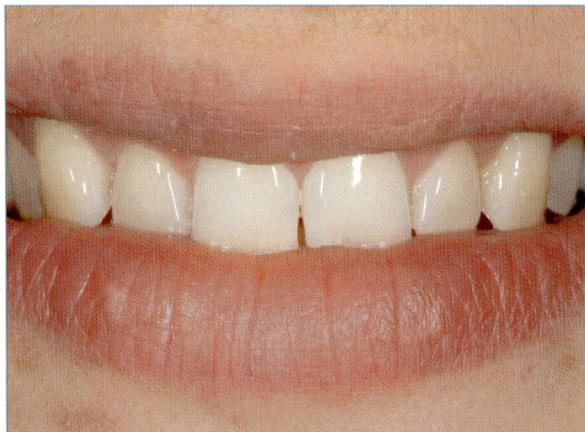

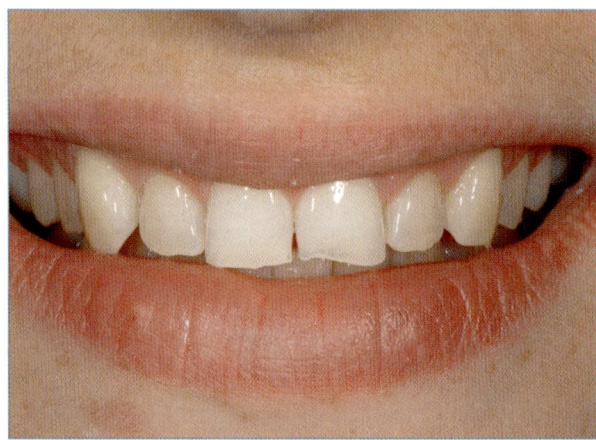

**Fig 6-6** The patient has her mouth slightly open. The contour of the lips follows the gingival borders of the teeth.

**Fig 6-7** At a wider opening of the lips, the chipped incisors and the abrasion at the left canine become visible.

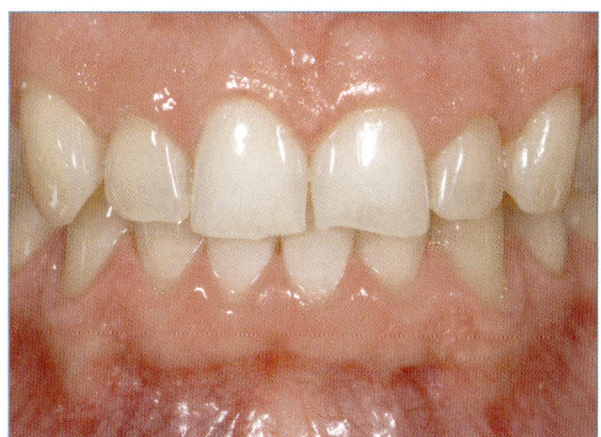

Fig 6-8  A frontal view at maximal intercuspidation gives additional information about the overbite of the patient.

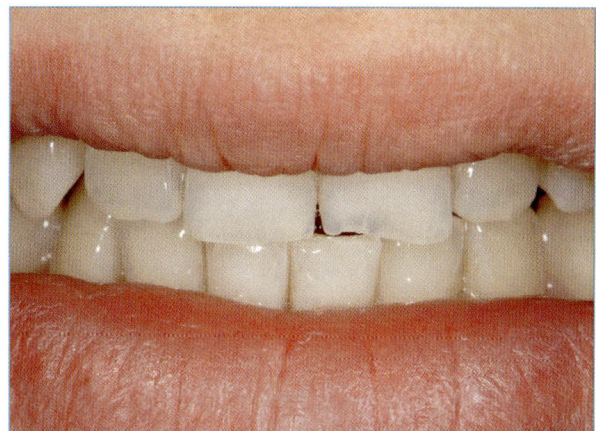

Fig 6-9  The patient finds the position of 'malfunction' that causes the abrasion of the anterior teeth.

## Treatment Planning: Esthetic Checklist

Digital photographs are an effective tool for discussion with the patient regarding the actual situation and the possible treatment options.

An individual smile analysis is performed with a series of images starting with a portrait and then focusing on the details (Figs 6-4 to 6-9). It is important to keep the overall appearance always in mind during the initial diagnostic phase.

At this point, the esthetic checklist (Fig 6-1) can be used to determine the necessary changes to enhance the dental setup of the patient. The two central incisors are too short and their form has been changed by abrasion. The maxillary left canine shows also signs of abrasion where the maxillary right canine is still intact. By lengthening the two central incisors and the maxillary left canine, the smile of the patient could be improved. To achieve maximum preservation of tooth structure and a predictable esthetic outcome, bonded composite build-ups are the first choice in young patients.

Before proceeding with the restoration of the involved teeth, it is mandatory to check the occlusal situation in the patient. The intraoral examination revealed the following situation, which can be also documented photographically while the patient is moving the mandible forward and to both sides to show the actual functional conditions (Figs 6-10 to 6-16). There

is canine guidance on the right and canine/incisor group guidance on the left side. On the right, there is an Angle class I and on the left an Angle class II. In addition, the mandibular arch shows tilted molars and crowding in the anterior area.

The functional analysis assists in understanding the reasons for the abrasions in the maxillary anterior teeth. In addition, the temporomandibular joint and muscles should be tested. This patient did not show any problems in these areas.

## Involve the Patient

At this stage, the treatment options are discussed with the patient. Building up the lost tooth structure is not possible without changing the positions of the teeth involved. This would lead to an invasive treatment with extensive veneer or crown preparations. Such restorations should never be considered in a relatively young patient without looking at treatment alternatives.

Repositioning the teeth before any reconstructive procedures would definitely be the preferred option in such a case.

The orthodontic treatment options were discussed with the patient. The main concern of an adult patient is the visibility of an orthodontic appliance. Invisalign uses a series of removable, clear aligners that are custom made, and this may be an option for some patients.[11,12]

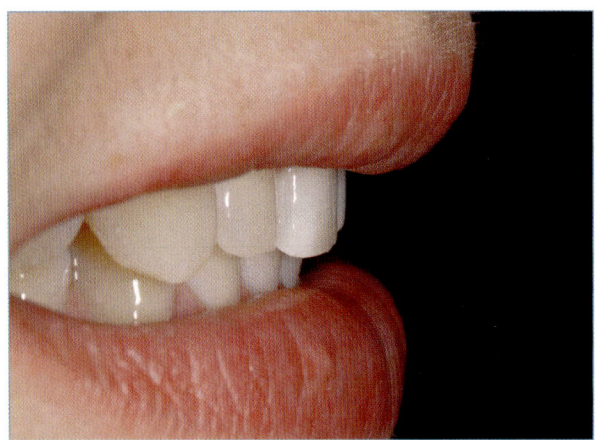

Fig 6-10  A lateral view at maximal intercuspidation gives additional information about the inclination/position of the anterior teeth.

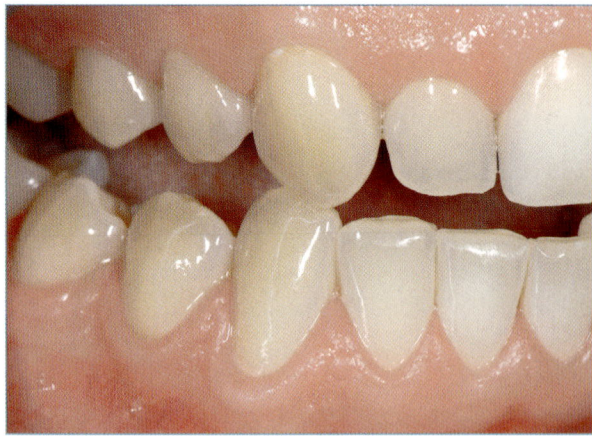

Fig 6-11  A functional analysis is performed, asking the patient to perform protrusive and lateral movements. Guidance can be checked as the patient performs a lateral movement to the right. Canine guidance can be seen here.

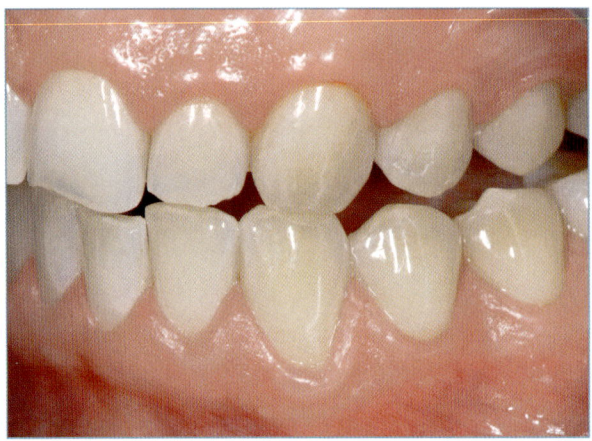

Fig 6-12  When the patient performs a lateral movement to the left, group guidance (canine, incisors) can be observed.

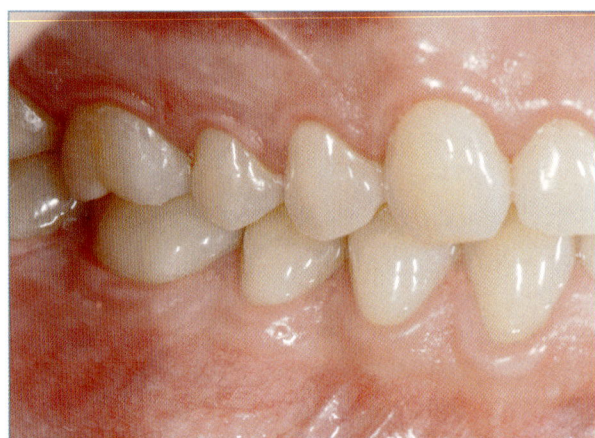

Fig 6-13  A lateral image of the right side shows the Angle class I.

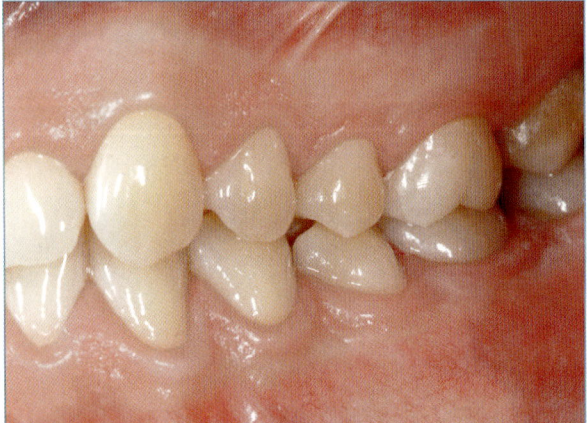

Fig 6-14  A lateral image of the right side shows the Angle class II.

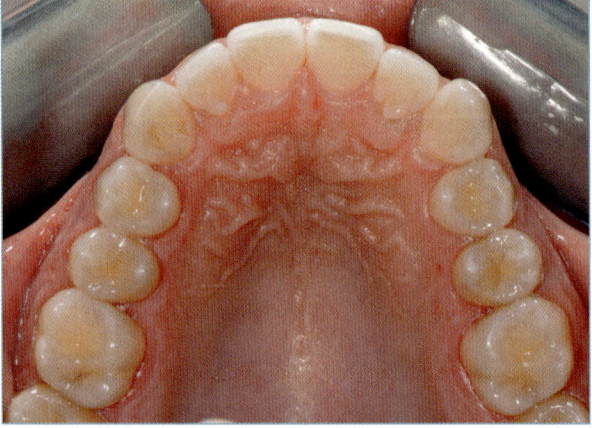

Fig 6-15  In the maxilla, the positions of the canines and premolars are not correct.

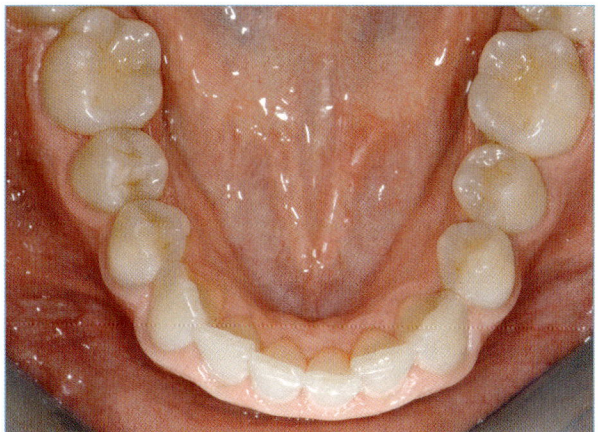

**Fig 6-16** The mandibular anterior teeth are crowded and the mandibular molars are tilted, showing the asymmetry already seen in the maxilla.

or smile design?', can be answered. Today's practice aims not only to restore function but also to create an enduring esthetic outcome. The most important goal in our treatment strategy is still to get our patients to feel comfortable with their personal appearance, including their smile. Nowadays, thanks to improved adhesive techniques, the indications for crowns have decreased and a more conservative approach may be proposed that will preserve tooth structure and postpone more invasive treatments until the patient is older. The dynamic character of oral structures must also be taken into consideration. Minimally invasive approaches will become increasingly important in our dental practice as our patients get older while retaining their natural dentition.

The classical approach using brackets offers a more effective way to solve the orthodontic problems within 9 months for this particular patient. As an option, the brackets could be placed at the lingual aspect or ceramic brackets could be bonded to the more visible maxillary teeth. The final decision was to use ceramic brackets in the maxilla and metal brackets in the mandible. The goal of the orthodontic treatment was to establish an Angle class I on both sides, eliminate the crowding in the mandibular arch and create the space necessary to restore the maxillary anterior with bonded restorations.

At the time of writing the patient is receiving orthodontic care.

This case shows the importance of a smile design based on functional principles so that, finally, there is the correct choice of the materials and technologies for a successful restoration for the patient in the long term.

# Conclusions

Static occlusal concepts established in the last century have been replaced with biomechanical approaches. The importance of occlusion, which was neglected in the 1990s with the flood of cosmetic dentistry, has been re-established and the question, 'functional reconstruction

# References

1. Schlott WJ. Form follows function. J Am Dent Assoc 1999;130:1562–1564.
2. Davis NC. Smile design. Dent Clin N Am 2007;51:299–318.
3. Belser UC. Esthetics checklist for the fixed prosthesis. Part II: Biscuit try-in In: Schärer P, Rinn LA, Kopp FR (eds) Esthetic Guidelines for Restorative Dentistry. Chicago, IL: Quintessence, 1982, pp.188–192.
4. Magne P, Belser UC. Bonded Porcelain Restorations in the Anterior Dentition: A Biomimetic Approach. Chicago: Quintessence, 2002.
5. Rufenacht CR. Fundamentals of Esthetics. Berlin: Quintessence, 1990, pp. 73, 80–82, 89, 94, 95, 125–127, 138.
6. Fradeani M. Esthetic Rehabilitation in Fixed Prosthodontics. Chicago, IL: Quintessence, 2004.
7. Keough B. Occlusion-based treatment planning for complex dental restorations: Part 1. Int J Periodontics Restorative Dent 2003;23:237–247.
8. Keough B. Occlusion-based treatment planning for complex dental restorations: Part 2. Int J Periodontics Restorative Dent 2003;23:325–335.
9. Magne P, Gallucci GO, Belser UC. Anatomic crown width/length ratios of unworn and worn maxillary teeth in white subjects. J Prosthet Dent 2003;89:453–461.
10. Sorenson DA. Form follows function: occlusion based rationale for esthetic dentistry. J Indiana Dent Assoc 1998;77:25–30.
11. Lagravère MO, Flores-Mir C. The treatment effects of Invisalign orthodontic aligners: a systematic review. J Am Dent Assoc 2005;136:1724–1729.
12. Maganzini AL. Outcome assessment of Invisalign and traditional orthodontic treatment and subsequent commentaries. Am J Orthod Dentofacial Orthop 2006;129:456.

# Root Canal Therapy versus Implant

Claus Löst

## Introduction

Lang in 2006 commented that 'Implants are a blessing for mutilated dentitions',[1] and even a convinced conservative clinician views implants as a valuable addition to the spectrum of dental treatment. While implants are an undisputed replacement for lost teeth or after mandatory extraction of teeth (e.g. after vertical root fracture), more extensive demands in the sense of 'early replacement of compromised teeth'[2,3] encounter resistance for various reasons and motivations. Spångberg complained that 'the value of the natural tooth has diminished dramatically among some clinicians' and anticipated a threat to the existence of his entire professional guild should practitioners continue to follow the trend of referring to implantologists instead of endodontists.[4] Some authors refer to medical questions that still surround extension beyond the already existing maximal therapeutical use of implants,[5] while others see the (still) valid self-image of the dental profession being threatened by aggressive marketing of manufacturers and distributors of implants, bone replacement grafts, growth factors and membranes.[6] Whatever the position, the discussion about 'early replacement of compromised teeth' has started[7,8] and endodontists (and periodontologists) find themselves abruptly in a position of

defence.[9,10] Since studies alone give no apparent proof of superiority of conservative dental treatment (e.g. by root canal therapy) over implants (see below), the American Association of Endodontists felt impelled to express 'flexibility', perhaps under economic pressure. In 2003, the American Association of Endodontists explained to its members that 'attacks' on the 'compromised' root canal-treated tooth from the community of implantologists were merely based on the commercial interest of manufacturers of implants or a handful of clinicians.[11] Meanwhile, a vast number of lectures and courses at the annual meetings of the association became devoted to the alternative 'implant' approach, and further educational courses on implantology are also part of their program. In the face of this area of economic conflict, and in order to curb competitive disadvantages, the American Association of Endodontists even decided to sacrifice its formerly strict, scientifically oriented definition of endodontic outcomes for 'softer' criteria,[12] according to which (as in many studies dealing with implants) the focus is on the mere 'survival function' of the tooth.

All these developments are signs of the lack of 'hard facts' and evidence base to support decisions for root canal therapy of a tooth and arguing against extraction of the tooth and possibly its replacement by an implant

– or the other way around. A decision-making algorithm[13] based on valid data remains an aspiration. This chapter will discuss the current thinking regarding root canal therapy and implants and will identify and evaluate the parameters that (consciously or subconsciously) will affect the decision: 'root canal therapy or implant?'

# Decision-Making Based on Studies on Treatment Outcome

Attempts to compare the quality of a root canal-treated tooth with that of an implant, generally or related to a certain clinical situation, are bound to fail if they merely compare success rates or prognoses established in clinical studies. There are a number of reasons for this. For example, a direct comparison of root canal treated teeth with implants requires specific situations that simply do not exist and could not be realised for methodological and ethical reasons. Indirect qualitative comparison of both therapies will be inconclusive because, among other things, there is a lack of good randomized controlled studies for either approach. A further reason is that differing criteria for outcome assessment are used. These will be discussed in more detail below.

## Outcome of Root Canal Treatment

Particularly in discussions of root canal treatment versus implants, the endodontic community refers to studies showing a success rate for root canal treatment of approximately 90%. An example of such a study is that of Sjögren and coworkers.[14] However, a summary report by Friedman[15] showed that the success rates of longitudinal studies range from 50% to 90%. Longitudinal clinical studies investigating the outcome of endodontic treatments published since the end of the 1990s have

been the subject of several systematic reviews (see the summary report by Ng and coworkers[16]). In this most recent review, the mean success rates of primary root canal treatment were between 31% and 96% 'based on strict criteria' and between 60% and 100% 'based on loose criteria'.[16] It was established that preoperative apical periodontitis, qualitatively bad root canal filling, overextension of root canal filling, and unsatisfactory coronal restoration were factors with negative influence on the results.[17]

In the context of this chapter, the following remarks and conclusions from the authors of the latter two papers are worth mentioning:[16,17]

◆ The studies selected for this meta-analysis only show a medium level of evidence.

◆ There are substantial variations in study characteristics (sample selection, definition of success, observation period, educational and experience background of operators etc.), which among other things complicates the pooling of data.

◆ Many of the selected studies depict relevant methodological shortcomings.

◆ The estimated pooled success rates of primary root canal treatment ranged between 68% and 85% when using strict criteria.

The conclusion that was drawn in these reviews was that the success rates of primary root canal treatment if critically assessed were lower than those occasionally claimed (see above), and that there is insufficient evidence from longitudinal studies conducted on root canal treatment to draw satisfactory conclusions. What remains to be added is that normally the success rates of non-surgical and surgical root canal re-treatments are lower than that for primary root canal treatment, but apart from this, the quality and the degree of evidence of studies in this area are the same as those discussed above for primary root canal treatment.[18]

## Outcome of Implant Therapy

Just as for advocates of root canal therapy, advocates of early replacement of compromised teeth by implants also like to refer to success rates of implant therapy that are 'mostly greater than 90% after five years'.[7] Here also the quality of the randomized controlled trials of oral implants published before the end of last century have been described as 'generally poor'.[19]

Newer studies, such as that of Roos-Jansåker and coworkers,[20] in which an overall success rate of more than 95% was reported, are also affected by similar methodological and other shortcomings. For example, in the study of Roos-Jansåker and coworkers,[20] 76 (26%) of the total of 294 patients scheduled for control visits (9- to 14-year follow up) could not or did not want to be integrated in the final control examination. While it should be stressed that loss of implants occurring before placement of the suprastructure was registered in the study (which was not the case in many other studies), it should also be mentioned that the study could be criticized for collecting data about the existence and degree of peri-implant lesions[21] but not considering these in the calculation of 'overall success rate'. Technical complications were also not considered. It must be asked if the term 'overall success rate' can realistically be used when important parameters such as biological and technical complications, which obviously carry numerical weight, are neglected.

## Outcome Studies in Root Canal Treatment and Implantology

The concept of evidence-based dentistry has been gaining recognition. However, attempting to discuss root canal treatment versus implant is fraught with difficulties when the best available clinical evidence is research papers:

- The quality of the available research papers is relatively low (see above).

- Successful outcome of treatment in endodontology is almost exclusively described by post-operative non-occurrence or resolution of pathological changes (healing), and in implantology it is predominantly depicted by survival rates.
- Survival rates without numerical data about intra- and post-operative biological and technical complications only partially describe the quality of the treatment procedures.
- Fewest data are available about implants in the indications where implants can be considered as an alternative to root canal treatment.
- No consideration has yet been taken of the potential influence of new techniques and materials in endodontology or of as the extension of indications and changes in implant design, material and procedures (immediate load implants) in implantology.
- To a large extent, it is not known whether the high survival rates achieved by experts and at certain centers can be generalized in implantology.

For the sake of completeness, it should be mentioned that a meta-analysis by Pjetursson et al.,[22] assessing the 5- and 10-year survival of implant-supported fixed dental protheses, showed peri-implantitis and soft tissue complications in 8.6% of the cases, cumulative incidence of connection-related complications in 7.3%, and suprastructure-related complications occurred in 14% of the cases at 5 years. Berglundh and coworkers criticized the meta-analysis in that the studies used in the analysis provided 'limited information regarding the occurrence of peri-implantitis'.[23] There is an increase in publications showing that previous experience of periodontitis correlates with an increased implant failure rate.[24–26]

The fact that most studies on success rate of dental implants use the survival of implants as reference parameter has prompted some of the endodontic community to cite or initiate studies on survival rates of root canal-treated teeth.[27–29] According to these, there is an insignificant difference in the mere survival rates of root canal-treated teeth and implants. This debate between

Fig 7-1a–f  Re-treatment in postendodontic disease, showing how endodontic treatment is defined and that saving a (compromised?) tooth can have a good prognosis.

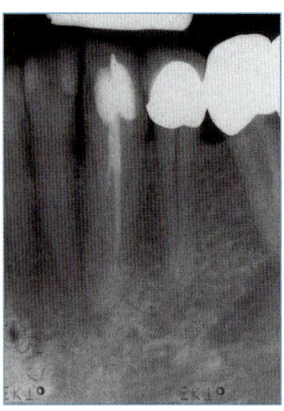
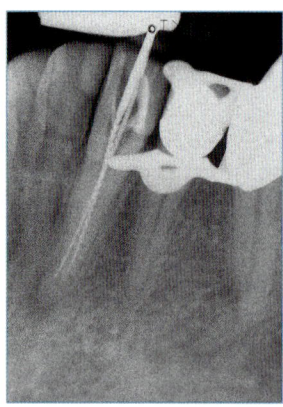
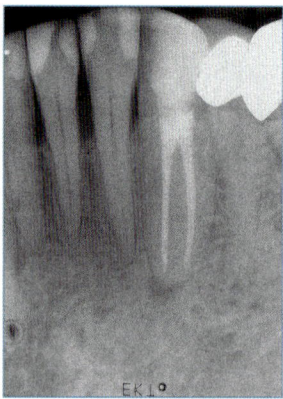
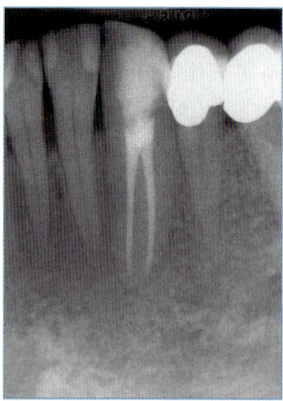

**(a)** Asymptomatic apical periodontitis in a mandibular cuspid in a 43-year-old patient that had received insufficient root canal treatment.

**(b)** Working length radiograph after accessing the full working length of both root canals.

**(c)** Radiograph of root canal filling after coronal restoration with bonded resin composite.

**(d)** Radiograph assessment almost 2 years after the root canal treatment, showing healing of the apical lesion.

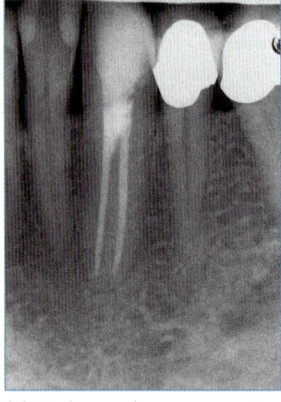
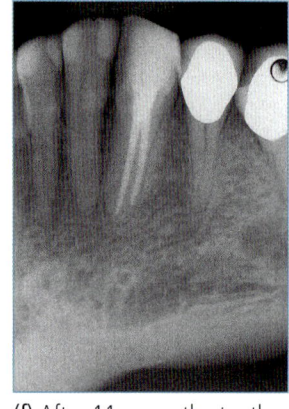

**(e)** Radiograph assessment 6 years after re-treatment.

**(f)** After 11 years, the tooth is asymptomatic without radiographic findings of disease (complete healing).

rates is absurd because the mere presence of the tooth is ensured regardless of whether there is root canal treatment. For root canal therapy, the only reasonable way of describing treatment success is to use terms such as healing and non-healing rates (Fig 7-1).[30]

# What Situations Might Demand a Decision between Root Canal Treatment and Implant?

the endodontology and implantology communities using the 'smallest common denominator' (survival or functionality) in outcome studies has the big disadvantage of not considering aspects of oral health (e.g. existence/non-existence of inflammation). To consider only survival rates in endodontology is even somewhat illogical: The reason for treating a tooth with an asymptomatic apical periodontitis is to eliminate intracanal infection and the inflammation resulting from it. Describing the success of therapy in the form of survival

In the context of a decision between root canal treatment and an implant, there are three different initial clinical situations that need to be differentiated.

♦ A tooth is in need of primary root canal treatment, endodontic re-treatment or endodontic surgery and is selected for a single-tooth restoration post-operatively (i.e. it is not to be integrated in prosthodontic work) (Figs 7-1 to 7-3). Here the practitioner, together with the patient, needs first of all to make a decision between endodontic therapy and extraction of the tooth based on consideration of numerous parameters. Only when the decision is in favor of extraction can the question be posed as to whether the loss of this one tooth could and should be compensated by an implant. Strictly speaking such cases are not even embedded in the question of 'root canal treatment or implant', unless the advising clinician attempts to alter the decision of the patient in favor of extraction by describing an implant as a desirable alternative, improving the quality of life in comparison with an endodontically treated tooth (this, the author feels, would be questionable ethical practice).

♦ A patient is requiring new prosthodontic work on one or more teeth in relevant strategic positions that need endodontic treatment and that show varying degrees of destruction and possibly the requirement for additional periodontal surgery. The consideration here might be whether to replace a compromised tooth by an implant.

♦ A patient requires prosthodontic replacement and one or more root canal-treated teeth in relevant strategic positions show varying degrees of destruction and/or are in need of non-surgical or surgical re-treatment and possibly additional periodontal surgery. Here, as well, the question might be posed as to whether the endodontically compromised tooth might not better be replaced by an implant.

The formulation of just these questions, which are generated from the daily practice routine, underlines the complexity encountered in counseling patients and that the corresponding answers can never be given based on clinical randomized studies alone, even when they are of high quality. At the least, the practitioner in agreement with the patient will always need to include case-, patient-, and clinician-specific aspects in the decision-making process in addition to referring to results of any (improved) outcome studies.

**Fig 7-2a–g**   The first molar of this 47-year-old patient with aggressive periodontitis is the last remaining molar on the left side of the maxilla. This is an example of long-term preservation of a 'compromised' tooth (root canal treatment plus root amputation).

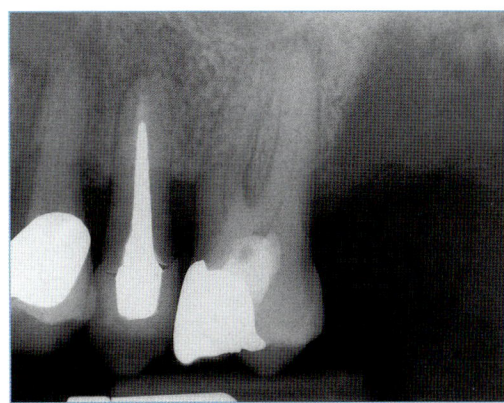

**(a)** The initial radiograph in 1983. The molar did not react to the cold test and there was through and through (mesiobuccal) furcal involvement.

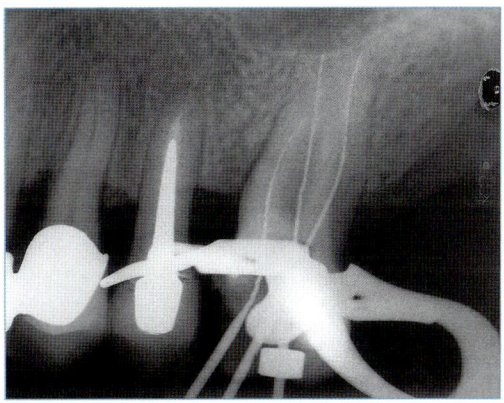

**(b)** The working length radiograph.

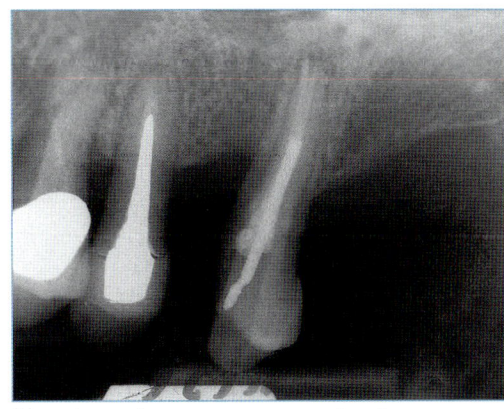

**(c)** Radiograph assessment 4 months after root canal treatment and 2 months after root amputation.

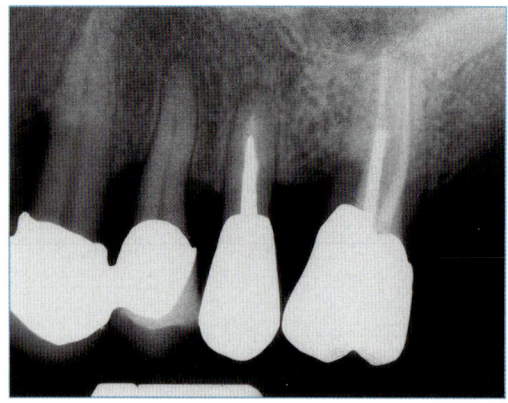

(d) Radiographic finding at 1 year after root canal treatment.

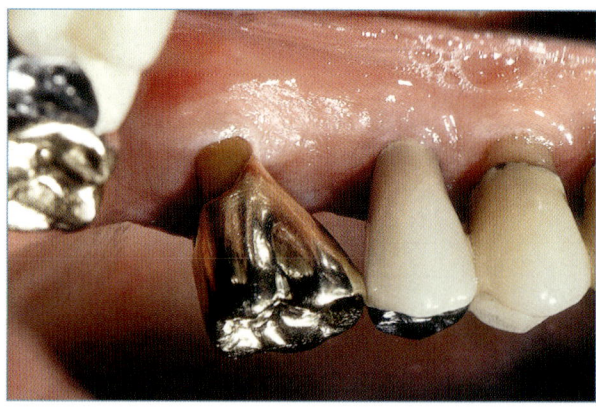

(e) Clinical situation 1 year after root canal treatment.

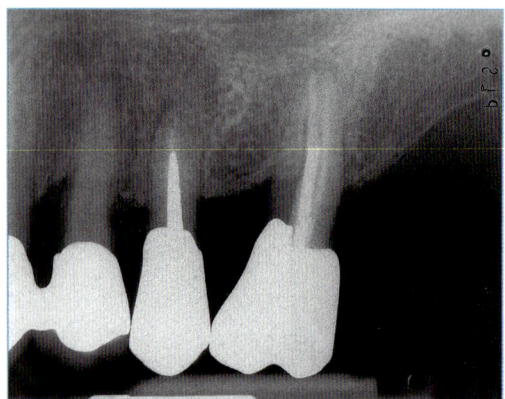

(f) Radiograph assessment at 13 years after treatment.

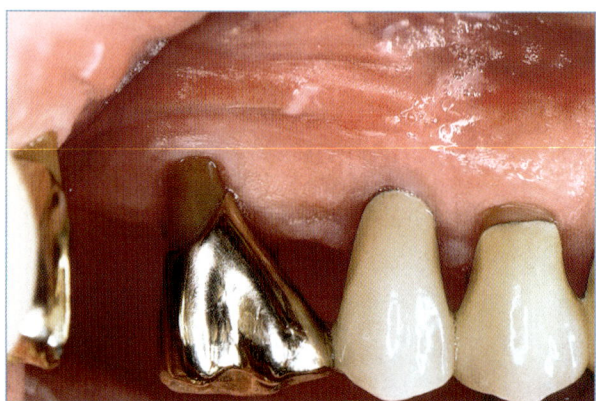

(g) Clinical situation at 13 years after treatment.

**Fig 7-3a–g** Example of the difficulty in achieving a dependable prognosis in individual cases for a tooth or implant. At the beginning of treatment, this 46-year-old female patient showed a history of aggressive periodontitis and at the time had symptomatic irreversible pulpitis in the first mandibular right molar.

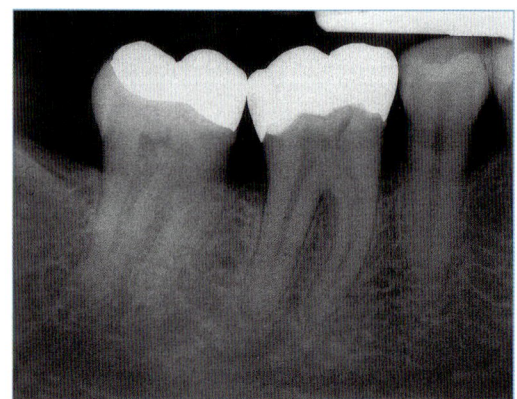

(a) Diagnostic radiograph prior to starting treatment.

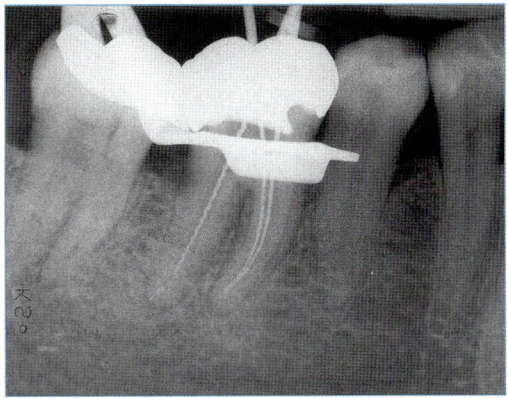

(b) Working length radiograph.

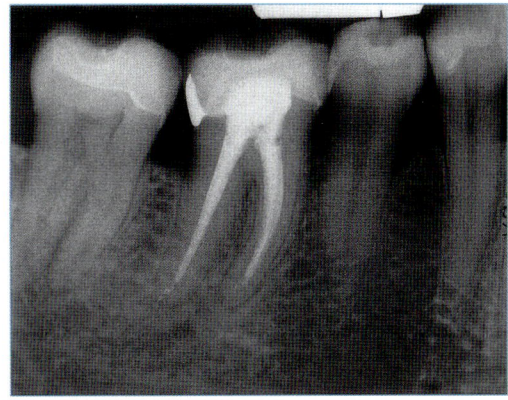

(c) Radiographic assessment 4 months after root canal treatment.

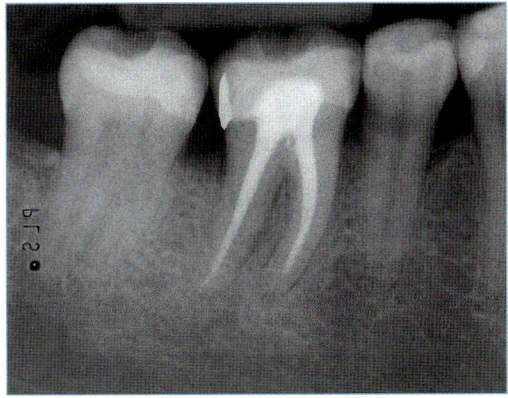

(d) Radiographic assessment 4½ years after root canal treatment.

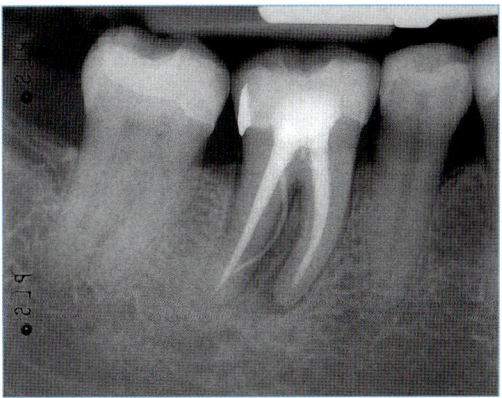

(e) Radiographic assessment with a pre-positioned gutta percha cone in a fistula located on the buccal side of the tooth 5½ years after endodontic therapy (after verification of a suspected vertical root fracture).

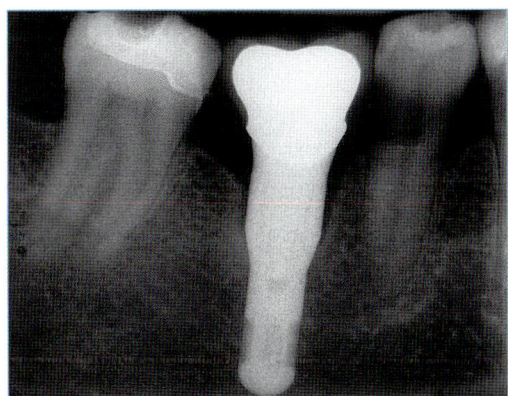

(f) Radiographic assessment of a single implant that was inserted *alio loco* as a replacement for a first molar 6 years before. There was pus emission after pressure to the peri-implant soft tissue.

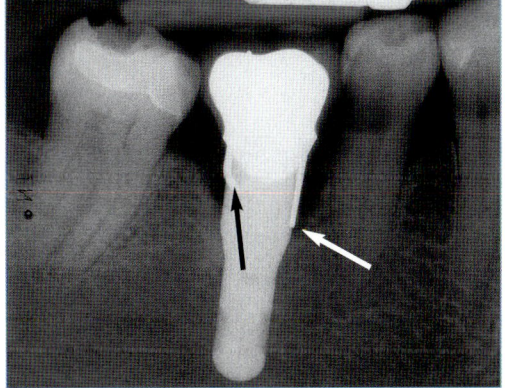

(g) A further 1½ years later, the radiograph shows peri-implant bone loss more clearly. Prior to the radiograph, a silver point was placed mesiolingually 9 mm subgingivally (white arrow). A loop of a second silver point (black arrow) becomes visible on the bottom of the buccal 'pocket' (8 mm deep). The implantologist recommended rinsing with chlorhexidine.

## Potential Parameters, in Addition to Outcome Studies, to be Considered in Decision-Making between Root Canal Treatment and Implant

The following factors have to be considered or clarified in connection with primary root canal treatment, endodontic retreatment, and endodontic surgery:

♦ expected degrees of difficulty of the treatment

♦ expertise of the clinician (referral to a specialist possible/advised?)

♦ eventuality of peri- or postendodontic complications, with possible impairment

♦ willingness of the patient to endure time-consuming and cost-intensive treatment in order to save teeth.

Factors that have to be taken into account or clarified when the replacement of endodontically treated (compromised) teeth by implants is considered include:

♦ Is the implant a possibility in that specific location?

♦ What is the degree of difficulty, possibly additional effort necessary (e.g. augmentation); is referral to a specialist possible/advised?

♦ Is the esthetic challenge manageable (area)?

♦ Does the patient have a medical history related to periodontitis?

♦ Are there other diseases, medications, habits (smoking) commonly related to poor survival rates of implants?

♦ Does the patient have the willingness and capability to get the necessary post-operative care?

♦ Does the patient have the willingness and capability to pay for the treatment, which is often (in comparison with root canal treatment) expensive, and also for any costs arising from possibly technical complications and for the necessary professional routine post-operative care of implants?

## Conclusions

The author has both a professional and an emotional affinity with conservative dentistry. However, all new developments in dentistry are welcomed, and this explicitly includes implants if they help to increase the quality of life of patients. There are several issues that lead to reluctance regarding the replacement of teeth with implants: peri-implantitis (with still unclear implications to general health), which in certain situations will make a series of additional treatments essential (Fig 7-3); the necessity for technical adjustments in many patients; and the necessity for post-operative care of implants in all patients. This reluctance is particularly relevant in light of the (open) question as to how the latter shall be achieved in the elderly and in patients well advanced in years (and whether the resulting financial burdens can still be met).

While the best strategies for selecting one treatment approach over another (such as root canal treatment versus implant) still have to be identified, responsible decision-making is possible now if the clinician- and patient-specific parameters discussed above are implemented.

## References

1. Lang NP. Wie wertvoll sind unsere Zähne? Parodontologie 2006;17:3–4.

2. Matosian GS. Treatment planning for the future: endodontics, post and core, and periodontal surgery – or an implant? J Calif Dent Assoc 2003;31:323–325.

3. Ruskin JD, Morton D, Krayazgan B, Amir J. Failed root canals: the case for extraction and immediate implant placement. J Oral Maxillofac Surg 2005;63:829–831.

4. Spångberg LSW. To implant or not to implant: that is the question. Oral Surg Oral Med Oral Pathol Oral Radiol Endod 2006;101:695–696.

5. Sanderink RBA, Saxer UP, Erne P. Implantate, Implantate, Implantate. Quintessenz 2008;59:217.

6. Kirchhoff W. Knochenprotektion, Strukturerhalt und medizinischer Vorteil von unversehrter Zahnhartsubstanz bei Implantattherapien? Marketing und medizinische Realitäten. ZMK 2007;23:573–579.

7. Heffernan M, Martin W, Morton D. Prognosis of endodontically treated teeth? Quintessence Int 2003;34:558–560.

8. Glickman GN. Editorial comment to Heffernan M, Martin W, Morton D, Prognosis of endodontically treated teeth? Quintessence Int 2003;34:560–561.

9. Trope M. Implant or root canal therapy: an endodontist's view. J Esthet Restor Dent 2005;17:139–140.

10. Balson M. The growing impact of implantology on endodontics. J Endod 2005;31:479–480.

11. American Association of Endodontists. AAE-Communiqué. The AAE monitors emergency trends from the field of implantology. Chigago, IL: American Association of Endodontists, May/June 2003.

12. American Association of Endodontists. AAE-Communiqué. AAE and Foundation approve definition of endodontic outcomes. Chigago, IL: American Association of Endodontists, Aug/Sept 2005.

13. Bader HJ. Treatment planning for implants versus root canal therapy: a contemporary dilemma. Implant Dent 2002;11:217–223.

14. Sjögren U, Hägglund B, Sundqvist G, Wing K. Factors affecting the long-term results of endodontic treatment. J Endod 1990;16:498–504.

15. Friedman S. Prognosis of initial endodontic therapy. Endod Topics 2002;2, 59–88.

16. Ng Y-L, Mann V, Rahbaran S, Lewsey J, Gulabivala K. Outcome of primary root canal treatment: systematic review of the literature, Part 1. Effects of study characteristics on probability of success. Int Endod J 2007;40:921–939.

17. Ng Y-L, Mann V, Rahbaran S, Lewsey J, Gulabivala K. Outcome of primary root canal treatment: systematic review of the literature, Part 2. Influence of clinical factors. Int Endod J 2008;41:6–31.

18. Cohn SA. Treatment choices for negative outcomes with non-surgical root canal treatment vs. surgical treatment vs. implants. Endod Topics 2005;11, 4–24.

19. Esposito M, Coulthard P, Worthington HV, Jokstad A. Quality assessment of randomized controlled trials of oral implants. Int J Oral Maxillofac Implants 2001;16:783–792.

20. Roos-Jansåker A-M, Lindahl C, Revert H, Revert S. Nine- to fourteen-year follow-up of implant treatment. Part I: implant loss and associations to various factors. J Clin Periodontol 2006;33:283–289.

21. Roos-Jansåker A-M, Lindahl C, Revert H, Revert S. Nine- to fourteen-year follow-up of implant treatment. Part II: presence of peri-implant lesions. J Clin Periodontol 2006;33:290–295.

22. Pjetursson BE, Tan K, Lang NP, Brägger U, Egger M, Zwahlen M. A systematic review of the survival and complication rates of fixed partial dentures (FPDs) after an observation period of at least 5 years. I. Implant-supported FPDs. Clin Oral Implants Res 2004:15;625–642.

23. Berglundh T, Persson L, Klinge B. A systematic review of the incidence of biological and technical complications in implant dentistry reported in prospective longitudinal studies of at least 5 years. J Clin Periodontol 2002;29(Suppl 3):197–212.

24. Outcome of implant therapy in relation to experienced loss of periodontal bone support. A retrospective 5-year study. Clin Oral Implants Res 2002:13;488–494.

25. Roos-Jansåker A-M, Revert H, Lindahl C, Revert S. Nine- to fourteen-year follow-up of implant treatment. Part III: factors associated with peri-implant lesions. J Clin Periodontol 2006;33:296–301.

26. Al-Zahrani MS. Implant therapy in aggressive periodontitis patients: a systematic review and clinicial implications. Quintessence Int 2008;39:211–215.

27. Fritz UB, Kerschbaum T. Langzeitverweildauer wurzelkanalgefüllter Zähne. Dtsch Zahnärztl Z 1999;54:262.

28. Alley BS, Kitchens GG, Alley LW, Eleazer PD. A comparison of survival of teeth following endodontic treatment performed by general dentists or by specialists. Oral Surg Oral Med Oral Pathol Oral Radiol Endod 2004;98:115–118.

29. Salehrabi E, Rotstein I. Endodontic treatment outcomes in a large patient population in the USA: an epidemiological study. J Endod 2004;30:846–850.

30. European Society of Endodontology. Quality guidelines for endodontic treatment: consensus report of the European Society of Endodontology. Int Endod J 2006;39:921–930.

# Tooth- or Implant-Supported Reconstructions in the Patient Susceptible to Periodontitis?

**8**

Giovanni E. Salvi and Søren Jepsen

## What does Susceptibility to Periodontitis Mean?

Periodontitis is characterized by inflammation of the periodontal tissues and subsequent destruction of the tooth-supporting structures, eventually leading to loss of the affected teeth.[1-3] Lesions in the periodontal tissues are clinically identified and diagnosed based on the presence of bleeding following probing of the periodontal pockets and by the reduced tissue resistance to pocket probing. These clinical signs ultimately develop as a result of tissue response to the chronic presence of a subgingival biofilm, leading to an immune inflammatory lesion, characterized by an abundance of polymorphonuclear leukocytes, immune cells, inflammatory mediators and cytokines, and loss of collagen in the gingival connective tissue adjacent to the root surface.[4-6] Although bacteria are necessary for periodontal disease to occur, a susceptible host is also needed. Individual susceptibility is assumed to be linked to the severity of gingival inflammation in response to bacterial plaque formation.[7]

While pathogenic microflora in the periodontal biofilm is the widely accepted cause of periodontitis, several genetic and environmental (i.e. smoking) and systemic (i.e. diabetes mellitus) risk factors have been identified with effects on the onset and progression of periodontitis.[8,9] Genetic variations in or near genes for cytokines could affect the systemic inflammatory response in patients with periodontitis and have been explored using a candidate gene approach as risk factors for periodontitis.[10] While several genetic polymorphisms have been associated with periodontal disease, at present there is insufficient evidence to support the use of genetic tests for risk assessment or to predict treatment response.[11] Furthermore, it has been convincingly demonstrated that smokers are much more likely than non-smokers to develop periodontitis and that smoking impairs the response of patients to periodontal treatment. In addition, the systemic effects of tobacco smoking on the periodontium are well understood.[12-14] Results from cross-sectional and prospective cohort studies have indicated that patients with type 1 diabetes and adults with type 2 diabetes have more severe periodontal disease than individuals without diabetes.[15,16] Although patients with well-controlled diabetes do not seem to be at increased risk of periodontal disease compared with people without diabetes, poorly controlled diabetes is clearly a risk factor for increased severity of periodontitis.[17]

## Maintenance of the Natural Dentition: Evidence for Successful Long-Term Periodontal Therapy

The main goal in the treatment of patients with periodontitis is to establish adequate infection control by reducing the bacterial infectious burden below the individual level for disease. The achievement of this goal involves several treatment phases.

1. *The establishment of optimal self-performed plaque control.* Oral hygiene instructions, motivation, and elimination of plaque retentive factors are prerequisites not only for disease prevention but also for successful treatment outcomes.[18–24]

2. *The suppression of the subgingival bacterial burden around periodontally affected teeth.* This can be can be successfully accomplished through non-surgical procedures.[25,26] Subgingival instrumentation of the root surfaces may involve manual and machine-driven debridement,[27,28] the use of lasers,[29,30] and the adjunctive use of local or systemic antimicrobial agents.[31–33] No additional benefit has been demonstrated for full-mouth treatment concepts.[34] In fact, similar short- and long-term effects on the subgingival biofilm were observed for quadrant scaling as for full-mouth scaling.[35]

3. *Access to the site of periodontal infection by a surgical approach.* This enables the proper instrumentation of deep sites and the correction of anatomical unfavorable features.[36] Access flap surgery can be more beneficial than scaling and root planing for probing pocket depth reduction in sites with deep pockets.[37] A surgical access is also required for regenerative procedures aiming at the (partial) reconstruction of the lost attachment apparatus. The clinical efficacy of periodontal regenerative procedures has been extensively evaluated in systematic reviews based on a large number of randomized controlled trials, mainly in intraosseous defects.[38–42] Whether combination procedures can further enhance regenerative outcomes

remains controversial.[42,43] Improvements for class II furcations following regenerative procedures have also been reported, but the evidence is more limited.[44,45] Even though results for regenerative procedures can be maintained on a long-term basis, at present there are only limited data on the long-term effects of periodontal regeneration on tooth survival.[46]

4. *Prevention of periodontal disease recurrence by regular monitoring and supportive periodontal therapy.*[47,48] Without continuous risk assessment and regular maintenance care, patients with previous disease predisposition are likely to experience further attachment loss.[47,49–51] It is well established that self-performed plaque control combined with compliance in maintenance care following active periodontal therapy represents an effective strategy for controlling gingivitis and periodontitis and, thus, limiting tooth mortality over extended periods of time.[48,52] Studies on patients treated for advanced periodontal disease and subsequently involved in a regular program of supportive periodontal therapy indicate an average incidence of tooth loss during a 10-year period of between 2 and 5%.[53–57] If teeth affected by periodontitis are treated adequately, then their prognosis appears to be equally as good as that for implant survival (see below). In addition, there is growing evidence that longitudinal bone loss at implants is positively associated with susceptibility for peridodontitis.

## Case Report

The clinical, periodontal, and radiographic characteristics of a 67-year-old patient diagnosed with advanced generalized chronic periodontitis with furcation involvement are presented in Figs 8-1 to 8-6. The patient wished to receive a comprehensive dental treatment including the use of fixed dental prostheses (FDPs) in both the mandible and the maxilla. After successful completion of non-surgical and surgical periodontal therapy, a prosthetic rehabilitation of the maxilla and the mandible involving the use of titanium oral implants was performed. Figures 8-7 to 8-11 illustrate the periodontal, peri-implant, and radiographic conditions after incorporation of tooth-, implant-, and tooth–implant-supported FDPs.

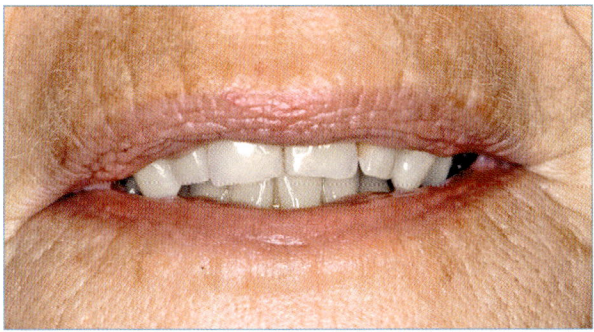

Fig 8-1 Extraoral front view of a 67-year-old patient before therapy.

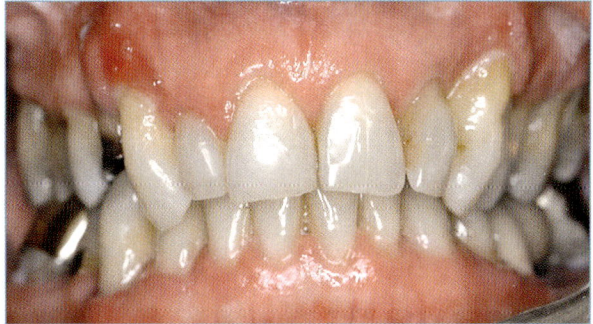

Fig 8-2 Intraoral front view at the initial examination. Teeth 13 and 23 present with pronounced buccal gingival recessions.

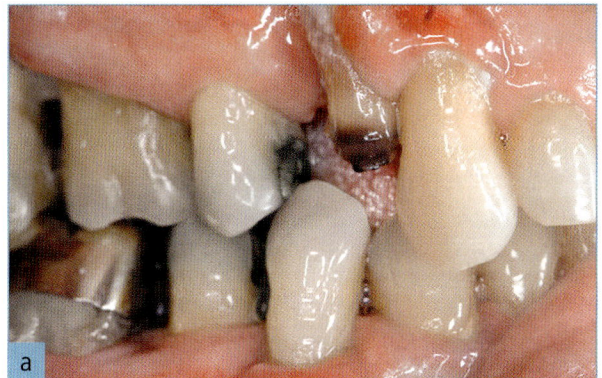

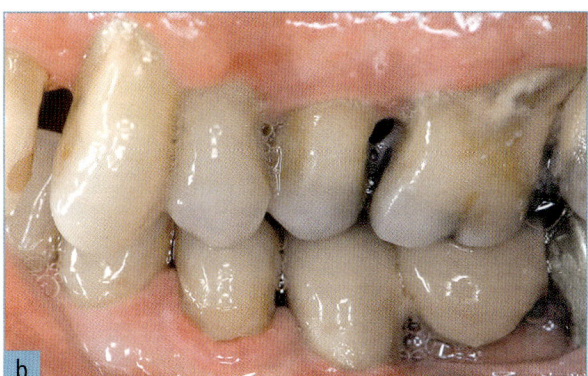

Fig 8-3a–b Lateral intraoral views at the initial examination. The marginal gingiva is inflamed around every tooth. Extensive plaque and calculus deposits are visible.

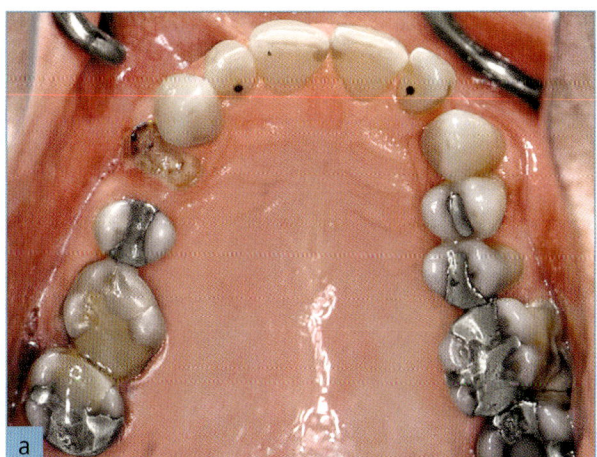

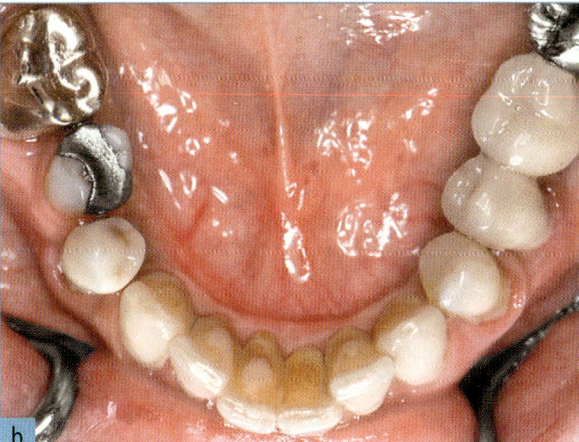

Fig 8-4a–b Occlusal views of the maxilla (a) and mandible (b) at the initial examination.

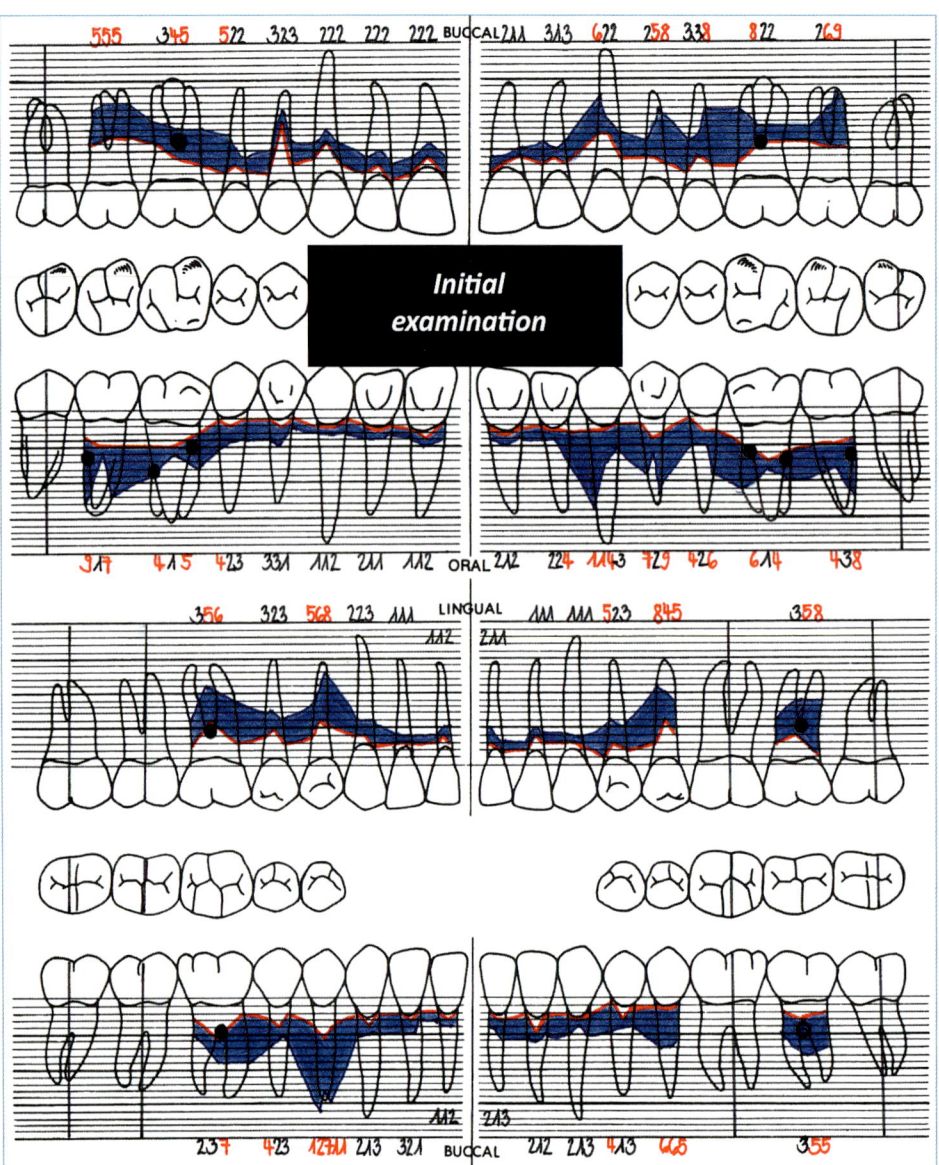

**Fig 8-5** Periodontal chart at the initial examination. The contour of the marginal gingiva is depicted by the red line. Pocket probing depths of ≤ 3 mm are marked in black and of ≥ 4 mm in red. Pocket probing depths up to 12 mm and gingival recessions up to 8 mm could be assessed.

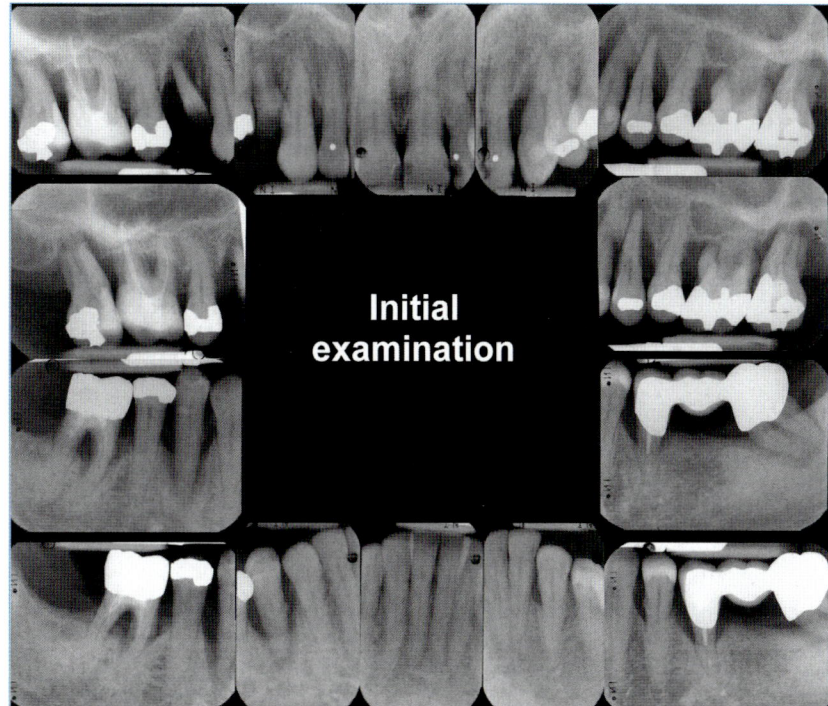

**Fig 8-6** Full-mouth intraoral periapical radiographs at the initial examination. A generalized horizontal bone loss with angular bony defects extending up to the apex is visible.

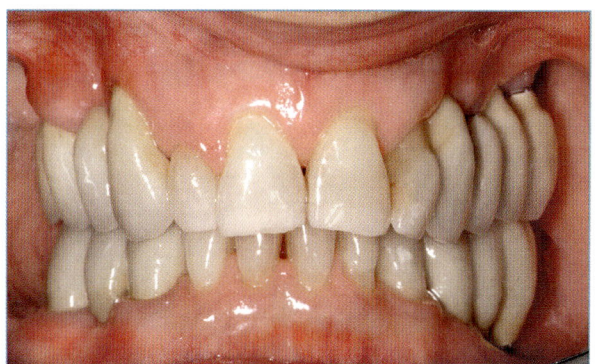

**Fig 8-7** Intraoral frontal view at the final examination after delivery of the fixed dental prostheses.

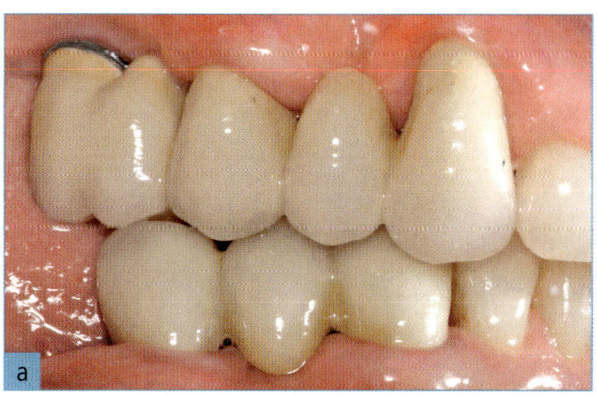
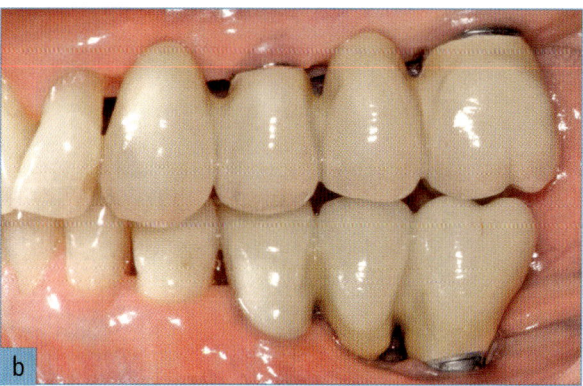

**Fig 8-8a–b** Lateral intraoral views at the final examination.

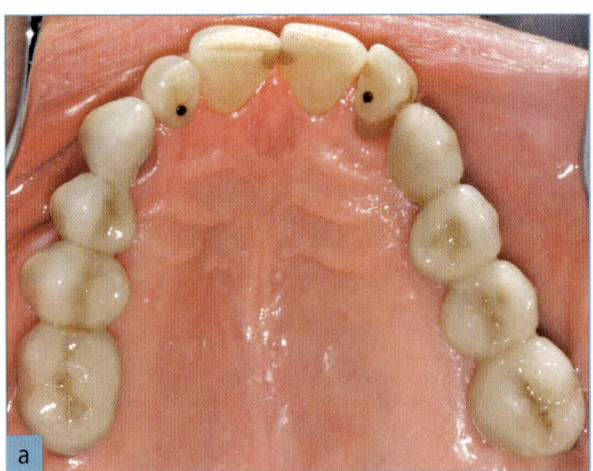
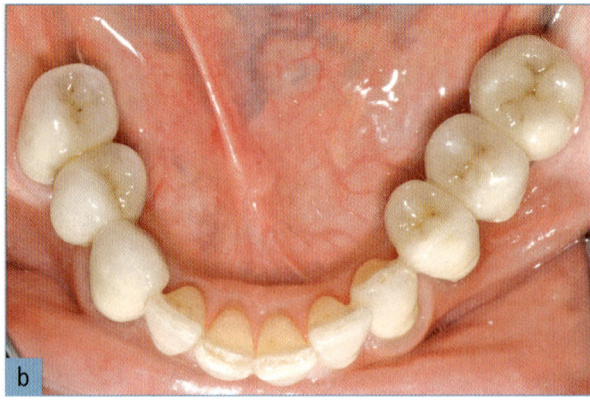

**Fig 8-9a–b** Occlusal views of the fixed dental prostheses at the final examination.

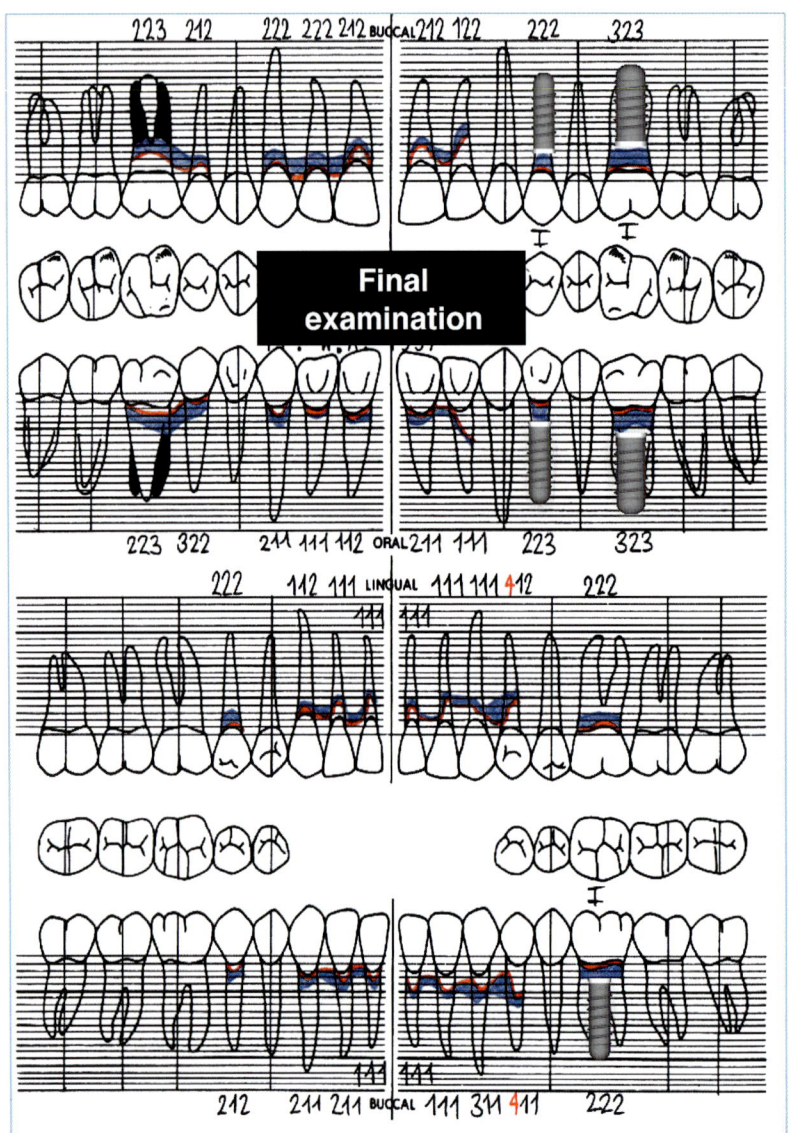

**Fig 8-10** Periodontal chart at the final examination. No pocket probing depths of ≥ 5 mm were recorded around natural teeth and oral implants.

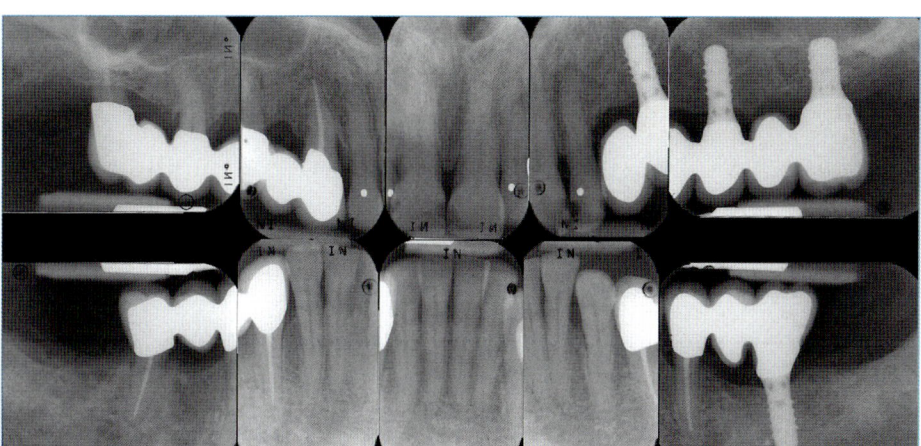

**Fig 8-11** Full-mouth intraoral periapical radiographs at the final examination showing the crestal bone levels around tooth-, implant-, and combined tooth–implant-supported fixed dental prostheses.

# To Extract or Not to Extract:

## Evidence for Tooth- or Implant-Supported Reconstructions in the Patient Susceptible to Periodontitis

The influence of gingival health or inflammation on tooth mortality is evident from analysis of data derived in a longitudinal study of the initiation and progression of periodontal disease that was conducted over a 26-year observation period in Oslo, Norway.[58] Teeth always surrounded with healthy gingival tissues had a 46 times lower risk of being lost than teeth with gingival tissues that always bled on probing.[58] In other words, teeth surrounded by gingival tissues that never bled on probing throughout the observation period displayed a cumulative survival rate of 99.5% at a tooth age of 51 years.[58]

In patients suffering from severe periodontal disease, only a few teeth may survive for use as abutments for prosthetic reconstructions. In order to restore periodontal health and function, a comprehensive treatment plan encompassing non-surgical and surgical periodontal therapy as well as prosthetic rehabilitation is needed.[59] The aim of a recently published systematic review was to assess survival rates and incidence of biological and technical complications of FDPs using abutment teeth with severely reduced, but healthy, periodontal tissue support.[60] The review showed that

teeth could be used as abutments for cross-arch FDPs with or without cantilevers despite advanced loss of periodontal tissue support. If indicated, hemisections or root amputations were performed for furcation-involved molars used as abutments, in order to eliminate plaque-retentive areas and facilitate self-performed plaque control. A high survival rate (93%) of furcation-involved and root-resected molars used as abutment teeth for FDPs was reported after an observation period of 10 years.[61] The estimated 10-year survival rate of 92.9% of FDPs in this systematic review[60] compares favorably with those of conventional FDPs (89.1%),[62] of combined tooth-implant-supported FDPs (82.1%),[63] and of FDPs with cantilevers (81.8%)[64] incorporated in patients without severely periodontally compromised dentitions.

It should be emphasized that oral rehabilitation of such patients with severe periodontal disease was carried out in phases, including non-surgical and surgical therapy followed by long-term maintenance care.[65]

Outcomes of clinical studies with at least 5 years of follow-up reporting on the use of oral implants for the prosthetic rehabilitation of partially edentulous patients susceptible to periodontitis are steadily increasing.[66–80] Collectively, findings from these studies in periodontally compromised patients demonstrated that the survival and success rates of implants and their suprastructures were not superior to those of natural abutment teeth and their reconstructions in patients who were treated for their periodontal disease. Hence, it can be concluded that the long-term prognosis of implants in periodontitis-susceptible patients is not any more favorable than that of teeth with healthy but reduced periodontal tissue support.

## Increased Risk for Failures and Complications Around Implants in the Patient Susceptible to Periodontitis

Periodontitis and peri-implantitis have been associated with the presence of key microbial pathogens. The reasons for increased susceptibility to biological complications around implants in patients with a history of chronic or aggressive periodontitis compared with those without such a predisposition may be related either to the biofilm accumulation in partially edentulous dentitions or to the host response to the bacterial challenge. Findings from several studies have showed that, in partially edentulous patients treated for periodontal disease and enrolled in a regular maintenance care program, the remaining dentition acts as a reservoir for the submucosal bacterial colonization around implants.[81–86]

Evidence presented in a recent systematic review[87] revealed that patients treated for periodontitis may experience more implant failures and biological complications than patients without periodontitis. Patient-based analysis from two long-term case series[72,76] included in this systematic review[87] demonstrated a statistically significant lower survival rate of implants installed in patients with treated periodontitis than in those without periodontitis. Similarly, lower implant success rates were reported for patients with treated periodontitis compared with those without periodontitis.[66,73,75] Finally, implant-based analysis showed a statistically significant higher incidence of peri-implantitis in patients with a history of periodontitis compared with those without periodontitis.[70,78] It should, however, be kept in mind that considerable differences in the prevalence of peri-implant lesions exist when comparing the long-term outcomes of patients enrolled[74] or not enrolled[77] in a supportive periodontal therapy program.

## Conclusion

Despite lower survival and success rates for such implants, the use of oral implants for the prosthetic rehabilitation of partially edentulous patients with a history of periodontitis can be recommended, provided that a regular supportive periodontal therapy program is implemented.

## Acknowledgement

We kindly thank Dr. B. Röthlisberger, Interlaken, Switzerland, for the clinical case documentation.

## References

1. Kinane DF. Causation and pathogenesis of periodontal disease. Periodontology 2001;25:8–20.
2. Page RC, Kornman KS. The pathogenesis of human periodontitis: an introduction. Periodontology 1997;14:9–11.
3. Pihlström BL. Periodontal diseases. Lancet 2005;19:1809–1820.
4. Page RC, Offenbacher S, Schroeder HE, Seymour GJ, Kornman KS. Advances in the pathogenesis of periodontitis: summary of developments, clinical implications and future directions. Periodontology 1997;14:216–248.
5. Madianos PN, Bobetsis YA, Kinane DF. Generation of inflammatory stimuli: how bacteria set up inflammatory responses in the gingiva. J Clin Periodontol 2005;32:57–71.
6. Nanci A, Bosshardt DD. Structure of periodontal tissues in health and disease. Periodontology 2006;40:11–28.
7. Trombelli L. Susceptibility to gingivitis: a way to predict periodontal disease? Oral Health Prev Dent 2004;2:265–269.
8. Kinane DF, Hart TC. Genes and gene polymorphisms associated with periodontal disease. Crit Rev Oral Biol Med 2003;14:430–449.
9. Kinane DF, Peterson M, Stathopoulou PG. Environmental and other modifying factors of the periodontal diseases. Periodontology 2006;40:107–119.
10. Loos BG, John RP, Laine ML. Identification of genetic risk factors for periodontitis and possible mechanisms of action. J Clin Periodontol 2005;32:159–179.

11. Shapira L, Wilensky A, Kinane DF. Effect of genetic variability on the inflammatory response to periodontal infection. J Clin Periodontol 2005;32:72–86.

12. Kinane DF, Chestnutt IG. Smoking and periodontal disease. Crit Rev Oral Biol Med 2000;11:356–365.

13. Palmer RM, Wilson RF, Hasan AS, Scott DA. Mechanisms of action of environmental factors: tobacco smoking. J Clin Periodontol 2005;32:180–195.

14. Johnson GK, Guthmiller JM. The impact of cigarette smoking on periodontal disease and treatment. Periodontology 2007;44:178–194.

15. Löe H. Periodontal disease. The sixth complication of diabetes mellitus. Diabetes Care 1993;16:329–334.

16. Taylor GW. Bidirectional interrelationships between diabetes and periodontal diseases: an epidemiologic perspective. Ann Periodontol 2001;6:99–112.

17. Salvi GE, Carollo-Bittel B, Lang NP. Effects of diabetes on periodontal and periimplant conditions. Update on association and risks. J Clin Periodontol 2008;35:(suppl 8): 398-409.

18. Axelsson P, Lindhe J. Effect of controlled oral hygiene procedures on caries and periodontal disease in adults. Results after 6 years. J Clin Periodontol 1981;8:239–248.

19. Dahlen G, Manji F, Baelum V, Fejerskov O. Putative periodontopathogens in 'diseased' and 'non-diseased' persons exhibiting poor oral hygiene. J Clin Periodontol 1992;19:35–42.

20. Katsanoulas T, Renee I, Attström R. The effect of supragingival plaque control on the composition of the subgingival flora in periodontal pockets. J Clin Periodontol 1992;19:760–765.

21. Magnusson I, Lindhe J, Yoneyama T, Liljenberg B. Recolonization of a subgingival microbiota following scaling in deep pockets. J Clin Periodontol 1984;11:193–207.

22. Needleman I, Suvan J, Moles DR, Pimlott J. A systematic review of professional mechanical plaque removal for prevention of periodontal diseases. J Clin Periodontol 2005;32:229–282.

23. van der Weijden GA, Hioe KP. A systematic review of the effectiveness of self-performed mechanical plaque removal in adults with gingivitis using a manual toothbrush. J Clin Periodontol 2005;32:214–228.

24. Westfelt E, Rylander H, Dahlén G, Lindhe J. The effect of supragingival plaque control on the progression of advanced periodontal disease. J Clin Periodontol 1998;25:536–541.

25. van der Weijden GA, Timmerman MF. A systematic review on the clinical efficacy of subgingival debridement in the treatment of chronic periodontitis. J Clin Periodontol 2002;29:55–71; discussion 90–91.

26. Hallmon WW, Rees TD. Local anti-infective therapy: mechanical and physical approaches. A systematic review. Ann Periodontol 2003;8:99–114.

27. Tunkel J, Heinecke A, Flemmig TF. A systematic review of efficacy of machine-driven and manual subgingival debridement in the treatment of chronic periodontitis. J Clin Periodontol 2002;29:72–81.

28. Walmsley AD, Lea SC, Landini G, Moses AJ. Advances in power driven pocket/root instrumentation. J Clin Periodontol 2008;35:(suppl 8): 22–38.

29. Krause F, Braun A, Brede O, Eberhard J, Frentzen M, Jepsen S. Evaluation of selective calculus removal by a fluorescence feedback-controlled Er:YAG laser in vitro. J Clin Periodontol 2007;34:66–71.

30. Schwarz F, Aoki A, Becker J, Sculean A. Laser application in non-surgical periodontal therapy. A systematic review. J Clin Periodontol 2008;35:(suppl 8): 29-44

31. Herrera D, Sanz M, Jepsen S, Needeman I, Roldan S. A systematic review on the effect of systemic antimicrobials as an adjunct to scaling and root planing in periodontitis patients. J Clin Periodontol 2002;29(Suppl 3):136–159.

32. Haffajee AD, Socransky SS, Gunsolley JC. Systematic anti-infective periodontal therapy. A systematic review. Ann Periodontol 2003;8:115–181.

33. Herrera D, Alonso B, Leon R, Roldan S, Sanz M. Antimicrobial therapy in periodontitis: the use of systemic antimicrobials against the subgingival biofilm. J Clin Periodontol 2008;35:(suppl 8): 45-66.

34. Eberhard J, Jervøe-Storm PM, Needleman I, Worthington H, Jepsen S. Full-mouth treatment concepts for chronic periodontitis: a systematic review. J Clin Periodontol 2008;35:591–604.

35. Jervøe-Storm PM, AlAhdab H, Semaan E, Fimmers R, Jepsen S. Microbiological outcomes of quadrant versus full-mouth root planing as monitored by real-time PCR. J Clin Periodontol 2007;34:156 163.

36. DeSanctis M, Murphy KG. The role of resective periodontal surgery in the treatment of furcation defects. Periodontology 2000;22:154–168.

37. Heitz-Mayfield LJ, Trombelli L, Heitz F, Needleman I, Moles D. A systematic review of the effect of surgical debridement vs non-surgical debridement for the treatment of chronic periodontitis. J Clin Periodontol 2002;29:92–102; discussion 160–162.

38. Murphy KG, Gunsolley JC. Guided tissue regeneration for the treatment of periodontal intrabony and furcation defects. A systematic review. Ann Periodontol 2003;8:266–302.

39. Needleman I, Tucker R, Giedrys-Leepser E, Worthington H. Guided tissue regeneration for periodontal intrabony defects: a Cochrane Systematic Review. Periodontology 2000;37:106–123.

40. Reynolds MA, Aichelmann-Reidy ME, Branch-Mays GL, Gunsolley JC. The efficacy of bone replacement grafts in the treatment of periodontal osseous defects. A systematic review. Ann Periodontol 2003;8:227–265.

41. Trombelli L, Heitz-Mayfield LJ, Needleman I, Moles D, Scabbia A. A systematic review of graft materials and biological agents for periodontal intraosseous defects. J Clin Periodontol 2002;29:117–135.

42. Trombelli L, Farina R. Clinical outcomes with bioactive agents alone or in combination with grafting or guided tissue regeneration. J Clin Periodontol 2008;35:(suppl 8):117-135.

43. Jepsen S, Topoll H, Rengers H, Heinz B, Teich M, Hoffmann T, et al. Clinical outcomes after treatment of intra-bony defects with an EMD/synthetic bone graft or EMD alone: a multicentre randomized-controlled clinical trial. J Clin Periodontol 2008;35:420–428.

44. Jepsen S, Eberhard J, Herrera D, Needleman I. A systematic review of guided tissue regeneration for periodontal furcation defects. What is the effect of guided tissue regeneration compared with surgical debridement in the treatment of furcation defects? J Clin Periodontol 2002;29(Suppl 3):103–116; discussion 160–162.

45. Jepsen S, Heinz B, Jepsen K, Arjomand M, Hoffmann T, Richter S, et al. A randomized clinical trial comparing enamel matrix derivative and membrane treatment of buccal class II furcation involvement in mandibular molars. Part I: Study design and results for primary outcomes. J Periodontol 2004;75:1150–1160.

46. Cortellini P, Tonetti MS. Long-term tooth survival following regenerative treatment of intrabony defects. J Periodontol 2004;75:672–678.

47. Axelsson P, Lindhe J. The significance of maintenance care in the treatment of periodontal disease. J Clin Periodontol 1981;8:281–294.

48. Axelsson P, Nyström B, Lindhe J. The long-term effect of a plaque control program on tooth mortality, caries and periodontal disease in adults. Results after 30 years of maintenance. J Clin Periodontol 2004;31:749–757.

49. Becker W, Becker BE, Berg LE. Periodontal treatment without mainte- nance. A retrospective study in 44 patients. J Periodontol 1984;55:505–509.

50. Cortellini P, Pini-Prato G, Tonetti M. Periodontal regeneration of human infrabony defects (V). Effect of oral hygiene on long-term sta- bility. J Clin Periodontol 1994;21:606–610.

51. Cortellini P, Paolo G, Prato P, Tonetti MS. Long-term stability of clini- cal attachment following guided tissue regeneration and conventional therapy. J Clin Periodontol 1996;23:106–111.

52. Fardal Ø, Johannessen AC, Linden GJ. Tooth loss during maintenance following periodontal treatment in a periodontal practice in Norway. J Clin Periodontol 2004;31:550–555.

53. Lindhe J, Nyman S. Long-term maintenance of patients treated for advanced periodontal disease. J Clin Periodontol 1984;11:504–514.

54. Yi SW, Ericsson I, Carlsson GE, Wenström JL. Long-term follow-up of cross-arch fixed partial dentures in patients with advanced periodontal destruction. Evaluation of the supporting tissues. Acta Odontol Scand 1995;53:242–248.

55. Rosling B, Serino G, Hellström MK, Socransky SS, Lindhe J. Longitudinal periodontal tissue alterations during supportive therapy. Findings from subjects with normal and high susceptibility to peri- odontal disease. J Clin Periodontol 2001;28:241–249.

56. König J, Plagmann H, Rühling A, Kocher T. Tooth loss and pocket probing depths in compliant periodontally treated patients: a retrospec- tive analysis. J Clin Periodontol 2002;29:1092–1100.

57. Karoussis IK, Müller S, Salvi GE, Heitz-Mayfield LJ, Brägger U, Lang NP. Association between periodontal and peri-implant conditions: a 10-year prospective study. Clin Oral Implants Res 2004;15:1–7.

58. Schätzle M, Löe H, Lang NP, Bürgin W, Ånerud Å, Boysen H. The clinical course of chronic periodontitis. IV. Gingival inflammation as a risk factor in tooth mortality. J Clin Periodontol 2004;31:1122–1127.

59. Nyman S, Lindhe J. Prosthetic rehabilitation of patients with advanced periodontal disease. J Clin Periodontol 1976;3:135–147.

60. Lulic M, Brägger U, Lang NP, Zwahlen M, Salvi GE. Ante's (1926) law revisited: A systematic review on survival rates and complications of fixed dental prostheses (FDPs) on severely reduced periodontal tissue support. Clin Oral Implants Res 2007;18: 63–72.

61. Carnevale G, Pontoriero R, di Febo G. Long-term effects of root-resec- tive therapy in furcation involved molars. A 10-year longitudinal study. J Clin Periodontol 1998;25:209–214.

62. Tan K, Pjetursson BE, Lang NP, Chan ESY. A systematic review of the survival and complication rates of fixed partial dentures (FPDs) after an observation period of at least 5 years. III. Conventional FPDs. Clin Oral Implants Res 2004;15:654–666.

63. Lang NP, Pjetursson BE, Tan K, Brägger U, Egger M, Zwahlen M. A systematic review of the survival and complication rates of fixed partial dentures (FPDs) after an observation period of at least 5 years. II. Combined tooth-implant-supported FPDs. Clin Oral Implants Res 2004;15:643–653.

64. Pjetursson BE, Tan K, Lang NP, Brägger U, Egger M, Zwahlen M. A systematic review of the survival and complication rates of fixed partial dentures (FPDs) after an observation period of at least 5 years. IV. Cantilever or extension FPDs. Clin Oral Implants Res 2004;15:667–676.

65. Lindhe J, Nyman S. The effect of plaque control and surgical pocket elimination on the establishment and maintenance of periodontal health. A longitudinal study of periodontal therapy in cases of advanced disease. J Clin Periodontol 1975;2:67–79.

66. Brocard D, Barthet P, Baysse E, Duffort JF, Eller P, Justumus P, et al. A multicenter report on 1022 consecutively placed ITI implants: a 7-year longitudinal study. Int J Oral Maxillofac Implants 2000;15:691–700.

67. Fugazzotto PA. A comparison of the success of root resected molars and molar position implants in function in a private practice: results of up to 15-plus years. J Clin Periodontol 2001;72:1113–1123.

68. Hardt CR, Gröndahl K, Lekholm U, Wennström JL. Outcome of implant therapy in relation to experienced loss of periodontal bone support: a retrospective 5-year study. Clin Oral Implants Res 2002;13:488–494.

69. Leonhardt Å, Gröndahl K, Bergström C, Lekholm U. Long-term fol- low-up of osseointegrated titanium implants using clinical, radiograph- ic and microbiological parameters. Clin Oral Implants Res 2002;13:127–132.

70. Karoussis IK, Salvi GE, Heitz-Mayfield LJA, Brägger U, Hämmerle CHF, Lang N. Long-term implant prognosis in patients with and with- out a history of chronic periodontitis: a 10-year prospective cohort study of the ITI® Dental Implant System. Clin Oral Implants Res 2003;14:329–339.

71. Baelum V, Ellegaard B. Implant survival in periodontally compromised patients. J Clin Periodontol 2004;75:1404–1412.

72. Evian CI, Emling R, Rosenberg ES, Waasdorp JA, Halpern W, Shah S, et al. Retrospective analysis of implant survival and the influence of periodontal disease and immediate placement on long-term results. Int J Oral Maxillofac Implants 2004;19:393–398.

73. Rosenberg ES, Cho SC, Elian N, Jalbout ZN, Froum S, Evian CI. A comparison of characteristics of implant failure and survival in peri- odontally compromised and periodontally healthy patients: a clinical report. Int J Oral Maxillofac Implants 2004;19:873–879.

74. Wennström JL, Ekestubbe A, Gröndahl K, Karlsson S, Lindhe J. Oral rehabilitation with implant-supported fixed partial dentures in peri- odontitis-susceptible subjects. A 5-year prospective study. J Clin Periodontol 2004;31:713–724.

75. Mengel R, Flores-de-Jacoby L. Implants in patients treated for general- ized aggressive and chronic periodontitis: a 3-year prospective longitu- dinal study. J Clin Periodontol 2005;76:534–543.

76. Roos-Jansåker AM, Lindahl C, Renvert H, Renvert S. Nine- to four- teen-year follow-up of implant treatment. Part I: Implant loss and asso- ciations to various factors. J Clin Periodontol 2006;33:283–289.

77. Roos-Jansåker AM, Lindahl C, Renvert H, Renvert S. Nine- to four- teen-year follow-up of implant treatment. Part II: Presence of peri- implant lesions. J Clin Periodontol 2006;33:290–295.

78. Roos-Jansåker AM, Renvert H, Lindahl C, Renvert S. Nine- to four- teen-year follow-up of implant treatment. Part III: factors associated with peri-implant lesions. J Clin Periodontol 2006;33:296–301.

79. Mengel R, Behle M, Flores-de-Jacoby L. Osseointegrated implants in subjects treated for generalized aggressive periodontitis: 10-year results of a prospective, long-term cohort study. J Clin Periodontol 2007;78:2229–2237.

80. Fardal Ø, Linden GJ. Tooth loss and implant outcomes in patients refractory to treatment in a periodontal practice. J Clin Periodontol 2008;35:733–738.

81. Leonhardt Å, Adolfsson B, Lekholm U, Wikström M, Dahlén G. A longitudinal microbiological study on osseointegrated titanium implants in partially edentulous patients. Clin Oral Implants Res 1993;4:113–120.

82. Mombelli A, Marxer M, Gaberthüel T, Grunder U, Lang NP. The microbiota of osseointegrated implants in patients with a history of periodontal disease. J Clin Periodontol 1995;22:124–130.

83. de Boever AL, de Boever, JA. Early colonization of non-submerged dental implants in patients with a history of advanced aggressive periodontitis. Clin Oral Implants Res 2006;17:8–17.

84. Quirynen M, Vogels R, Peters W, van Steenberghe D, Naert I, Haffajee AD. Dynamics of initial subgingival colonization of 'pristine' peri-implant pockets. Clin Oral Implants Res 2006;17:25–37.

85. Fürst MM, Salvi GE, Lang NP, Persson GR. Bacterial colonization immediately after installation on oral titanium implants. Clin Oral Implants Res 2007;18:501–508.

86. Salvi GE, Fürst MM, Lang NP, Persson GR. One-year bacterial colonization patterns of Staphylococcus aureus and other bacteria at implants and adjacent teeth. Clin Oral Implants Res 2008;19:242–248.

87. Ong CC, Ivanovski S, Needleman I, Retzepi M, Moles DR, Tonetti MS, et al. Systematic review of implant outcomes in treated periodontitis subjects. J Clin Periodontol 2008;35:38–62.

# The Missing Tooth – Replacement with a Tooth-Supported or Implant-Supported Reconstruction?

*9*

Bjarni E. Pjetursson

## Introduction

Clinicians routinely in daily practice face the challenge of making fast and difficult decisions. These are mostly influenced by paradigms dictated by basic dental education and many years of clinical practice. In the early 1980s, treatment planning in reconstructive dentistry was much simpler, and the treatment options to restore edentulous spans were restricted to conventional and cantilever tooth-supported fixed dental prostheses (FDPs) or removable dental prostheses. With the emergence of new techniques, the number of options to restore edentulous gaps has increased substantially.

Today, when planning a fixed reconstruction, the first decision to be made is the type of reconstruction: a tooth-supported (conventional or cantilever), combined tooth–implant-supported, or solely implant-supported reconstruction; FDPs or single crowns (SCs).

Decisions like these should be evidence-based, but the question remains whether or not the practice of evidence-based treatment planning is possible in prosthetic dentistry. Ideally, treatment decisions should be based on comparative studies with the highest level of evidence, randomized controlled clinical trials, or on well-performed systematic reviews and meta-analysis of the available evidence.[1-3]

At present there is only one randomized controlled clinical trial that compares survival and success of reconstructions of different design. This Swedish trial compared combined tooth–implant-supported FDPs and solely implant-supported FDPs.[4-7] The trial included 23 patients with residual dentition in the mandible and complete maxillary dentures. Patients with two edentulous sites in the mandible were randomly selected for an FDP incorporation supported by either two implants (control) or by one abutment tooth and one implant (test). Over a 10-year observation period, 2 of 23 test implants and 5 of 46 control implants were lost during function. There was no significant difference between test and control sites and it was concluded that the combination of teeth and implants in FDPs may be recommended as a predictable and reliable treatment alternative for reconstruction of the posterior mandible.

However, this study clearly did not have the necessary power to detect smaller but clinically relevant differences in the proportion of lost implants. With the two groups of 23 and 46 implants, this study had a power of 43% to detect a 10% versus 30% difference in the proportion of implants lost. The size needed for an effective trial can be illustrated by the following. To detect a clinically relevant difference in the annual rate of loss of reconstructions of 1% versus 2% with 80%

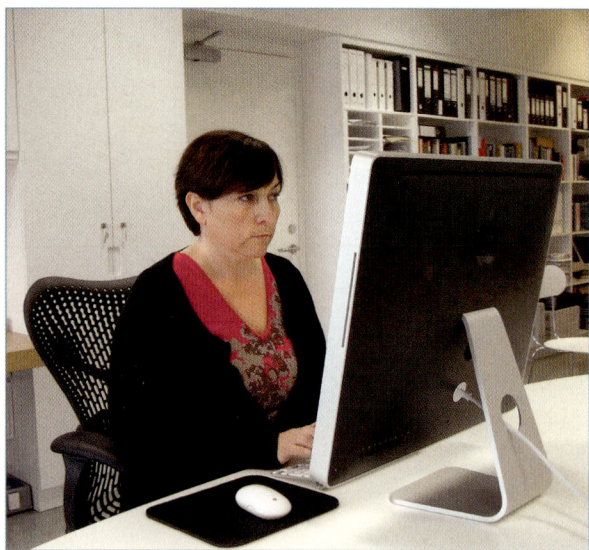

**Fig 9-1** More and more patients get information regarding dental implants over the internet.

impact on the survival and risk assessment of fixed reconstructions, for use in treatment planning for standard cases.

## Step 1: The Patient's Perception

Today, patients can get information regarding dental treatment from a number of different sources, such as the internet (Fig 9-1). Some implant companies started to advertise treatment options directly to patients. Slogans like 'teeth in an hour' or 'beautiful teeth now' are directed to possible customers. However, most patients still get information regarding dental treatment from dental professionals or from friends and relatives. In the early 1990s, implant treatment was not as common, but most patients who are middle age or older now will know someone who has undertaken implant treatment. It appears that implant treatment is usually well accepted by patients, as shown in a 10-year prospective study which concluded that more than 90% of the patients were satisfied with the implant therapy performed and would be willing to undergo implant therapy again if necessary.[8] The cost associated with implant therapy was also considered to be justified.

### Cost of Treatment
In most European countries, the cost of an implant-supported SC is similar to the cost for a three-unit tooth-supported FDP. Brägger and coworkers in a retrospective study evaluated the economic aspects of a single-tooth replacement in Switzerland.[9] The total cost of treatment and the chair time needed were evaluated for a group of 37 patients with 41 tooth-supported three-unit FDPs and a group of 52 patients with 59 implant-supported SCs. The total cost of treatment was 3939 ± 766 Swiss francs for a tooth-supported three-unit FDP compared with 3218 ± 512 Swiss francs for an implant-supported SC. The authors concluded that the implant-supported SC showed better cost effectiveness than the tooth-supported FDP.

power and at a significance level of 5%, a two-arm study would need to randomize approximately 1060 patients in 1 year and to follow them for at least 4 years, resulting in a total study time of 5 years. With a longer follow-up of about 10 years, it would be sufficient to randomize 500 patients. For a scenario comparing annual rate of loss of reconstructions of 0.5% versus 2.5%, 5- or 10-year follow-up studies would need to randomize 260 and 130 patients, respectively. This is clearly a difficult task.

Studies in the dental literature reporting on tooth-supported and implant-supported FDPs are, unfortunately, mostly observational studies and single-center case cohorts. As there are no studies providing the highest level of evidence (randomized controlled clinical trials) on this issue, and only a few studies have reported on the longevity of reconstructions on implants, evidence-based treatment planning in prosthetic dentistry is difficult. Because of this lack of evidence in the dental literature to guide in choosing between different types of reconstruction, clinicians, unfortunately, must continue to rely on clinical experience and 'gut' feeling.

The aim of this chapter is to discuss the available evidence and other factors that affect treatment planning, and also to identify the various parameters that

If, however, one or both teeth adjacent to the edentulous space require new restorations, the cost effectiveness of a tooth-supported three-unit FDP is significantly better.

## The Treatment Time

The total treatment time is another factor that can influence the treatment plan. If the edentulous ridge is healed and the treatment has to be completed in a very short time, tooth-supported FDP is the treatment of choice. Originally, it was suggested that a waiting time of 3 months for the mandible and 6 months for the maxilla was needed prior to loading of dental implants.[10] With new surface technology, the healing time of dental implants is significantly shorter,[11] but the total treatment time for implant-supported SCs is still at least 2 months in a standard situation.

After tooth extraction, the treatment time for tooth-supported FDPs could be prolonged to 4 or 5 months, or until complete healing of the edentulous ridge is reached. In patients where soft tissue grafting is utilized, the treatment time is also significantly longer and could extend to 6 months or more. For implant-supported SCs where simultaneous bone augmentation procedure is necessary, the total treatment is usually prolonged to 4 to 6 months. Moreover, when two-stage sinus floor elevations or two-stage lateral bone augmentations are needed, the total treatment time could even extend to a year, which could favor tooth-supported reconstructions if time is an important factor.

The mean total treatment times for tooth-supported FDPs and implant-supported SCs were evaluated in a retrospective study.[9] The mean treatment time for the implant-supported SCs was almost twice as long as for the tooth-supported FDPs: $5.9 \pm 3.3$ months and $3.2 \pm 2.6$ months, respectively.

Consequently, tooth-supported FDPs would be the treatment of choice if treatment time is a major consideration, as less time is needed.

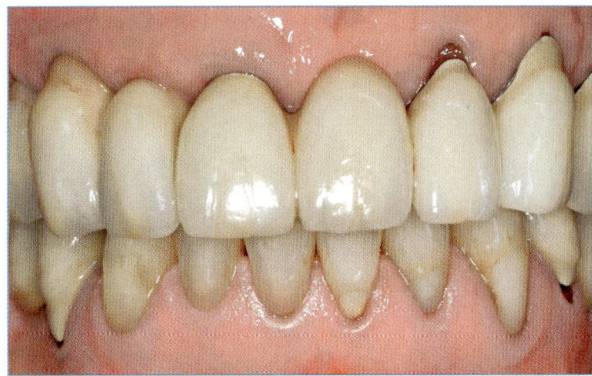

**Fig 9-2** Gingival recession on teeth 22 and 23, resulting in a supragingivally placed crown margin and compromised esthetics.

## Esthetics

To restore a missing tooth in the esthetic zone remains a difficult challenge, whether with tooth-supported or implant-supported reconstructions. The esthetic results depend both on the color and form of the reconstruction and on the position and form of the soft tissue around the tooth.

There are not many studies that have evaluated the esthetic outcome of tooth-supported FDPs and the stability of the soft tissue below the pontic area. A longitudinal study observed that 40% of original subgingivally placed restorative margins became supragingival and were exposed after 5 years (Fig 9-2).[12]

Several authors stated that soft-tissue recessions can be expected during the first 3–6 months in function for implant-supported SCs;[13,14] following which, the soft tissue is stable as long as there is no infection around the implant.

Although esthetic outcome has become a main focus of interest in partially edentulous patients, the esthetic appearance of the implant-supported SCs was evaluated in only 7 out of 26 studies included in a systematic review addressing implant-supported SCs.[15] The cumulative rate of crowns having unacceptable or semi-optimal esthetic appearance was 8.7%. This result is difficult to interpret because of a lack of standardized esthetic criteria and the fact that the esthetic outcome was

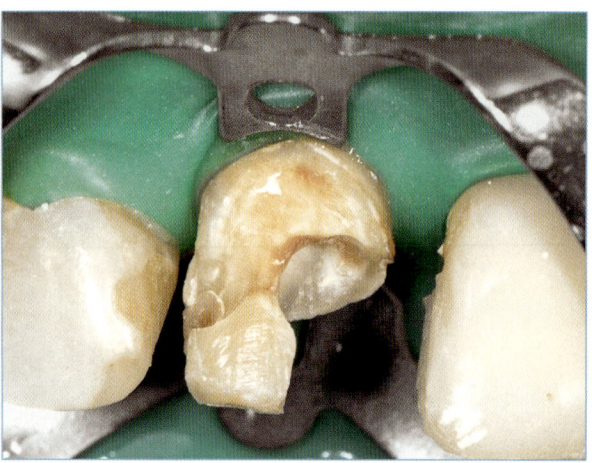

**Fig 9-3** A compromised tooth with significant amount of lost substance. This tooth can be restored with a fiber-reinforced composite resin post and composite resin build-up to support a single crown. However, this tooth would not be a good abutment for a fixed partial prosthesis.

evaluated by either dental professionals or the patients. Hence, there is a need for widely accepted and reproducible esthetic scores, not only for the evaluation of teeth but also for the soft tissues around the implant.[16]

In situations where the neighboring teeth would profit from a crown esthetically, a tooth-supported reconstruction would be the most appropriate treatment choice. Otherwise, it is difficult to make a distinction between tooth-supported or implant-supported reconstructions on esthetic grounds.

### The Provisional Phase

For tooth-supported FDPs, the fabrication of a provisional reconstruction is usually simple; these have high acceptance by the patients and are comfortable to wear. Provisional reconstructions that have a similar form to the final reconstruction can be used during the whole treatment time. However, provisional removable dentures have to be used during the healing period for dental implants. Patients often have problems adapting to them, and time needed for adjustment and repairs is substantial.

If the ease of the provisional phase is considered alone, the tooth-supported reconstructions would be the treatment of choice.

### Long-Term Survival

When planning a fixed reconstruction, the different treatment options have to be discussed with the patient, who must be informed about the estimated survival of the reconstruction and the possible risk factors. Different treatment options have various documented longevities, and biological as well as technical risks have to be considered during treatment planning.

## Step 2: The Neighboring Teeth

One of the determining factors in whether to plan a tooth-supported or an implant-supported reconstruction is the status of the teeth situated next to the edentulous gap.

### Amount of Remaining Tooth Structure

For a tooth-borne reconstruction, the condition of the abutment teeth must be evaluated. If a tooth is intact or has only a small restoration, it is definitely more appropriate to leave it intact rather than preparing it as a FDP abutment. Hence, in situations with intact neighboring teeth, implant-supported reconstructions or resin-bonded bridges (RBBs) with minimal tooth preparations would be the treatment of choice.

However, if a tooth is compromised by substantial loss of tooth substance or by periodontal or endodontic conditions, it might be more sensible for the tooth to be free-standing and not used as a FDP abutment.

A build-up is usually necessary to be able to maintain teeth that have lost a substantial amount of tooth substance. This can be accomplished using cast post and core or by utilizing fiber-reinforced composite resin post and composite resin build-up. These teeth are not as strong as intact teeth (Fig 9-3) and should, if possible, not be used as FDP abutments but rather be left as SCs. Moreover, if a SC is the treatment of choice and an all-ceramic crown is to be used to restore the tooth, bonding techniques could be utilized for the build-up as well as for the restoration. An ideal FDP abutment would be a tooth that is in a good condition but would still profit from the FDP-abutment crown because of caries, fillings, esthetics, and so on.

## Endodontic Aspects

If the neighboring teeth have incomplete endodontic treatment, they should be left as single standing units rather than being used as FDP abutments, unless successful re-treatment of the root canal can be accomplished without any complications. It has been shown in several studies that the success of endodontic re-treatment is, on average, not very high. A prospective study evaluated the success of endodontic re-treatment for 452 teeth in 425 patients over 2 years.[17] The teeth were divided into a group consisting of teeth with no significant anatomical changes of the root canal morphology and a second group with modified root canal morphology after the initial treatment. The success rate ranged from 28% to 100% depending on the reason for the endodontic failure. The best results were obtained where the reason for re-treatment was underfilling of the canal with gutta-percha or cement with no alteration of the root-canal morphology. If the reason for endodontic re-treatment was stripping, internal or external transportation, calcification, perforation, apical resorption, internal resorption or apical stop, the success rate ranged from 28% to 76%.[17] This makes these teeth questionable for use as FDP abutments. In a longitudinal study from the University of Bergen, Norway, 112 endodontically re-treated roots were followed for up to 27 years after endodontic treatment.[18] The authors observed that persistent periapical radiolucencies disappeared in some cases after more than 10 years. In other teeth, where no radiolucencies were seen in the first decade after treatment, periapical radiolucencies appeared after 10 to 17 years. Therefore, the authors suggested that persistent asymptomatic periapical radiolucencies should not be classified as failures. Though endodontically treated teeth with small asymptomatic periapical lesions should not be extracted, they should preferably be left single standing and not be used as FDP abutments as there is increased risk that they may flare up over time.

## Periodontal Aspects

The neighboring teeth must also be evaluated from the periodontal point of view. Tooth mobility per se is not a contraindication for using teeth as FDP abutments. Teeth with reduced but healthy periodontium can certainly be used as abutment teeth despite increased mobility. However, teeth with residual pockets of 5 mm or more and teeth with furcation involvement Class II or more should not be used as FDP abutments[19] because of the increased risk of periodontal progression.[20,21] The ratio between bone loss evaluated on periapical radiographs and the age of the patient can also be used as an indicator for periodontal risk.[22] For example, a 30-year-old patient who has lost 30% of bone support has a ratio of 1 and is classified as a high-risk patient. However, a 60-year-old patient with the same amount of bone support would only have a ratio of 0.5 and would be classified as a medium-risk patient. Hence, a tooth that would not be used as an abutment tooth in the younger patient might be considered as an abutment tooth in the older patient.

A longitudinal study that evaluated the maintenance of periodontal attachment levels in prosthetically treated patients with gingivitis or moderate chronic periodontitis 5 to 17 years after therapy concluded that there was no significant difference regarding loss of attachment between reconstructed abutment teeth and non-reconstructed control teeth.[23]

# Step 3: Evaluation of the Edentulous Gap

Based on limited evidence, it has been suggested that a minimal distance between a tooth and a dental implant should be 1.5 mm.[24]

The risk for bone loss increases if the bone wall between the root and the implant is < 1.5 mm. This means that at least 6 mm of bone in the mesiodistal direction is needed for a narrow 3.3 mm implant but at least 7 mm of bone is needed in the premolar and molar area where standard 4 mm or wider implants are pre-

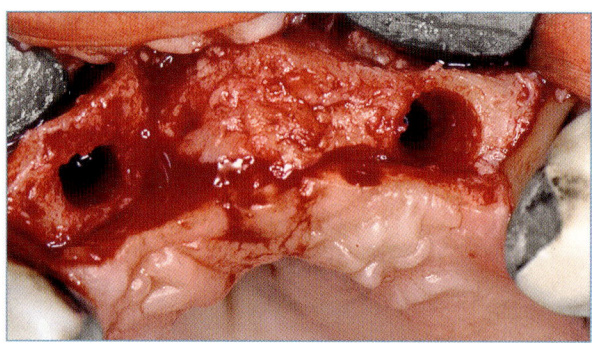

**Fig 9-4** The ITI Consensus Conference in 1998 suggested that a minimal bone wall of 0.7 mm was needed buccally and orally for standard implant placement.[26]

ferred. If this condition is not fulfilled, tooth-supported reconstructions where dimensions of the neighboring teeth can be altered via prosthetic means are indicated. Another treatment option would be to increase the size of the edentulous gap with orthodontic tooth movements. However, it must always be kept in mind that the width of the edentulous gap should be measured at the bone level and not at the contact point of the neighboring teeth.

The interocclusal distance needed for a tooth-supported pontic is dependent on the height of the neighboring teeth. It has been suggested that a minimal height for the walls of the prepared tooth should be at least 3–4 mm with less than 10 degree convergent, translating into a minimal height of the reconstruction of 5–6 mm.[25]

For implant-supported reconstruction, the minimal height of abutments for cemented reconstruction is 4 mm, translating into a reconstruction of 5–6 mm depending on the material used. For screw-retained reconstruction, the height of the abutment, including the occlusal screw, is approximately 4 mm, giving a minimal height of the reconstruction similar to that of the cemented reconstruction. In situations with limited interocclusal space, implant-supported reconstruction may be preferred owing to the risk of loss of retention of a tooth-supported reconstruction. With loss of retention in tooth-supported FDPs, there is an increased risk of caries of the abutment teeth. This might cause the

loss of the abutment and even the loss of the whole reconstruction. As for implant-supported reconstructions, loss of retention and occlusal screw loosening are usually minor complications that can be solved with a simple procedure.

## Step 4: The Complexity of Implant Placement

Prior to treatment planning, the edentulous site has to be examined. For implant-borne reconstructions, the ease of implant placement affects the treatment decision. Is there adequate bone volume for standard implant placement or is there a need for complicated bone augmentation procedures, which will increase the cost and duration of treatment?

There is, however, limited evidence on how much bone width is really needed for a standard implant placement and to maintain the bone surrounding the implant. This question needs to be addressed with large studies utilizing three-dimensional radiographic imaging to evaluate the long-term stability of the buccal and oral bone walls. Based on expert opinions at the ITI Consensus Conference 1998, it was suggested that the minimal bone width for placement of an implant with a diameter of 3.3 mm was 4.8 mm, and that the minimal width for placement of an implant with a diameter of 4.1 mm was 5.5 mm.[26] This translated to a minimal thickness of 0.7 mm for the buccal as well as the oral bone wall (Fig 9-4). If this is not achievable, then some kind of bone augmentation is required.

A systematic review examined the survival of implants in bone sites augmented with barrier membranes (guided bone regeneration) in partially edentulous patients and concluded that the survival rates varied between 79% and 100%.[27] However, the majority of the studies covered in the review indicated more than 90% survival after at least 1 year in function, and the survival rate was similar to those generally reported for implants placed conventionally into sites without need for bone augmentation.

## The Posterior Maxilla

Implant placement in the posterior maxilla remains a challenge. The soft bone and the reduced bone volume owing to alveolar bone resorption and pneumatization of the sinus cavity make it more difficult to place implants to support dental prostheses.

Several treatment options have been utilized in the posterior maxilla to overcome the problem of inadequate bone quantity. The most conservative treatment option would be to place short implants to avoid entering the sinus cavity. Even for placement of short implants, however, there is still a need for at least 6 mm of residual bone height. A recent review prepared for the Consensus Meeting of the European Association of Osseointegration included eight studies on rough textured implants.[28] The authors concluded that the survival and success rates of short implants was comparable to those obtained with longer implants provided that surgical preparation was related to bone density, rough textured implants were used, and the operators' surgical skills were well developed. However, it must be kept in mind that the implants considered short in this review were mainly 8, 9, and 10 mm long. There is still limited evidence that short implants of 6 mm or less will perform well in the posterior maxilla.

In patients with appropriate residual bone height, minor augmentation of the sinus floor can be accomplished via the trans-alveolar approach using the osteotome technique.[29,30] A systematic review has evaluated the success of sinus floor elevation and the survival of implants inserted in combination with sinus floor elevation using a trans-alveolar approach.[31] Based on the meta-analysis, the estimated survival rate after 3 years in function was 92.8%. Furthermore, the subject-based analysis revealed an estimated annual failure of 3.71%, translating to 10.5% of the subjects experiencing implant loss over 3 years.

The authors concluded that the survival rate of implants placed in trans-alveolar sinus floor augmentation sites are comparable to those in non-augmented sites, especially if this is limited to sites with a preoperative bone height of 5 mm or more. This technique is

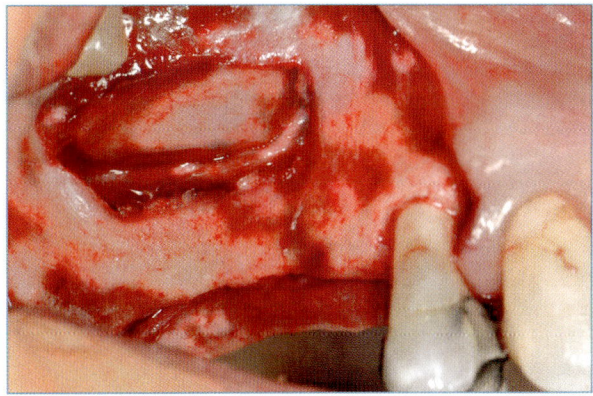

**Fig 9-5**  A two-stage sinus floor elevation, using the lateral approach, is probably the most invasive treatment option in the posterior maxilla.

predictable, with low incidence of complications during the treatment and post-operatively.

The most invasive treatment option in the posterior maxilla is the one- or two-stage sinus floor elevation with lateral approach (Fig 9-5). A recent systematic review has evaluated the survival of implants inserted in combination with sinus floor elevation using a lateral approach and included 48 studies with over 12 000 implants.[32] Based on the meta-analysis, the estimated survival rate after 3 years in function was 90.1%. However, when only studies that used rough-surface implants were included, the survival rate increased to 96.4% after the same observation period.

Most edentulous areas in the maxilla can be restored with implant-supported reconstructions if the following methods are mastered: the use of short implants and sinus floor elevation via a trans-alveolar or lateral approach.

Standard implant placement is usually well accepted by patients.[8] If implants are placed with simultaneous guided bone regeneration (Fig 9-6) or sinus floor elevation using the trans-alveolar technique, there is usually increased post-operative trauma, the cost of treatment is more, and the treatment time is usually 4 to 8 weeks longer than standard implant placement. Based on limited evidence, this treatment is still well accepted by the patients and more than 9 out of 10 patients treated in

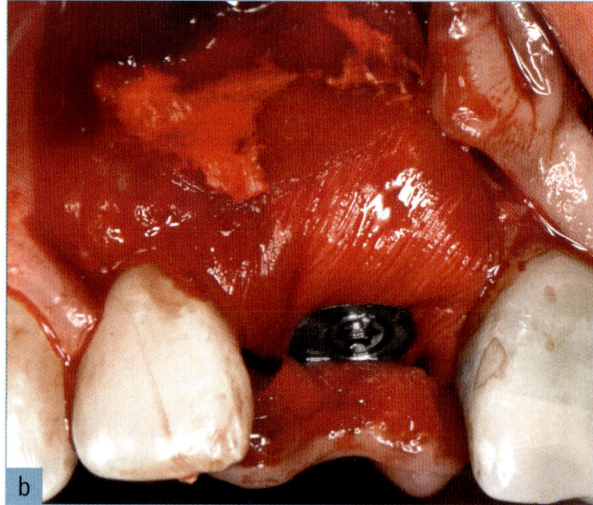

Fig 9-6a–b   (a) Guided bone regeneration performed simultaneously with implant insertion. (b) Collagen membrane is used to hold the grafting material in place.

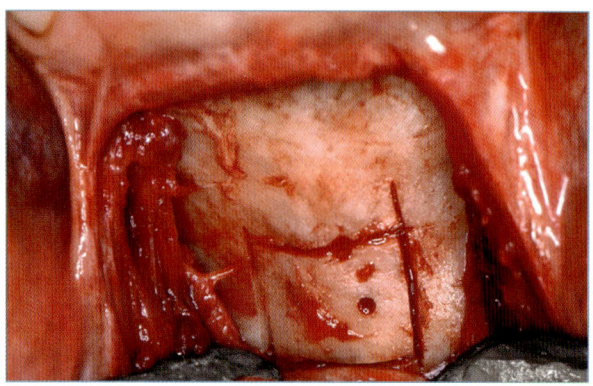

Fig 9-7   Bone harvesting usually causes more trauma to the patient than bone regeneration procedures per se.

this way would be ready to undergo this treatment again, if necessary.[33] However, if major bone augmentations are needed, the treatment is much more complex. The post-operative trauma is significantly more, especially if there is need for autogenous bone harvesting (Fig 9-7). For example, if bone is harvested from the hip, it can take patients several months to fully recover after the procedure. Moreover, in the two-stage bone augmentation procedures, the treatment time is at least 6 months longer than standard implant placement and the cost of treatment is also significantly higher.

In patients where complex two-stage bone augmentation procedures are needed, other treatment options, such as tooth-supported reconstructions or a shortened dental arch, should be given serious thought. The work of Käyser and coworkers showed that patients maintain adequate (50–80%) chewing capacity with a premolar occlusion.[34]

# Step 5: The Estimated Longevity of the Reconstructions

Another very important factor in treatment planning is to estimate the long-term survival of the reconstructions. The question remains whether the good results seen for tooth-borne reconstructions can be transferred to implant-borne reconstructions, as the use of natural teeth and implants as abutments differ in important ways.

A series of systematic reviews based on consistent inclusion and exclusion criteria have been produced by Pjetursson and coworkers.[15,35–39] These have summarized the available information on survival and success rates and the incidence of biological and technical complications of conventional FDPs,[37] cantilever FDPs,[38] combined tooth–implant-supported FDPs,[36] and solely implant-supported FDPs,[35] as well as implant-supported SCs[15] and RBBs.[39] These reviews have been updated and completed in a recent systematic review[40] based on the relevant literature sourced up to July 2006.

In the absence of randomized controlled clinical trials, this series of systematic reviews was based on prospective or retrospective cohort studies. The additional inclusion criteria for study selection were that:

♦ the studies had a mean follow-up time of 5 years or more
♦ the included patients had been examined clinically at the follow-up visit; that is, publications based on patient records only, on questionnaires, or interviews were excluded
♦ the studies reported details on the characteristics of the suprastructures.

*Survival* was defined as the reconstruction remaining *in situ* at the follow-up examination visit irrespective of its condition. *Success* was defined as the reconstruction remaining unchanged and not requiring any intervention during the entire observation period.

Failure and complication rates were calculated by dividing the number of events (failures or complications) by the total exposure time of the reconstruction.

The event rates for reconstructions were calculated by dividing the total number of events by the total reconstruction exposure time in years. For further analysis, the total number of events was considered to be Poisson distributed for a given sum of reconstruction *exposure-years*, and Poisson regression with a logarithmic link function and *total* exposure time per study as an offset variable was used.[41,42]

The meta-analysis of the included studies from the dental literature indicated an estimated 5-year survival rate of 93.8% for conventional tooth-supported FDPs, 91.4% for cantilever FDPs, 95.2% for solely implant-supported FDPs, 95.5% for combined tooth–implant-supported FDPs, 94.5% for implant-supported SCs, and 87.7% for RBBs (Table 9-1). Moreover, after 10 years of function, the estimated survival decreased to 89.2% for conventional FDPs, to 80.3% for cantilever FDPs, to 86.7% for implant-supported FDPs, to 77.8% for combined tooth–implant-supported FDPs, to 89.4% for implant-supported SCs, and to 65% for RBBs (Table 9-2).

Based on the results of the systematic reviews, planning of prosthetic rehabilitations should preferentially include conventional end-abutment tooth-supported FDPs, solely implant-supported FDPs or implant-supported SCs. Only for reasons of anatomical structures or patient-centered preferences, and as a second option, should cantilever tooth-supported FDPs, combined tooth–implant-supported FDPs or RBBs be chosen.

## Step 6: Assessment of Risk Factors

Finally, risk factors, such as biological and technical complications, must be taken into account as these complications are frequent despite the high survival of FDPs.[35–38]

Biological complications for tooth-supported reconstructions include dental caries, loss of pulp vitality, and periodontal disease progression. Biological complications for implant- and combined tooth–implant-supported reconstructions are characterized by processes affecting the supporting tissues.

Technical complications for tooth-supported reconstructions include loss of retention, abutment tooth fractures, and fractures or deformations of the framework or veneers (Fig 9-8). Technical complications for implant- and combined tooth–implant-supported reconstructions include mechanical damage of implants, implant components, and/or the suprastructures; this includes fractures of the implants, fracture of screws or abutments, loss of retention, fractures or deformations of the framework or veneers, loss of the screw access hole restoration, and screw or abutment loosening.

Despite the high survival rates, 38.7% of the patients with implant-supported FDPs had some complications during the 5-year observation period,[35] compared with 15.7% for conventional FDPs,[37] 20.6% for cantilever FDPs,[37] and 19.2% for RBBs.[39]

**Table 9-1** Summary of annual failure rates, relative failure rates and 5-year survival estimates

| Type of reconstruction | Total number of reconstructions | Total exposure time (years) | Mean follow-up time (years) | Estimated annual failure rate (% [95 % CI]) | 5-year survival summary estimate (% [95 % CI]) |
|---|---|---|---|---|---|
| Conventional FDPs | 2088 | 11 998 | 5.7 | 1.28 (0.64–2.59) | 93.8 (87.9–96.9) |
| Cantilever FDPs | 432 | 2 112 | 5.2 | 1.80 (1.15–2.82) | 91.4 (86.9–94.4) |
| Implant-supported FDPs | 1384 | 6 880 | 5 | 0.99 (0.64–1.52) | 95.2 (92.7–96.8) |
| Tooth–implant supported FDPs | 199 | 976 | 5 | 0.92 (0.50–1.70) | 95.5 (91.9–97.5) |
| Implant-supported single crowns | 465 | 2 280 | 5 | 1.14 (0.76–1.70) | 94.5 (91.8–96.3) |
| Composite resin-bonded FDPs | 1374 | 8 241 | 6 | 2.61 (1.68–4.06) | 87.7 (81.6–91.9) |

CI, confidence intervals; FDP, fixed dental prosthesis.

**Table 9-2** Summary of annual failure rates, relative failure rates and 10-year survival estimates

| Type of reconstruction | Total number of reconstructions | Total exposure time (years) | Mean follow-up time (years) | Estimated annual failure rate (% [95 % CI]) | 10-year survival summary estimate (% [95 % CI]) |
|---|---|---|---|---|---|
| Conventional FDPs | 1218 | 10 446 | 11.9 | 1.14 (0.48–2.73) | 89.2 (76.1–95.3) |
| Cantilever FDPs | 239 | 2 229 | 10.9 | 2.20 (1.70–2.84) | 80.3 (75.2–84.4) |
| Implant-supported FDPs | 219 | 1 889 | 10 | 1.43 (1.08–1.89) | 86.7 (82.8–89.8) |
| Tooth-implant supported FDPs | 72 | 517 | 10 | 2.51 (1.54–4.10) | 77.8 (66.4–85.7) |
| Implant-supported single crowns | 69 | 623 | 10 | 1.12 (0.45–2.32) | 89.4 (79.3–95.6) |
| Composite resin-bonded FDPs | 51 | 464 | 9.1 | 4.31 (2.63–6.66) | 65.0 (51.4–76.9) |

CI, confidence intervals; FDP, fixed dental prosthesis.

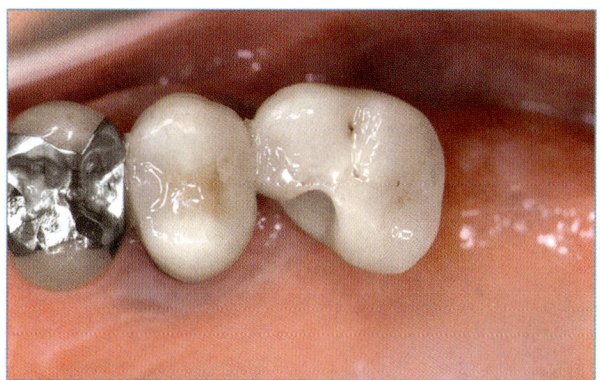

**Fig 9-8**  Ceramic fracture of a zirconium-based ceramic crown. The zirconium coping is intact, but the feldspar ceramic fractured after only 1 week of function.

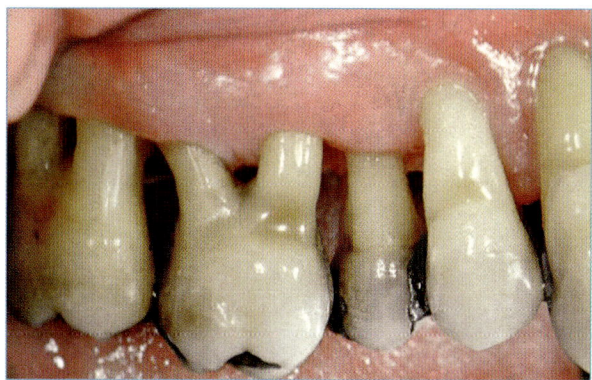

**Fig 9-9**  All molars and premolars here are seriously compromised by periodontal disease. However, these teeth have no other risk factors and had been maintained for 12 years when this picture was taken. *(Courtesy of Dr Jürg Schmid, Ilanz, Switzerland.)*

For conventional tooth-supported FDPs, the most frequent complications were biological complications such as caries and loss of pulp vitality. The incidence of technical complications was significantly higher for implant-supported reconstructions than for tooth-supported FDPs. The most frequent technical complications were fractures of the veneer material (ceramic fractures or chipping), abutment or screw loosening, and loss of retention. For RBBs, the most frequent complication was debonding.

## Step 7: Multiple Risk Factors

Last, but not least, the concept of multiple risk factors must be considered. If a tooth has a 100% chance of surviving the next 10 years from a periodontal point of view, it can be said to have a risk of survival of 1.0. If a tooth is endodontically compromised and has only an 80% chance of survival for endodontic reasons, it would get a value for tooth survival of 0.8.

Combined risks are multiplied. For example, if a tooth has an 80% chance of survival based on periodontal reasons and an 80% chance of survival based on endodontic reasons, the combined survival risk for the tooth is only 0.64 (0.8 x 0.8), meaning that the chance of this tooth surviving the next 10 years is only 64%. It must be understood that the value of a compro-

mised tooth decreases dramatically when it has combined or multiple risk factors.

For the clinician, this means that a seriously compromised tooth from an endodontic standpoint, such as a tooth with internal resorption, should only be kept if it is not compromised periodontally, with adequate tooth structure and not requiring complicated reconstructions afterwards. The same would apply for a tooth that is seriously compromised by periodontal disease (Fig 9-9). It is only worth keeping such a tooth if it is not endodontically compromised and does not need complicated and expensive reconstruction.

# Evidence-Based Treatment Planning of Standard Clinical Situations

For the present discussion, it is assumed that the dentition presented with endodontically and periodontally healthy teeth. Teeth that were considered irrational to treat for whatever reason were extracted prior to decision making for the prosthetic reconstruction of the dentition. Hence, the clinical situation was evaluated prior to replacing teeth that were already missing.

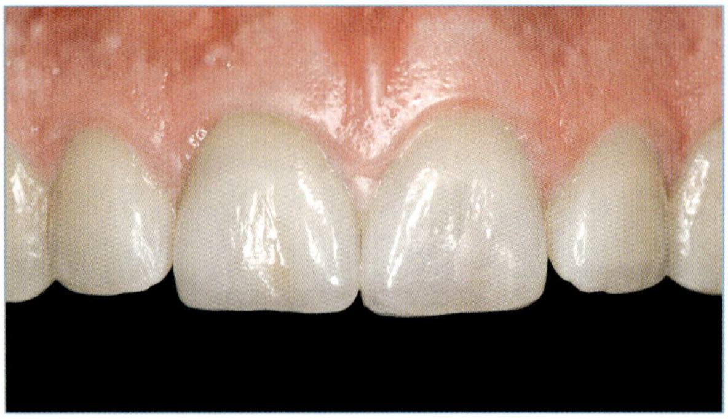

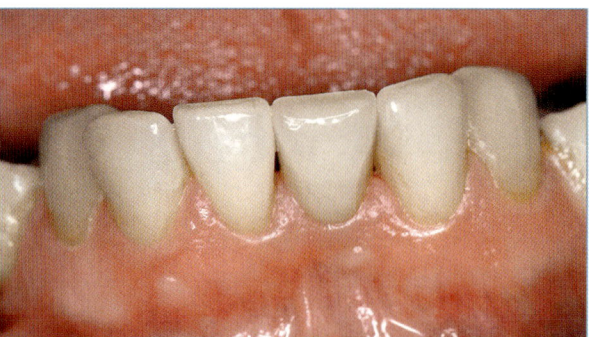

**Fig 9-10** A young patient who lost her maxillary right central incisor (tooth 11) in a bicycle accident. The edentulous space was restored with a screw-retained implant-supported single crown.

**Fig 9-11** A patient with a congenitally missing mandibular central incisor. After orthodontic treatment, the edentulous space was restored with a screw-retained implant-supported single crown.

## Single Tooth Gaps in the Anterior Maxilla

In areas of esthetic priority, single tooth replacement is faced with the challenges to achieve an illusion close to nature. In this respect, it is important to identify esthetic parameters such as heights and extension of smile lines, tissue biotype, tooth characteristics, and so on. These factors may have higher priority in determining the choice of treatment modality than the longevity of the reconstruction per se.

However, based on the evidence of the systematic reviews discussed above, the missing tooth is replaced preferably by an implant-supported SC (annual failure rate, 1.12%)[15] provided that the adjacent teeth are intact and in perfect condition (Fig 9-10). This represents the most conservative and most 'biological' treatment option. However, if the adjacent teeth are severed or in need of being restored, the conventional FDP is to be preferred (annual failure rate, 1.14%).[37] Based on longevity and cost, the two options are similar, with 10-year survival rates of 89.4% and 89.2% for implant-supported SCs and conventional FDPs, respectively.[40] An RBB should be considered as a second option as it has a higher annual failure rate at 5-year follow-up (2.61%) and an even higher annual failure rate after 10 years (4.31%).[39]

## Single Tooth Gaps in the Anterior Mandible

Esthetic aspects usually have lower priority in the anterior mandible than in the maxilla. Yet the anterior mandible has important functional roles, particularly for speech. While choosing the treatment option for optimal functional outcomes, both an implant-supported SC (Fig 9-11) and a conventional FDP may be chosen. However, it must be kept in mind that the preparation of mandibular incisors presents a serious risk for pulp vitality. Consequently, whenever the bone morphology and volume allow the placement of an implant, the implant-supported SC should be preferred. Beyond this, issues discussed for the anterior maxilla may also apply. The RBB is often chosen when economic and space issues play a role. However, such RBBs should only be placed on teeth with favorable jaw relations, adequate periodontal support, and intact enamel.

## Single Tooth Gaps in the Posterior Region

In the posterior region, functional aspects dominate the decision-making process. Moreover, the condition of the adjacent teeth is crucially important. If these are intact or only repaired with minimally invasive restorations, it is preferable not to prepare these as abutments. Again, an implant-supported SC is the first choice and

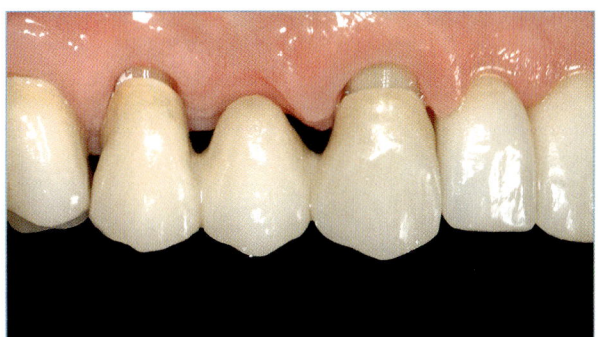

**Fig 9-12** A patient with a missing maxillary first premolar. As both adjacent teeth required reconstructions, the edentulous space was restored with a three-unit conventional tooth-supported fixed dental prosthesis. The soft tissue in the edentulous space was conditioned with a provisional prosthesis to provide optimal esthetic, as visualized by the incomplete seating of the fixed dental prosthesis prior to cementation.

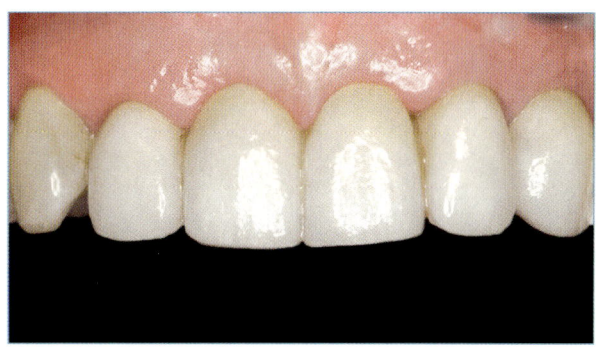

**Fig 9-13** A female patient who lost all her maxillary incisors through periodontal disease. Two implants were placed in the positions 12 and 22 and the edentulous span was restored with a four-unit implant-supported fixed dental prosthesis.

represents the most tissue-preserving treatment. The conventional FDP should only be chosen if the adjacent teeth require reconstructions (Fig 9-12). RBBs yield an annual rate of debonding of 5.17% in the posterior region[39] and, therefore, are not recommended.

## Multiple Missing Adjacent Teeth in the Anterior Maxilla

In addition to the issues discussed for single gaps in the anterior maxilla, functional as well as esthetic aspects have to be considered if multiple teeth are missing. In situations with, for example, four missing incisors, the volume of soft tissues and bone has to be analyzed. The placement of two non-adjacent implants may be the first choice of treatment provided that both soft tissue and bone volumes are adequate (Fig 9-13). However, the decision may be influenced by the morbidity encountered with advanced augmentation procedures. In favoring conventional FDP over implant-supported FDP, the extension and the retention aspects of the FDPs have to be analyzed. The use of more than one abutment adjacent to a large edentulous space may increase the risk of complications. The implant-supported FDP is a smaller reconstruction but it has slightly poorer longevity data, the implant-supported FDPs exhibiting an annual failure rate of 1.43%[35,40] compared

with 1.14% for conventional FDP.[37,40] The 10-year survival is also slightly lower for implant-supported FDPs (86.7%)[35,40] compared with conventional FDPs (89.2%).[37,40]

## Multiple Missing Adjacent Teeth in the Anterior Mandible

Similar aspects govern the decision-making process in the anterior mandible as in the anterior maxilla, although the risks for complications with the incorporation of conventional FDPs (Fig 9-14) appear to be lower than in the maxilla. Tissue volume and morphology of the alveolar bone may, however, dictate the necessity for augmentation procedures, which are difficult to perform and often have unpredictable outcomes. Therefore, unfavorable morphological conditions may preclude the possibility of an otherwise preferred implant-supported reconstruction. Evidence for the incorporation of multiunit RBBs in the anterior mandible is lacking.[39]

## Multiple Missing Adjacent Teeth in the Posterior Region (Bounded Saddle)

While in the past implant-supported reconstructions were not considered as a predictable treatment for large edentulous gaps, today these may preferably be recon-

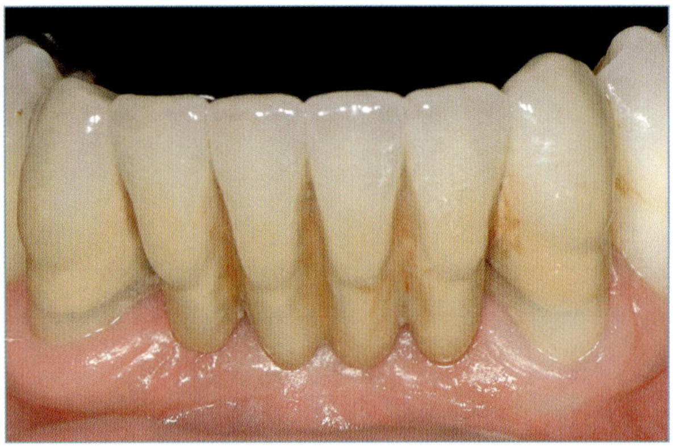

**Fig 9-14**  A smoker who lost all mandibular incisors through periodontal disease. Implant placement would only be possible with lateral bone augmentation (two stages). As the canines had good periodontal support, the edentulous space was restored with a six-unit tooth-supported fixed dental prosthesis extending from 43 to 33.

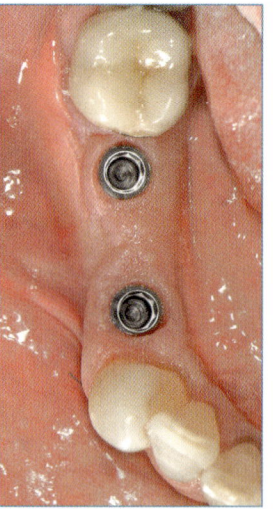

**Fig 9-15**  A patient with three missing teeth in the fourth quadrant. Instead of inserting a long-span tooth-supported fixed dental prosthesis from tooth 43 to 47, the edentulous space was restored by a three-unit fixed dental prosthesis-supported by two implants.

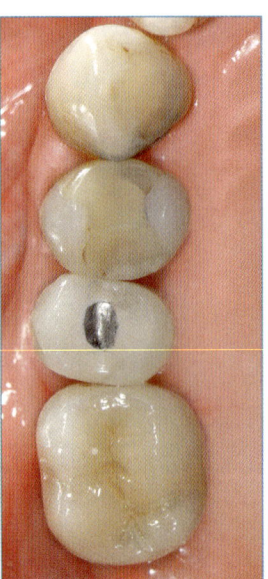

**Fig 9-16**  A female patient who had lost tooth 16 through a vertical root fracture. She was not satisfied with a shortened dental arch. Hence, an implant was placed in position 16 and after a healing period of 8 weeks it was restored with a cemented crown. This improved the subjective chewing capacity of the patient.

structed with implant-supported FDPs (Fig 9-15). The shorter extension of the implant-supported FDP usually avoids many of the biomechanical risks encountered with long-span conventional FDPs. Against this, the incidence of technical complications such as ceramic fractures or chipping is generally higher for implant-supported reconstructions than for tooth-supported reconstructions: annual complication rates of 1.84% and 0.59%, respectively.[40]

## Free-End Situation with Missing Molars

The treatment options available to replace missing molars with fixed reconstructions are implant-supported SC or tooth-supported cantilever FDP. The former presents with a very favorable annual failure rate (only 1.12%),[15] while the latter has a higher annual failure rate (2.20%).[38] It is evident that the implant-supported SC (Fig 9-16) is preferred over the tooth-supported cantilever FDP provided the bone morphology favors implant placement. If the adjacent teeth of the free-end distal-extension are to be crowned, the tooth-supported cantilever FDP may be chosen. However, it must be realized that non-vital endodontically treated terminal abutments present with an increased risk for tooth fractures compared with vital cantilever abutments.[43,44]

Prior to choosing a treatment option for missing molars, an evaluation of the subjective chewing capacity and the functional needs of the patient regarding molar replacement has to be made. Shortened dental arches with bilateral premolar occlusion provide a reasonable and individually optimal restricted treatment goal in many patients,[45–47] presenting an option where no prosthetic reconstruction is needed.

## Free-End Situation with Missing Premolars and Molars

Where there is a free-end situation with missing premolars and molars, increasing chewing comfort is a desire in most patients. In addition to the options discussed above for the free-end situation with missing molars, tooth–implant-supported FDPs, solely implant-supported FDPs, and multiple implant supported SCs may be considered. From a longevity point of view, the first options include solely implant-supported prostheses such as implant-supported FDPs (Fig 9-17) and multiple implant-supported SCs. These have annual failure rates of 1.43%[15,40] and 1.12%,[40] respectively, based on the 10-year data. As a second option, tooth-supported cantilever FDPs and combined tooth–implant-supported FDPs may be considered. These have annual failure rates of 2.20%[40] and 2.51%,[36,40] respectively.

It is evident that aspects other than longevity and complication rates may dominate the decision-making process. For example, anatomical situations may dictate choosing the second-option treatments.

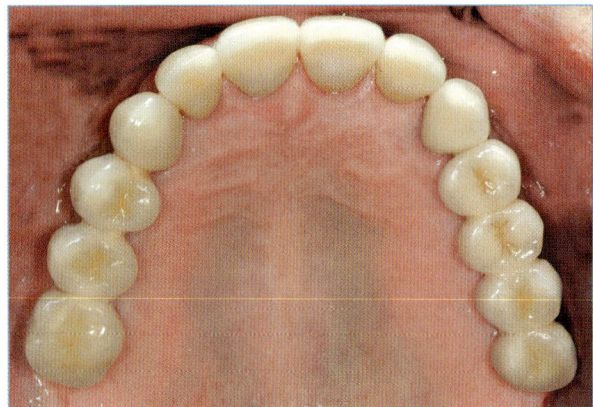

**Fig 9-17**  Several years ago, the patient lost all his premolars and molars in the maxilla. He had difficulties adjusting to a removable dental prosthesis. Bilateral sinus floor elevations were performed, and five implants were placed to support one 3-unit- and one 4-unit FDP.

# Conclusions

For conventional tooth-supported FDPs, the most frequent complications reported are biological complications such as caries and loss of pulp vitality. For cantilever FDPs, the incidence of biological complications is similar to that of conventional FDPs. Technical complications such as loss of retention and material fractures are, however, more frequent.

For implant-supported reconstructions, the incidence of biological complications, such as mucositis and peri-implantitis, is similar for solely implant-supported, combined implant–tooth-supported FDPs, and implant-supported SCs. Fractures of the veneer material (ceramic fractures), abutment or screw loosening, and loss of retention are the most frequently reported technical complications. Fractures of the veneer material are more frequent in studies reporting on gold–acrylic resin reconstructions than those for metal–ceramic reconstructions.

The incidence of complications is substantially higher in implant-supported than in tooth-supported reconstructions. This, however, does not necessarily imply that the possibilities for corrective measures are more cumbersome.

Although a variety of subjective and objective aspects heavily influence the choice of treatment modalities, the knowledge of survival and complication rates of various reconstructions based on long-term studies certainly help in optimizing the decision process.

# References

1. Egger M, Smith GD. Meta-analysis: Potentials and promise. BMJ 1997;315:1371–1374.
2. Egger M, Smith GD, Sterne JA. Uses and abuses of metaanalysis. Clin Med 2001;1:478–484.
3. Egger GD, Smith GD, Altmann DG (eds). Systematic Reviews in Health Care: Meta-analysis in Context, 2nd edn, Ch 3: Problems and limitations in conducting systematic reviews. London: BMJ Publishing Group, 2001.
4. Åstrand P, Borg K, Gunne J, Olsson M. Combination of natural teeth and osseointegrated implants as prosthesis abutments: a 2-year longitudinal study. Int J Oral Maxillofac Implants 1992;6:305–312.

5. Gunne J, Åstrand P, Ahlén K, Borg K, Olsson M. Implants in partially edentulous patients. A longitudinal study of bridges supported by both implants and natural teeth. Clin Oral Implants Res 1992;3:49–56.

6. Olsson M, Gunne J, Åstrand P, Borg K. Bridges supported by free-standing implants versus bridges supported by tooth and implant: a five-year prospective study. Clin Oral Implants Res 1995;6:114–121.

7. Gunne J, Åstrand P, Lindh T, Borg K, Olsson M. Tooth–implant and implant supported fixed partial dentures: a 10-year report. Int J Prosthodont 1999;12:216–221.

8. Pjetursson BE, Karoussis I, Lang NP, Brägger U. Patients' perception for implant therapy: ten years following installation of ITI dental implants. Clin Oral Implants Res 2005;16:185–193.

9. Brägger U, Krenander P, Lang NP. Economic aspects of single-tooth replacement. Clin Oral Implants Res 2005;16:335–341.

10. Brånemark PI, Hansson BO, Adell R, Breine U, Lindström J, Hallén O, et al. Osseointegrated implants in the treatment of the edentulous jaw. Experience from a 10-year period. Scand J Plast Reconstr Surg Suppl 1977;16:1–132.

11. Bornstein MM, Schmid B, Belser UC, Lussi A, Buser D. Early loading of non-submerged titanium implants with a sandblasted and acid-etched surface. 5-year results of a prospective study in partially edentulous patients. Clin Oral Implants Res 2005;16:631–638.

12. Valderhaug J, Heloe LA. Oral hygiene in a group of supervised patients with fixed prostheses. J Periodontol 1977;48:221–224.

13. Grunder U. Stability of the mucosal topography around single-tooth implants and adjacent teeth: 1-year results. Int J Periodontics Restorative Dent 2000;20:11–17.

14. Small PN, Tarnow DP. Gingival recession around implants: a 1-year longitudinal prospective study. Int J Oral Maxillofac Implants 2000;15:527–532.

15. Jung RE, Pjetursson BE, Glauser R, Zembic A, Zwahlen M, Lang NP. A systematic review of the 5-year survival and complication rates of implant-supported single crowns. Clin Oral Implants Res 2008;19:119–130

16. Furhauser, R, Florescu, D, Benesch, T, Haas, R, Mailath, G, Watzek, G. Evaluation of soft tissue around single-tooth implant crowns: the pink esthetic score. Clin Oral Implants Res 2005;16:639–644.

17. Gorni FG, Gagliani MM. The outcome of endodontic retreatment: a 2-yr follow-up. J Endodont 2004;30:1–4.

18. Molven O, Halse A, Fristad I, MacDonald-Jankowski D. Periapical changes following root-canal treatment observed 20–27 years postoperatively. Int Endod J 2002;35:784–790.

19. Hamp SE, Nyman S, Lindhe J. J. Periodontal treatment of mutilated teeth. Results after 5 years. J Clin Periodontol 1975; 2:126 –135.

20. Matuliene G, Pjetursson BE, Salvi GE, Schmidlin K, Brägger U, Zwahlen M, et al. Influence of residual pockets on progression of periodontitis and tooth loss: Results after 11 years of maintenance. J Clin Periodontol 2008;35:685–695.

21. Carnevale G, Cairo F, Tonetti MS. Long-term effects of supportive therapy in periodontal patients treated with fibre retention osseous resective surgery. II: tooth extractions during active and supportive therapy. J Clin Periodontol 2007;34:342–348.

22. Tonetti MS, Lang NP. Periodontal risk assessment (PRA) for patients in supportive periodontal therapy (SPT). Oral Health Prev Dent 2003;1:7–16.

23. Moser P, Hammerle CH, Lang NP, Schlegel-Bregenzer B, Persson R. Maintenance of periodontal attachment levels in prosthetically treated patients with gingivitis or moderate chronic periodontitis 5–17 years post therapy. J Clin Periodontol 2002;29:531–539.

24. Andersson B, Odman P, Lindvall AM, Brånemark PI. Cemented single crowns on osseointegrated implants after 5 years: results from a prospective study on CeraOne. Int J Prosthodont 1998;11:212–218.

25. Maxwell AW, Blank LW, Pelleu GB Jr. Effect of crown preparation height on the retention and resistance of gold castings. Gen Dent 1990;38:200–202.

26. Buser D, von Arx T, ten Bruggenkate C, Weingart D. Basic surgical principles with ITI implants. Clin Oral Implants Res 2000;11(Suppl 1):59–68.

27. Hämmerle CHF, Jung RE, Feloutzis A. A systematic review of the survival of implants in bone sites augmented with barrier membranes (guided bone regeneration) in partially edentulous patients. J Clin Periodontol 2002;29(Suppl 3):226–231; discussion 232–233.

28. Renouard F, Nisand D. Impact of implant length and diameter on survival rates. Clin Oral Implants Res 2006;17(Suppl 2), 35–51.

29. Summers RB. Maxillary implant surgery: the osteotome technique. Comped Cont Educ 1994;15:152–162.

30. Rosen PD, Summers R, Mellado JR, Salkin LM, Shanaman RH, Marks MH, et al. The bone-added osteotome sinus floor elevation technique: multicenter retrospective report of consecutively treated patients. Int J Oral Maxillofac Implants 1999;14:853–858.

31. Tan WC, Lang NP, Zwahlen M, Pjetursson BE. A systematic review of the success of sinus floor elevation and survival of implants inserted in combination with sinus floor elevation. Part II: transalveolar technique. J Clin Periodontol 2008;35(Suppl):241–254.

32. Pjetursson BE, Tan WC, Zwahlen M and Lang NP. A systematic review of the success of sinus floor elevation and survival of implants inserted in combination with sinus floor elevation. Part I: lateral approach. J Clin Periodontol 2008;35(Suppl):216–240.

33. Pjetursson BE, Rast C, Brägger U, Zwahlen M, Lang NP. Maxillary sinus floor elevation using the osteotome technique with or without grafting material. Part I: implant survival and patient's perception. Clin Oral Implants Res 2009;19:in press.

34. Käyser AF. Shortened dental arches and oral function. JOral Rehabil 1981;8:457–462.

35. Pjetursson BE, Tan K, Lang NP, Brägger U, Egger M, Zwahlen, M. A systematic review of the survival and complication rates of fixed partial dentures (FDPs) after an observation period of at least 5 years. I. Implant supported FDPs. Clin Oral Implants Res 2004;15:625–642.

36. Lang NP, Pjetursson BE, Tan K, Brägger U, Egger M, Zwahlen M. A systematic review of the survival and complication rates of fixed partial dentures (FDPs) after an observation period of at least 5 years. II. Combined tooth-implant supported FDPs. Clin Oral Implants Res 2004;15:643–653.

37. Tan K, Pjetursson BE, Lang NP, Chan ESY. A systematic review of the survival and complication rates of fixed partial dentures (FDPs) after an observation period of at least 5 years. III. Conventional FDPs. Clin Oral Implants Res 2004;15:654–666.

38. Pjetursson BE, Tan K, Lang NP, Brägger U, Egger M, Zwahlen M. A systematic review of the survival and complication rates of fixed partial dentures (FDPs) after an observation period of at least 5 years. IV. Cantilever or extensions FDPs.Clin Oral Implants Res 2004;15:667–676.

39. Pjetursson BE, Tan WC, Tan K, Brägger U, Zwahlen M, Lang NP. A systematic review of the survival and complication rates of resin-bonded bridges after an observation period of at least 5 years. Clin Oral Implants Res 2008;19:131–141

40. Pjetursson BE, Brägger U, Lang NP, Zwahlen M. Comparison of survival and complication rates of tooth supported fixed partial dentures and implant supported fixed partial dentures and single crowns. Clin Oral Implants Res 2007;18(Suppl 3):97–113.

41. Kirkwood BR, Sterne JAC (eds). Essential Medical Statistics. Ch 24: Poisson regression. Oxford: Blackwell Science, 2003.

42. Kirkwood BR, Sterne JAC (eds). Essential Medical Statistics. Ch 26: Survival analysis: displaying and comparing survival patterns. Oxford: Blackwell Science, 2003.

43. Nyman S, Lindhe J. A longitudinal study of combined periodontal and prosthetic treatment of patients with advanced periodontal disease. J Periodontol 1979;50:163–169.

44. Hämmerle CH, Ungerer MC, Fantoni PC, Brägger U, Bürgin W, Lang NP. Long-term analysis of biologic and technical aspects of fixed partial dentures with cantilevers. Int J Prosthodont 2000;13:409–415.

45. Käyser, AF. Shortened dental arches and oral function. J Oral Rehabil 1981;8:457–462.

46. Fontijn-Tekamp FA, Slagter AP, van der Bilt A, van't Hof MA, Witter DJ, Kalk W et al. Biting and chewing in overdentures, full dentures, and natural dentitions. J Dent Res 2000;79:1519–1524.

47. Kanno T, Carlsson GE. A review of shortened dental arch concept focusing on the work by the Käyser/Nijmegen group. J Oral Rehabil 2006;33:850–862.

# The Free-End Situation – Restore with Partial Removable Dental Prosthesis, Cantilever Fixed Dental Prosthesis, Implant-Supported Crowns or Fixed Dental Prosthesis?

Stefan Holst and Hans Geiselhöringer

## Introduction

The rate of edentulism among the elderly is continually decreasing, and it is anticipated that, by 2010, 75-year-old patients will most likely have, on average, more than 16 residual teeth. Despite the success of preventive treatment and prophylaxis in recent years, the need for prosthetic treatment because of loss of teeth will continue to increase in relation to the age of the patient, particularly for partial edentulism.

A shortened dental arch or distal free-end situation is defined as a dentition with intact anterior teeth and a reduction of occluding pairs of posterior teeth affecting the premolars and/or molars.[1] The consensus is that masticatory efficiency decreases with the number of lost teeth. However, although some authors assert that occlusal stability is at risk after loss of posterior support because of various phenomena (migration of teeth, increased number of occlusal contacts, increased vertical and horizontal overlap, increased tooth mobility, and over-eruption of unopposed teeth), such statements lack firm scientific evidence,[2–5] and it has been reported that a shortened dental arch with three to four occluding pairs of posterior teeth can provide durable occlusal stability. It appears that minor migration of teeth occurs after extractions but teeth will end in stable occlusions

with time.[6] One study revealed that the risk of moderate-to-severe over-eruption of non-opposed molars was relatively low with 24% of posterior teeth present, and that tilting of molars without mesial adjacent teeth was rare in the maxilla and occurred more frequently in the mandible.[7] When evaluating the long-term survival of teeth adjacent to treated or untreated posterior-bounded edentulous spaces, teeth restored with fixed dental prosthesis (FDPs) had a 10-year survival estimate of 92% compared with spaces that remained untreated (81% survival of adjacent teeth); use of partial removable dental protheses (RDPs) resulted in only a 56% survival rate.[8]

A recent review stated that, although there is no linear relationship between tooth loss and dysfunction of the masticatory system, some evidence indicates that a shortened dental arch involving nine to ten pairs of occluding teeth (including the anterior dentition) assures masticatory function, occlusal support, and dental arch stability for most elderly people.[9] Dietary intake for people with this level of oral function is unchanged. Reduction in the number of occlusal units below this level is likely to result in impaired mastication, altered food choices, and reduced oral health related to quality of life.[9]

# Current Therapeutic Options

Therapeutic treatment options have significantly changed in recent years. Although initially the prosthetic armamentarium comprised primarily RDPs or cantilevered FDPs, the introduction of dental implants into everyday routine and their continued improvement has expanded treatment alternatives considerably. Recently, computer-aided design and manufacturing (CAD/CAM) technology has added new possibilities and indicate future trends.

In general, the patient and the clinician can choose between two basic treatment options: either RDPs or FDPs are fabricated for patients with shortened dental arches. An RDP can be retained by either clasps or by extracoronal attachments or it can be designed as an overdenture retained by telescopic copings. An FDP, by comparison, can be tooth retained (cantilevered FDP), supported by an implant–tooth pair, or retained solely with an implant.

The decision for one specific treatment choice depends on the patient's intra- and extraoral clinical situation (remaining and opposing dentition, periodontal status, available hard and soft tissues), the patient's expectations and financial means, and the experience and preferences of the restorative team of clinician and dental technician. When deciding on a treatment option, both the patient and the clinician must be aware of the advantages, limitations, and shortcomings of each method, because there is no single 'best technique' available today.

An extensive review has analyzed the prevalence of prosthetic dental restorations and the frequencies of FDPs and RDPs in the adult populations of several European countries.[10] Although several epidemiological studies were available, the authors concluded that it was difficult to compare the frequencies of dental restorations in different countries because of large variations in study designs. They noted that the selection of fixed or removable restorations depended to a great extent on the patient's age and the number of missing teeth, as well as on socioeconomic factors. The analysis also revealed that the frequency of oral implants is increasing but remains relatively low (2-4%).[10]

In terms of technological advancements and materials, CAD/CAM technology has already had a considerable impact in various areas of dentistry and will continue to do so in the foreseeable future. The technology was introduced to dentistry in the 1970s and is now applied to a broad range of materials, from non-precious alloys to titanium and high-strength ceramic materials. Advantages related to material and manufacturing processes will promote the continuous adoption of CAD/CAM systems over conventional casting techniques. The CAD/CAM technology offers several benefits compared with conventional framework fabrication, including excellent precision, material homogeneity, individual customized design, and ease of fabrication. At the same time, industrialized fabrication methods guarantee standardized quality, reduce cost-intensive manual labor, and provide cost efficiency in the dental laboratory and practice. Application of homogeneous biocompatible materials minimizes material incompatibilities and corrosive phenomena arising from dissimilar metal alloys and interfaces between cast and machined components. Until a few years ago, this technology allowed only fabrication of crown copings, small, three-unit FDPs, or single implant abutments.

New hardware and software refinements and high-strength ceramics have led to the introduction of systems allowing the design and fabrication of FDP frameworks exceeding three units, as well as of bar superstructures for implant-retained restorations. However, CAD/CAM technology is not solely limited to the fabrication of crowns, FDPs, or implant superstructures; research also focuses on alternative techniques for fabrication of RDP frameworks with rapid prototyping technology or laser sintering methods.

# Partial Removable Dental Prostheses

Because of the multitude of influencing variables precluding comparison of results, it is impossible to draw any conclusions from available scientific data about the estimated success rates and long-term clinical survival of RDP designs, abutment teeth survival, and different attachment systems. Restoration of the severely shortened mandibular dental arch has traditionally been carried out with uni- or bilateral free-end RDPs. A review of the prevalence and quality of RDPs indicated that RDPs are still used in all age cohorts, including young adults, in spite of a decline in tooth loss. However, a large number of RDPs have been found to have defects.[11] Although these dentures are provided to restore appearance and masticatory function, they may adversely affect the remaining natural teeth. A number of longitudinal studies have reported an increased incidence of caries and periodontal breakdown when RDPs are worn.[12,13] This outcome becomes especially relevant for elderly patients, for whom there is growing evidence for an association between wearing clasp-retained RDPs and developing root-surface caries.[14–16]

In addition, the biological cost associated with the use of RDPs is offset by several reports indicating a low prevalence of use for mandibular bilateral free-end RDPs. According to these findings, 30–50% of patients never or only occasionally wear their dentures. These patients prefer continued function with a severely shortened lower arch, despite apparent limitations, rather than the use of an RDP.[13,17–19] Treasure and coworkers[20] stated that, given this situation and considering the increasing number of elderly patients with natural teeth, alternative treatment options must be considered. Research has shown that adults who are dentally compromised have poorer diets, but evidence also suggests that although the use of RDPs improves masticatory function and efficacy it does not influence dietary intake.[21,22]

The replacement of absent molar teeth is not necessarily required for a patient's perception of adequate masticatory function. Adequate function was associated with having at least two occluding pairs of posterior teeth on each side of the dental arch.[1]

## Longevity of Partial Removable Dental Prostheses

In terms of the type of attachment for RDPs, there are three basic restorative options available: clasp-retention, double-crown/telescopic-coping, or precision-attachment retention.

Although clasp-retained dentures were shown to have a markedly lower frequency of failures than double-crown systems, the calculated repair costs per event during the observation time were more than twice as high for the former.[23] Studies have shown that teeth adjacent to bounded edentulous spaces restored with an RDP have poor survival estimates (less than 60%) after 10 years.[8]

For abutment teeth with a double crown with clearance fit, the risk of tooth loss was 4% after 5 years and 15% after 10 years for rigid support, and 10% and 24%, respectively, for resilient support.[24]

The survival probability after 5 years was reported to be 95.1% for the telescope-retained RDPs and 95.3% for the abutment teeth. No denture with more than four abutments required replacement. However, approximately 65% of all telescopic dentures required maintenance in the functional period to a varying degree.[25] Despite the high adjustment rates, it was concluded that an RDP retained by telescopic crowns on the residual dentition is an acceptable option to a conventional clasp-retained RDP. Recently, the application of CAD/CAM technology to fabricate primary crowns for telescopic-retained FDPs has become more and more popular. Ease of fabrication, excellent biocompatibility of available materials, and high precision will lead to continued and increased use of such methodology (Figs 10-1 and 10-2).

A clinical investigation of precision-attachment-retained RDPs over a 3-year period showed that 80% of

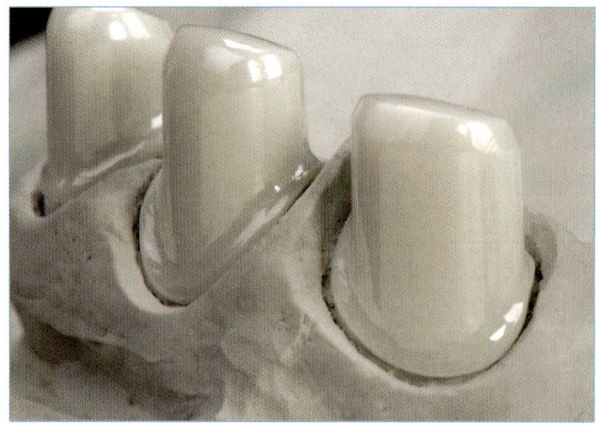

**Fig 10-1** The versatility of the computer-aided design and manufacturing (CAD/CAM) systems allows for easy fabrication of different restorative solutions, from single tooth restorations on natural teeth to large-span fixed dental prosthesis frameworks on implants or teeth. CAD/CAM-generated telescopic copings are an excellent alternative to conventional cast copings (Procera Zirconia, Nobel Biocare, Glattbrugg, Switzerland).

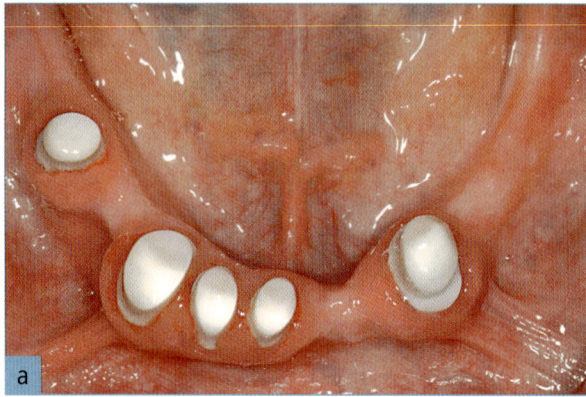

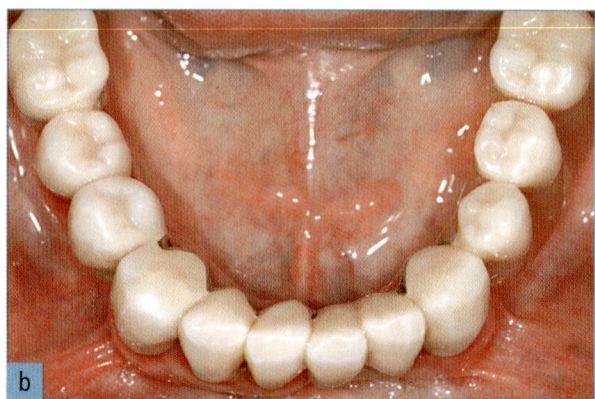

**Fig 10-2a–b** (a) Intraoral occlusal view of a mandibular residual anterior dentition with two distal free-end situations and cemented computer-aided designed and manufactured zirconia copings. (b) The inserted overdenture. (Dentist: Dr. M. Göllner)

the prostheses were functioning well.[26] However, other studies have found failure rates between 35% and 40% after 5 years of clinical use and only a 30.1% survival rate after 8 years.[27] According to longitudinal studies, the lack of success of extracoronal attachments must be attributed primarily to biological and then to technical factors.[28,29] In terms of long-term clinical success, the authors suggest that at least two abutment teeth be splinted when precision attachments are being used[30] and selective adaptation of friction elements is necessary (Figs 10-3 and 10-4).

## Outlook for Removable Solutions

It is unlikely that future developments will eliminate the current biological and technical problems common to RDPs after years of clinical use, such as caries in the abutment tooth, periodontal problems, abutment loosening, or fractures. However, new technology and the implementation of CAD/CAM technology in these areas will increase productivity and reduce the costs of time-consuming framework fabrication procedures. Several techniques are available for the fabrication of frameworks. Scanning of the definitive cast is already performed with a multitude of different optical and tactile scanner systems, with excellent precision. Virtual design of the desired framework followed by techniques such as rapid prototyping or laser sintering will be implemented on a larger scale soon.[31] Laser sintering can be applied on a broader basis as an industrialized process to fabricate non-precious alloy or titanium frameworks directly from CAD data. Other developing techniques are rapid prototyping processes, which may

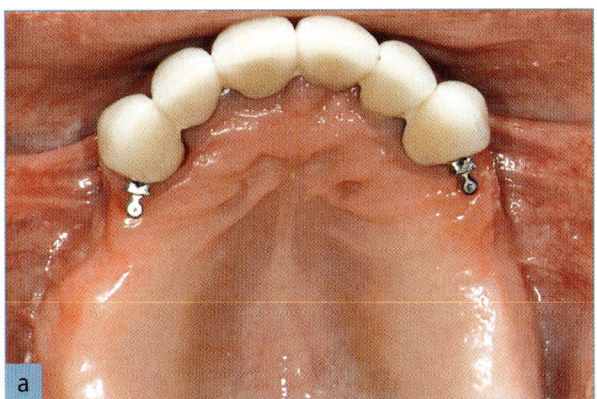

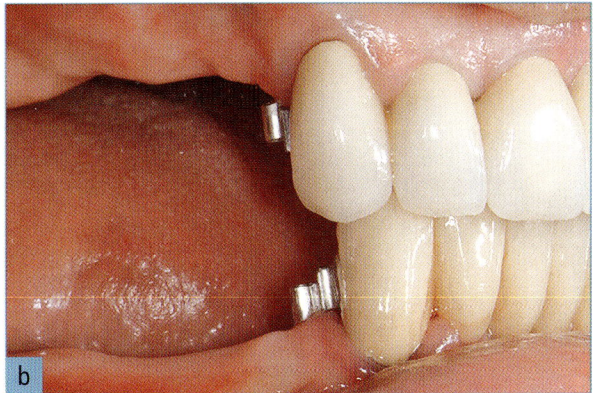

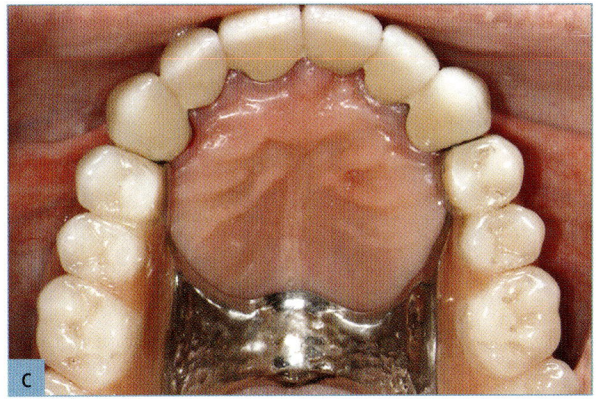

**Fig 10-3a–c** Intraoral occlusal (**a**) and lateral (**b**) views of a maxillary residual dentition restored with a fixed dental prosthesis and distal precision attachments (Mini SG Plus, Cendre Metaux Group, Biel, Switzerland). (**c**) Occlusal view of an inserted partial removable dental prosthesis retained by precision attachments.

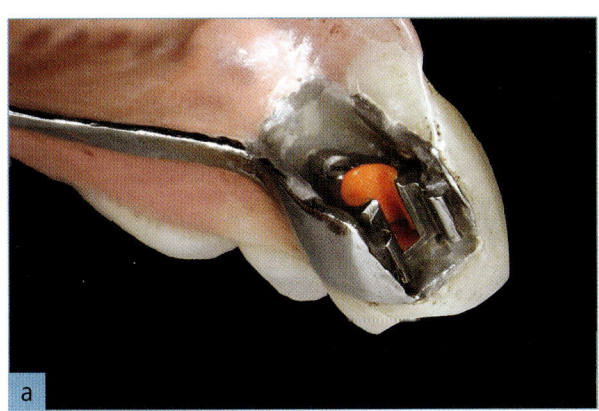

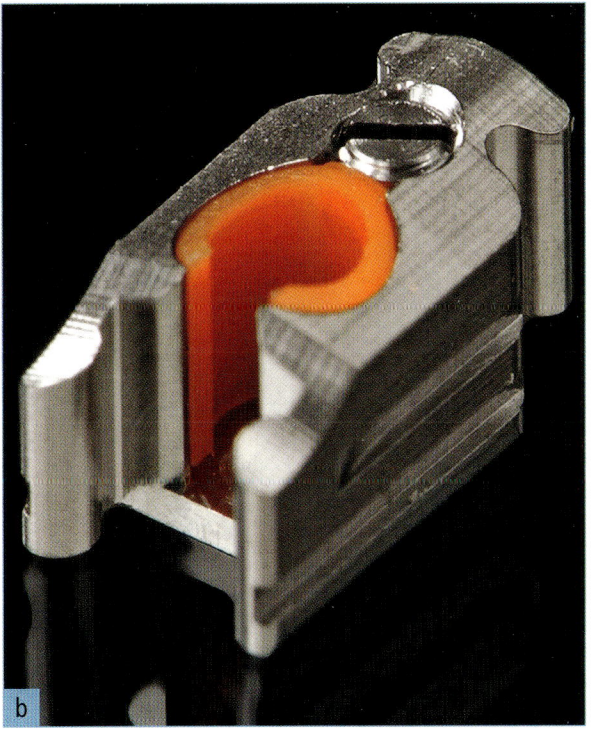

**Fig 10-4a–b** Continuous clinical function leads to wear and subsequent loss of retention (**a**), but this can easily be compensated by using adjustment screws or exchange of plastic inserts, which provide different degrees of retention (**b**) even after years.

be more appropriate in certain CAD/CAM fabrication methods than milling the thin-walled, complex shapes typical of RDP frameworks.[32]

# Fixed Dental Prostheses

The use of fixed prostheses rather than conventional removable prostheses to restore part of the maxillary or mandibular dentition offers the advantage of less bulk, a more normal contour, and in many situations a more profound effect on patient acceptance. The most cost-efficient and easy-to-realize solution, cantilevered resin-bonded FDPs, have shown acceptable survival rates in several studies.[33–35] When comparing long-term success rates of RDPs and cantilever FDPs, a 50% survival rate after 10 years is realistic for RDPs and this simply cannot compete with results reported for cantilever FDPs. In a meta-analysis, cantilever FDPs were calculated to have a 5-year survival of 91.4% and a 10-year survival of 80.3%.[36] Other studies have found up to six-fold higher incidences of caries in RDP groups after 5 years in comparison with distal free-end FDPs.[12,37,38]

## Tooth-Retained Fixed Dental Prostheses

A cantilever is defined as an FDP that has an abutment or abutments at one end with the other end of the pontic remaining unattached. This setup can potentially be biomechanically destructive to the tooth structures if it is not adequately designed or is overextended.

A recent systematic review[29] assessed survival rates and incidences of biological and technical complications of FDPs with or without the incorporation of cantilever units on abutment teeth with severely reduced but healthy periodontal tissue support.[39] The authors concluded that the estimated 10-year survival rates compared favorably with those of FDPs incorporated in patients without severely periodontally compromised dentition.[39] These results were also supported by other publications, which estimated a 10-year survival rate of 89.1% for conventional[40] and 81.8% for cantilever[41] FDPs.

## Implant-Retained Fixed Dental Prostheses

On the basis of studies used for a systematic review, planning of prosthetic rehabilitations for distal free-end situations should preferentially include conventional end-abutment tooth-supported FDPs, solely implant-supported FDPs, or implant-supported single crowns. Only for reasons of anatomical limitations or patient-specific preferences and as a second option should the choice be cantilever tooth-supported FDPs or FDPs supported by a combination of implants and teeth.[36]

Dental implants have become an integral part of dentistry. Scientific research and everyday clinical experience have led to new techniques and improved materials. Conceptual changes have taken place from initial reports of integration of titanium into bone through to principles such as 'letting the restoration be the guide', and to immediate loading protocols and soft tissue preservation techniques for improved esthetic results.[42–44]

Patient demands for improved function, long-term stability, and esthetics are constantly increasing, and success is not defined by mere osseointegration of the implant. Multiple biological, functional, and biomechanical aspects must be addressed, and potential problems must be identified preoperatively. Factors having a direct influence on success or failure include the amount of available alveolar ridge, the soft tissue type, the correct positioning of the implant in all three dimensions, the design and material of the implant abutment, and selection of the definitive crown.[44,45] Contingent on the initial clinical situation, the practitioner is challenged with an array of treatment options that must carefully be considered to provide the patient with the best solution. The primary decision is the choice between a screw-retained or cemented solution and whether or not to splint multiple implants.

## Tooth–Implant-Retained Fixed Dental Prostheses

The cantilever resin-bonded FDP on natural teeth in distal free-end situations essentially extends but maintains a shortened dental arch. Prior to the introduction of dental implants, this outcome was sufficient to achieve a general improvement in appearance and function of shortened dental arches.[46] To reduce costs, the clinical alternative of tooth–implant-supported FDPs is applied in many cases. Although some studies report sufficient and predictable clinical success rates,[47–49] research clearly reveals that a rigid connection between tooth and implant is necessary, rather than a non-rigid connection, if a prosthesis is connected to both tooth and implant.[50–54] These studies illustrate the fact that there are manifold biological and functional interactions that have yet to be fully explained for tooth–implant-supported FDPs, as demonstrated by intrusion of the abutment teeth where there are non-rigid connections.[52,53] Based on these studies, it must be assumed that, after 5 years, approximately 10% of the tooth–implant-supported FDPs will have been subjected to at least one technical modification such as renewal, reintegration, repair of veneer fracture, or fracture of frame. After as few as 3 years, connection-related complications (abutment or occlusal screw loosening, loss of cementation) occurred in approximately 8% of patients.[48] The high incidence of intrusion and non-scheduled patient visits suggest that alternative treatments that avoid connecting implants to teeth may be indicated.[52]

A review of the literature found that survival rates of implants and reconstructions in FDPs supported by combined tooth-implants were lower than those reported for FDPs solely supported by implants.[41] Therefore, planning of prosthetic rehabilitation may preferentially include solely implant-supported FDPs. However, anatomical aspects, patient-centered issues, and risk assessments of the residual dentition may still justify reconstructions supported by combined tooth-implants. It was evident from the present review of the literature that such combination support for FDPs has not been studied to a great extent and that there is a definitive need for more longitudinal studies examining these reconstructions (Figs 10-5 and 10-6).

## Future Choice of Retention for Fixed Dental Prostheses

In the future, implant-retained FDPs or single crowns to restore shortened dental archs will become the predominant form of restoration. The clinical success rates, the high predictability, and a reduction of costs, as well as the implementation of implantology into dental school curricula, will lead to more-frequent and sooner implant placement when a tooth is deemed non-restorable. When high occlusal loads are applied in the posterior region, high stresses on the restoration result. Depending on the amount of lost vertical bone height and the length of the implant, varying crown-to-implant ratios may result. Although it has been stated that the crown-to-implant ratio cannot exceed 1, this assertion does not correspond to clinical reality in many instances because of atrophy of the alveolar ridges after periodontal breakdown or long-time edentulism. Studies have shown no crestal bone loss in situations where biomechanically unfavorable non-axial loading forces were applied to a restoration, which is similar to the forces observed in high crown-to-implant ratios.[55] In fact, those implant restorations with higher crown-to-implant ratios showed a statistically significant lower crestal bone loss over time. This biological phenomenon does not preclude possible mechanical problems, such as recurrent screw loosening or screw fractures, which may result if a long cantilever arm exists.

To reduce risk factors such as overload, crestal bone loss, and component and metal fatigue, splinting multiple dental implants has been recommended in the prosthetic rehabilitation of implants placed in the posterior jaw, especially where there is immediate loading.[56–59] The use of single units, however, offers a more comfortable prosthetic approach by eliminating additional laboratory steps and improving fit of the framework and access for oral hygiene. The clinical success of this approach is supported by several authors, who suggest that single-implant restorations can be a viable option for the rehabilitation of the posterior jaw.[60–63] Nevertheless, when a large crown-to-implant ratio is unavoidable, splinting of the implant restorations can

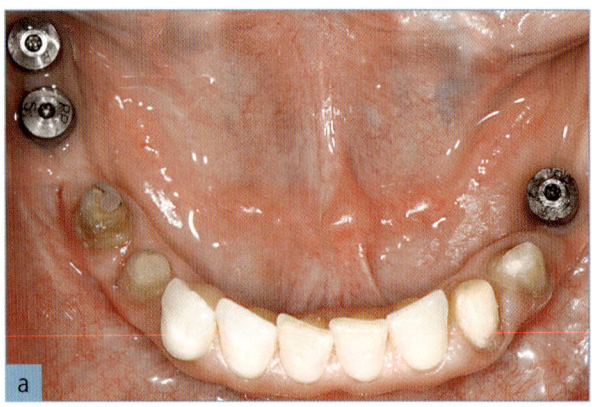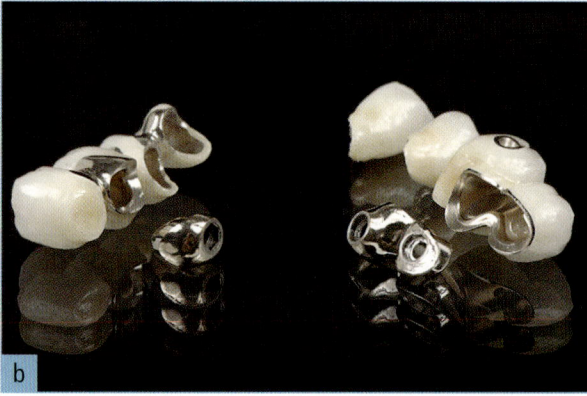

**Fig 10-5a–b**  Prior to the advancements in computer-aided design and manufacturing (CAD/CAM), cast nobel alloy abutments were considered the gold standard for implant-retained fixed dental prostheses. With the introduction of high-strength oxide ceramics such as zirconia, these materials and CAD/CAM techniques are used routinely because of their advantages over casting techniques.

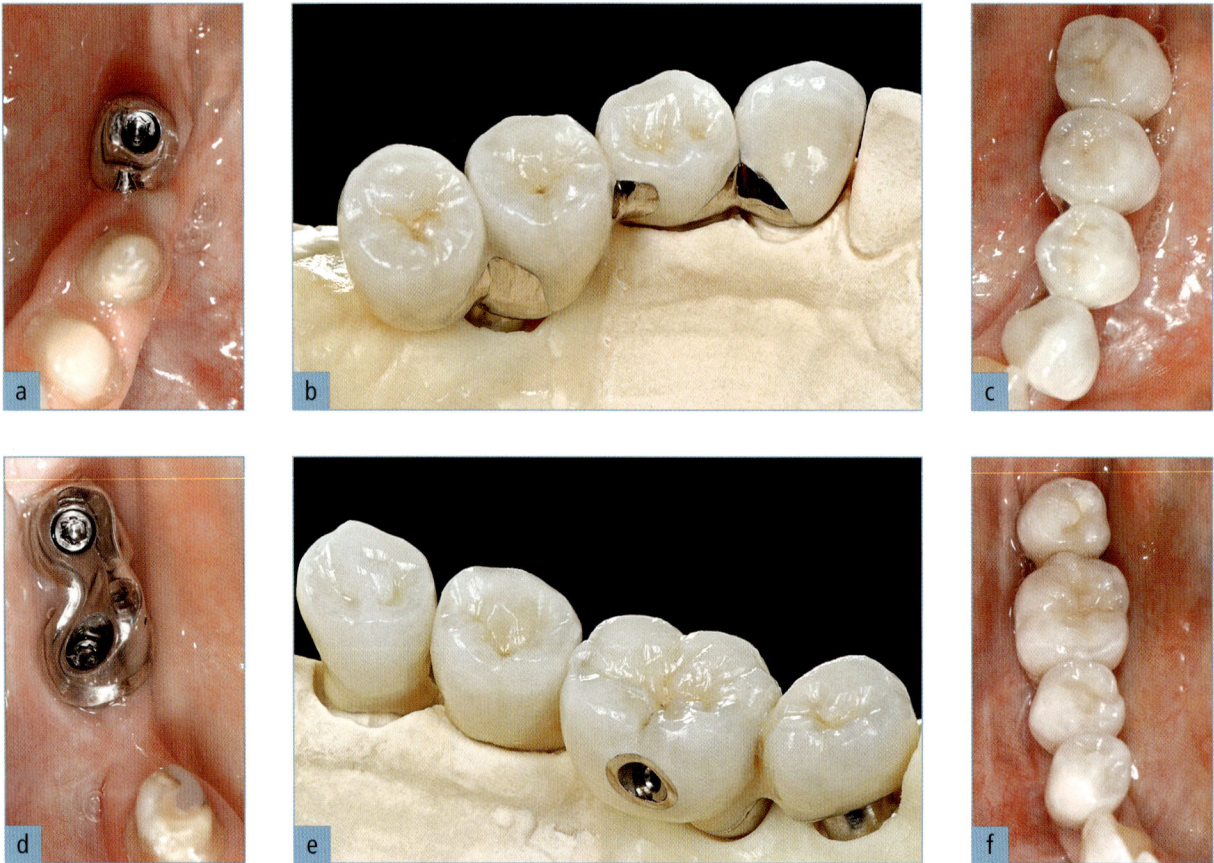

**Fig 10-6a–f**  **(a–c)** If an implant needs to be connected to natural teeth, a rigid connection is mandatory. **(d–f)** Cast solutions are still the material of choice if the fixed dental prostheses are retained by horizontal screws. (Technician: Mr M Bergler)

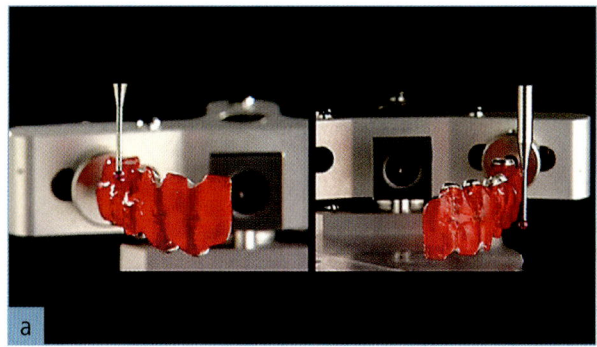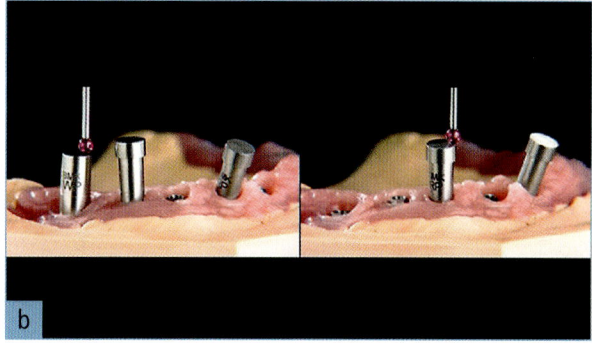

**Fig 10-7a–b** **(a)** Tactile scanning (Procera Forte Scanner, Nobel Biocare) of an implant framework. **(b)** The resin mock-up is scanned from both the occlusal and intaglio surface, followed by scanning of the implant position on the definitive cast. Scanning with a probe ensures precise data matching.

provide a better distribution of the occlusal forces among the implants.[56] The major drawback, which favors single or small-unit restorations, has always been the difficulty in achieving proper fit of casted frameworks. Today, CAD/CAM-generated FDP frameworks on implants provide an excellent clinical solution in distal free-end situations, with unrivaled biocompatibility and precision of fabricated components (Fig. 10-7). The advantages of these frameworks are similar to those that apply to single-implant abutments, described above. Specific attention must be directed to the proper design of these frameworks to achieve optimal support for the porcelain veneering materials.

## Abutment Material

The abutment design and the material to restore an implant-retained single-tooth or an implant-retained FDP must fulfill some basic requirements. Today, multiple abutment types are available. Various studies have demonstrated successful application of ceramic and titanium abutments in terms of acceptable soft tissue and marginal bone stability. A study has examined different abutment materials and their influence on soft tissue barriers surrounding dental implants.[64] Results revealed that the type of material used affected both the height and the quality of the tissue. Titanium and ceramic abutments permitted the formation of a mucosal attachment, while gold alloy and metal-ceramic abutments led to soft tissue recession and crestal bone resorption.[64]

Similar findings were observed in studies *in vitro*, which confirmed the finding of reduced plaque and bacterial adhesion on titanium or zirconia abutments.[65,66]

Despite superior fracture strengths of metal-ceramic crowns cemented on to titanium abutments, compared with all-ceramic crowns cemented on to ceramic abutments, the use of all-ceramic materials is increasing rapidly. Ceramic abutments have an excellent esthetic potential when associated guidelines are meticulously followed, and they offer biocompatibility and long-term stability. The first all-ceramic abutments were available in only one size. Their disadvantages were the time-consuming preparation in the laboratory and finishing in the dental office and the risk of microcracks, which could result in fracture during preparation or placement. Currently, the most promising and interesting material for abutment manufacturing is zirconia. Stabilized zirconium oxide ($ZrO_2$) is a highly biocompatible ceramic material.[67–69] It provides strength values that allow application in any location of the mouth and, despite few long-term clinical data, ongoing studies are providing encouraging results (Fig 10-8).

## Abutment Manufacturing

The clinician may choose between two abutment types for implant-retained FDPs: prefabricated or customized abutments. The primary objectives must always be support of the surrounding tissues, optimal design to support the restoration without impairing hygiene mainte-

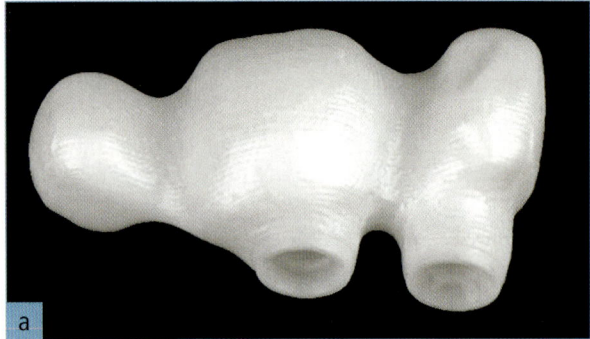

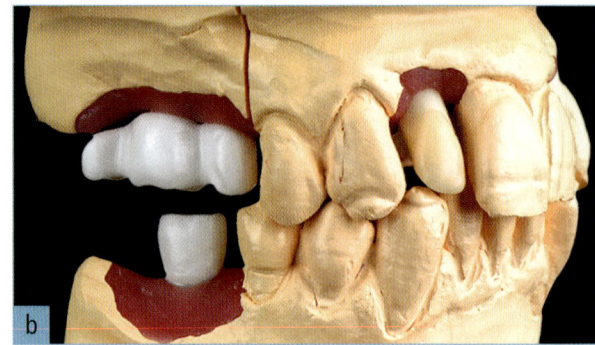

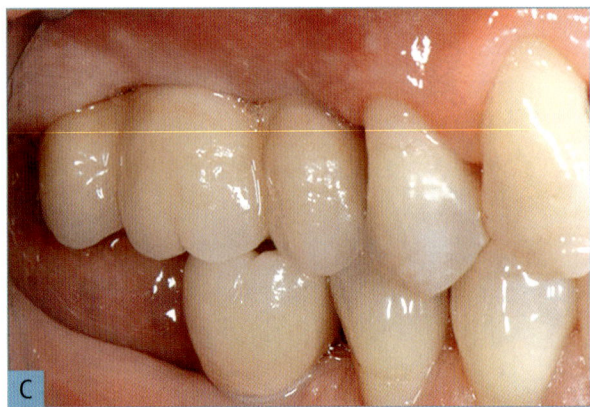

**Fig 10-8a–c** The outstanding biocompatibility of zirconia makes it the material of choice for implant abutments in close contact with the surrounding tissues. Even in patients with periodontitis, zirconia minimizes plaque and bacterial accumulation on the surfaces and provides soft tissue stability. **(a)** Material properties of yttria-stabilized zirconium oxide allow fabrication of distal extensions. **(b,c)** Versatility of the systems allows fabrication of implant-retained single-tooth restorations or multiunit fixed dental prosthesis frameworks (Procera Implant Bridge Zirconia, Nobel Biocare) with maximum precision and ease of fabrication.

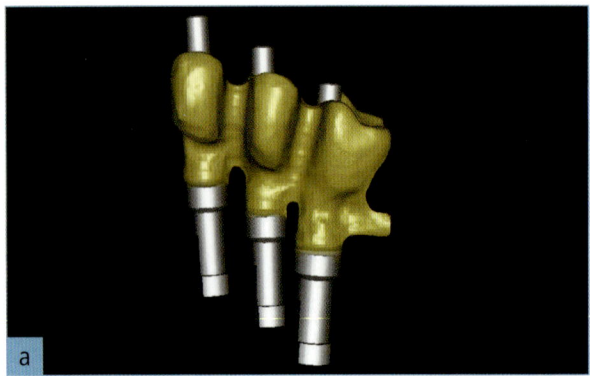

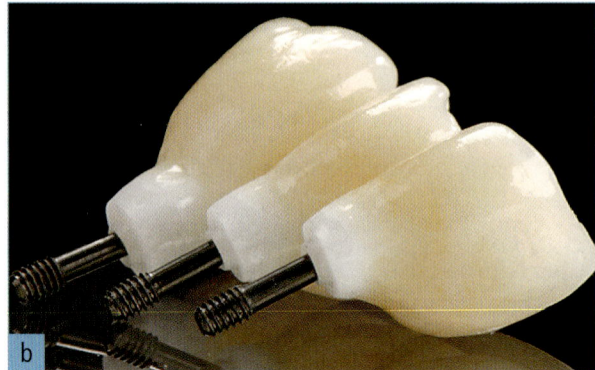

**Fig 10-9a–b** **(a)** Virtual design (Procera Software 2.0) of the implant-retained framework provides maximum support of the veneering ceramics without the need for major adjustments after milling and sintering. **(b)** The optimal tissue adaptation to zirconia is especially beneficial in situations with deep implant placement.

nance, and anatomical design to allow for proper support of the veneering ceramics. These can only be achieved if the abutment is custom made. Again, the advantage of CAD/CAM-machined abutments is their material homogeneity and material properties, individual custom design, and ease of fabrication (Fig 10-9). Their application can avoid problems such as incorrect abutment selection, and concerns about dissimilar metals and interfaces between cast and machined components can be eliminated. Because no controlled clinical trials are currently available to define acceptable microgaps that do not compromise restoration longevity and implant survival, meticulous and accurate implant prosthodontic procedures and the appropriate use of advanced laboratory techniques are recommended to obtain a precise fit.

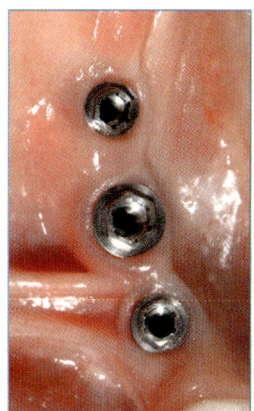

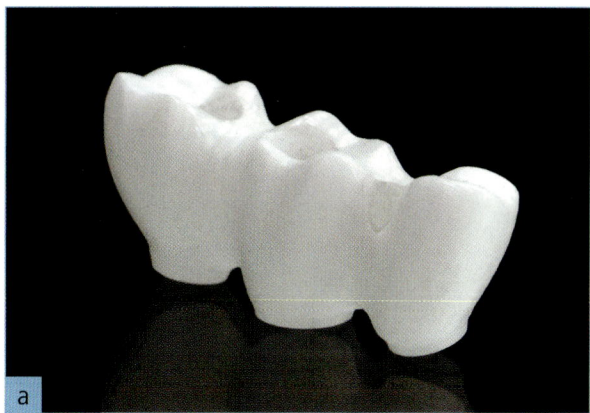

**Fig 10-10** Intraoral occlusal view of three dental implants after tooth extraction to restore the distal free end.

**Fig 10-11a–b** (a) A zirconia superstructure prior to veneering that was custom-made using computer-aided design and manufacturing. Anatomical design of the framework ensures adequate support of the veneering ceramics and improves long-term clinical success. (b) Procera Implant Bridge can be used on different implant systems and platforms (internal or external) and be veneered with any porcelain that meets the coefficient of thermal linear expansion of zirconia.

## Screw-Retained Crown versus Cemented Crown

Whether an implant-retained crown or FDP is cemented or the abutment–crown complex is screw retained depends on the preference of the clinician and the positioning of the implant. If the screw access is favorable (in the central fossae of a posterior molar or premolar), a screw-retained restoration may be fabricated. Porcelain is directly fired on to the abutment, and the abutment–crown complex can be screwed onto the implant. This type of restoration offers the possibility for retrieval or retightening, and for reassessing the abutment screw. Another advantage is the absence of cement between the abutment and the crown. Possible complications of such restorations may be chipping of the ceramic veneering owing to the discontinuous porcelain, which can be easily corrected. Cement-retained restorations on individual ceramic abutments not only allow

compensation of misaligned implants but also can be treated like natural teeth. If a screw-retained abutment is chosen, the height of the interproximal crown margin should be located just below the gingival margin to allow for complete removal of cement, because the presence of cement may compromise soft tissue health.[67,44]

Fabrication is easier for cement-retained prostheses than for screw-retained prostheses because traditional prosthetic techniques can be applied and there is no need for special training of laboratory technicians. The main disadvantage of cemented prostheses is the difficulty of retrievability. Both types of prosthesis – screw retained and cemented – present certain advantages and disadvantages. The clinician, therefore, should be aware of the limitations and disadvantages of each type in order to select the appropriate method for a given clinical situation (Figs 10-10 to 10-14).

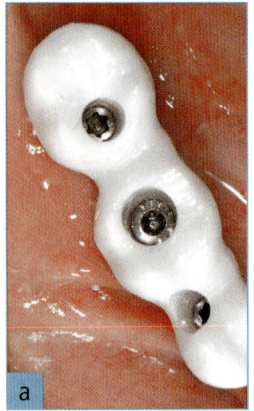
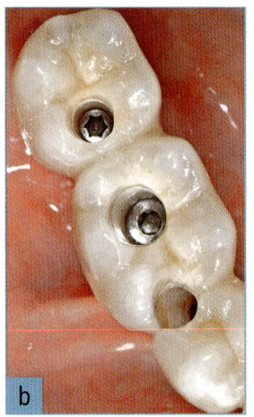

**Fig 10-12a–b** The properties of zirconia allow fabrication of restorations according to patient's expectations and financial means. **(a)** Implants may be restored with a screw-retained zirconia fixed dental prosthesis (Procera Implant Bridge Zirconia). **(b)** This is directly veneered with porcelain. *(Courtesy of Zenline Dental, Bruchköbel)*

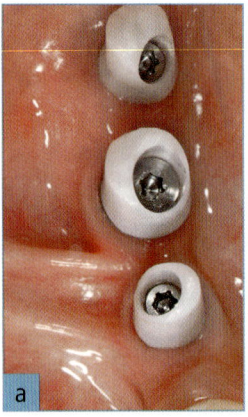
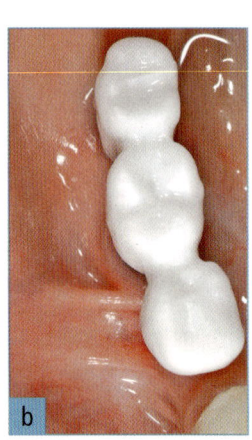
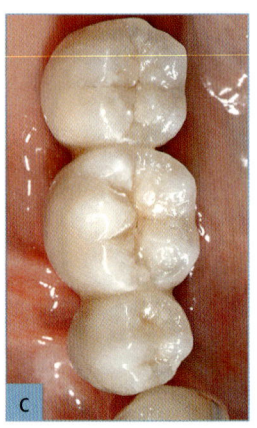

**Fig 10-13a–c** An alternative treatment solution is the insertion of single zirconia abutments **(a)** for cementation of single crowns or a fixed dental prosthesis **(b,c)**. *(Courtesy of Zenline Dental, Bruchköbel)*

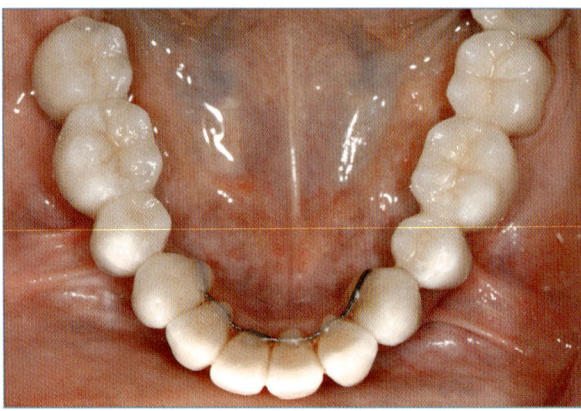

**Fig 10-14** Both solutions, screw or cement retained, provide maximum precision, material homogeneity, and biocompatibility for the patient. (Technician: E.A. Hegenbarth)

In an extensive overview of clinical complications with implants and implant prostheses, Goodacre and coworkers[70] found that approximately 22% of all prosthetic interventions were related to screw loosening or screw fractures, followed by problems with the veneering ceramic materials. These results must be regarded with caution, however, because studies were included from as early as 1981. Because of the dramatic improvements in both implant and prosthetic options and techniques, as well as the increase in knowledge, these overviews must be regarded with care. A trend to improvement can be clearly seen in terms of the prevalence of screw loosening. The authors found an average screw loosening of 6% up to 45% with single-implant crowns. The overall average was 25% screw loosening for single-implant-retained crowns, but when the authors assessed the six most recent studies, this fell to 8%, indicating a substantial improvement with new screw design.

## Outlook for Fixed Solutions

Today, the number of abutments or retainers can be increased by means of dental implants, which facilitate the desired treatment option in many instances. If more teeth have to be replaced and financial means are a limiting factor, a removable restoration may be favored over fixed restorations, which become more expensive with an increasing number of units. The prognosis for the potential abutment teeth will also influence this decision-making process. In addition to these clinical and economic aspects, other factors that influence decision making include the clinician's level of training and/or specialization and personal preferences. However, the introduction of industrialized fabrication processes into dentistry, such as CAD/CAM technology, centralized fabrication of frameworks, three-dimensional treatment planning for implant therapy, and new materials for bone reconstruction, will considerably reduce the costs of highly predictable and long-term stable clinical results with dental implants.

The complete virtual treatment from surgical planning to restorative realization will be the major trend of the future. Not only will the clinician and technician be able to visualize the final treatment outcome prior to initiation of treatment but also CAD/CAM technology will allow realization of multiple types of restoration. New material development and the improvement and understanding of currently used ones will continue.

## Acknowledgements

The authors would like to express their gratitude to Dr. A. Felderhoff and Prof. Dr. E. Nkenke for conducting the surgeries, Mr M. Bergler, University of Pennsylvania, for fabricating the restoration of Figs 10-5 and 10-6, and to Zenline Dental, Bruchköbel, for fabricating the restorations shown in Figs 10-11–10-14.

# References

1. Käyser AF. Shortened dental arches and oral function. J Oral Rehabil 1981;8:457–462.
2. Southard TE, Southard KA, Stiles RN. Factors influencing the anterior component of occlusal force. J Biomech 1990;23:1199–1207.
3. Johansson A, Haraldson T, Omar R, Kiliaridis S, Carlsson GE. An investigation of some factors associated with occlusal tooth wear in a selected high-wear sample. Scand J Dent Res 1993;101:407–415.
4. Martinez-Canut P, Carrasquer A, Magán R, Lorca A. A study on factors associated with pathologic tooth migration. J Clin Periodontol 1997;24:492–497.
5. Mohl ND. Introduction to occlusion. In: Mohl ND, Zarb GA, Carlsson GE, Rugh JD (eds). A Textbook of Occlusion. Chicago: Quintessence, 1988:15–23.
6. Witter DJ, Creugers NHJ, Kreulen CM, de Haan AFJ. Occlusal stability in shortened dental arches. J Dent Res 2001;80:432–436.
7. Kiliaridis S, Lyka I, Friede H, Carlsson GE, Ahlqwist M. Vertical position, rotation, and tipping of molars without antagonists. Int J Prosthodont. 2000;13:480–486.
8. Aquilino SA, Shugars DA, Bader JD, White BA. Ten-year survival rates of teeth adjacent to treated and untreated posteriorbounded edentulous spaces. J Prosthet Dent 2001;85:455–460.
9. Gotfredsen K, Walls AWG. What dentition assures oral function? Clin Oral Implants Res 2007;18(Suppl 3):34–45.
10. Zitzmann NU, Hagmann E, Weiger R. What is the prevalence of various types of prosthetic dental restorations in Europe? Clin Oral Implants Res 2007;18(Suppl 3):20–33.
11. Hummel SK, Wilson MA, Marker VA, Nunn ME. Quality of removable partial dentures worn by the adult US population. J Prosthet Dent 2002;88:37–43.
12. Budtz-Jorgensen E, Isidor F. A 5-year longitudinal study of cantilevered fixed dental prosthesis compared with removable partial dentures in a geriatric population. J Prosthet Dent 1990;64:42–47.
13. Miyamoto T, Morgano SM, Kumagai T, Jones JA, Nunn ME. Treatment history of teeth in relation to the longevity of the teeth and their restorations: outcomes of teeth treated and maintained for 15 years. J Prosthet Dent 2007;97:150–156.
14. Wright PS, Hellyer PH, Beighton D, Heath R, Lynch E. Relationship of removable partial denture use to root caries in an older population. Int J Prosthodont 1992;5:39–46.
15. Steele JG, Walls AW, Murray JJ. Partial dentures as an independent indicator of root caries risk in a group of older adults. Gerodontology 1997;14:67–74.
16. Nevalainen MJ, Närhi TO, Ainamo A. A 5-year follow-up study on the prosthetic rehabilitation of the elderly in Helsinki, Finland. J Oral Rehabil 2004;31:647–652.
17. Wetherell JD, Smales RJ. Partial denture failures: a long-term clinical survey. J Dent 1980;8:333–340.
18. Jepson NJA, Thomason JM, Steele JG. The influence of denture design on patient acceptance of partial dentures. Br Dent J 1995;178:296–300.
19. Kapur KK, Deupree R, Dent RJ, Hasse AL. A randomized clinical trial of two basic removable partial denture designs. Part I: Comparisons of five-year success rates and periodontal health. J Prosthet Dent 1994;72:268–282.

20. Treasure E, Kelly M, Nuttall N, Nunn J, Bradnock G, White D. Factors associated with oral health: a multivariate analysis of results from the 1998 Adult Dental Health survey. Br Dent J. 2001;190:60–68.

21. Papas AS, Palmer CA, Rounds MC, Russell RM. The effects of denture status on nutrition. Spec Care Dent 1998;18:17–25.

22. Gunne J. Masticatory ability in patients with removable dentures. A clinical study of masticatory efficiency, subjective experience of masticatory performance and dietary intake. Swed Dent J Suppl 1985;27:1–107.

23. Hofmann E, Behr M, Handel G. Frequency and costs of technical failures of clasp- and double crown-retained removable partial dentures. Clin Oral Invest 2002;6:104–108.

24. Wenz HJ, Hertrampf K, Lehmann KM. Clinical longevity of removable partial dentures retained by telescopic crowns: outcome of the double crown with clearance fit. Int J Prosthodont. 2001;14:207–213.

25. Wöstmann B, Balkenhol M, Weber A, Ferger P, Rehmann P. Long-term analysis of telescopic crown retained removable partial dentures: survival and need for maintenance. J Dent 2007;35:939–945.

26. Zajc D, Wichmann M, Reich S, Eitner S. A prefabricated precision attachment: 3 years of experience with the Swiss Mini-SG system. A prospective clinical study. Int J Prosthodont 2007;20:432–434.

27. Studer SP, Mäder C, Stahel W, Schärer P. A retrospective study of combined fixed-removable reconstructions with their analysis of failures. J Oral Rehab 1998;25:513–526.

28. Owall B. Precision attachment-retained partial dentures. Part 1: Technical long-term study. Int J Prosthodont 1991;4:249–253.

29. Owall B. Precision attachment-retained removable partial dentures. Part 2: Long-term study of ball attachments. Int J Prosthodont 1995;8:21–26.

30. Altay OT, Tsolka P, Preiskle HW. Abutment teeth with extracoronal attachments: the effects of splinting on tooth movement. Int J Prosthodont 1990;3:441–448.

31. Williams RJ, Bibb R, Eggbeer D, Collis J. Use of CAD/CAM technology to fabricate a removable partial denture framework. J Prosthet Dent 2006;96:96–99.

32. Williams RJ, Bibb R, Rafik T. A technique for fabricating patterns for removable partial denture frameworks using digitized casts and electronic surveying. J Prosthet Dent 2004;91:85–88.

33. Hussey DL, Linden GJ. The clinical performance of cantilevered resin-bonded bridgework. J Dent 1996;24:251–256.

34. Hämmerle CH, Ungerer MC, Fantoni PC, Brägger U, Bürgin W, Lang NP. Long-term analysis of biologic and technical aspects of fixed dental prosthesis with cantilevers. Int J Prosthodont 2000;13:409–415.

35. Thomason JM, Moynihan PJ, Steen N, Jepson NJ. Time to survival for the restoration of the shortened lower dental arch. J Dent Res 2007;86:646–650.

36. Pjetursson BE, Brägger U, Lang NP, Zwahlen M. Comparison of survival and complication rates of tooth supported fixed dental prostheses (FDPs) and implant supported FDPs and single crowns (SCs). Clin Oral Implants Res 2007;18(Suppl 3): 97–113.

37. Wagner B, Kern M. Clinical evaluation of removable partial dentures 10 years after insertion: success rates, hygienic problems, and technical failures. Clin Oral Invest 2000;4:74–80.

38. Jepson NJ, Moynihan PJ, Kelly PJ, Watson GW, Thomason JM. Caries incidence following restoration of shortened dental arches in a randomized controlled trial. Br Dent J 2001;191:140–144.

39. Lulic M, Brägger U, Lang NP, Zwahlen M, Salvi GE. Ante's (1926) law revisited: a systematic review on survival rates and complications of fixed dental prostheses (FDPs) on severely reduced periodontal tissue support. Clin. Oral Impl. Res 18 (Suppl 3), 2007; 63–72.

40. Tan K, Pjetursson BE, Lang NP, Chan ES. A systematic review of the survival and complication rates of fixed dental prosthesis (FDPs) after an observation period of at least 5 years. Clin Oral Implants Res 2004;15:654–666.

41. Pjetursson BE, Tan K, Lang NP, Brägger U, Egger M, Zwahlen M. A systematic review of the survival and complication rates of fixed dental prosthesis (FDPs) after an observation period of at least 5 years. Clin Oral Implants Res 2004;15:667–676.

42. Branemark PI, Adell R, Breine U, Hansson BO, Lindstrom J, Ohlsson A. Intra-osseous anchorage of dental prostheses. I. Experimental studies. Scand J Plast Reconstr Surg 1969;3:81–100.

43. Garber DA. The esthetic dental implant: letting restoration be the guide. J Am Dent Assoc 1995;12:319–325.

44. Belser UC, Schmid B, Higginbottom F, Buser D. Outcome analysis of implant restorations located in the anterior maxilla: a review of the recent literature. Int J Oral Maxillofac Implants 2004;19(Suppl):30–42.

45. Block M, Finger I, Castellon P, Lirettle D. Single tooth immediate provisional restoration of dental implants: techniques and early results. J Oral Maxillofac Surg 2004;62:1131–1138.

46. Witter DJ, de Haan AF, Käyser AF, van Rossum GM. A 6-year follow-up study of oral function in shortened dental arches. Part II: Craniomandibular dysfunction and oral comfort. J Oral Rehabil 1994;21:353–366.

47. Kindberg H, Gunne J, Kronström M. Tooth- and implant-supported prostheses: a retrospective clinical follow-up up to 8 years. Int J Prosthodont 2001;14:575–581.

48. Nickenig HJ, Spiekermann H, Wichmann M, Andreas SK, Eitner S. Survival and complication rates of combined tooth-implant-supported fixed and removable partial dentures. Int J Prosthodont 2008;21:131–137.

49. Lindh T. Should we extract teeth to avoid tooth-implant combinations? J Oral Rehabil 2008;35(Suppl 1):44–54.

50. Lindh T, Dahlgren S, Gunnarsson K, Josefsson T, Nilson H, Wilhelmsson P, et al. Tooth-implant supported fixed prostheses: a retrospective multicenter study. Int J Prosthodont 2001;14:321–328.

51. Naert IE, Duyck JA, Hosny MM, van Steenberghe D. Freestanding and tooth-implant connected prostheses in the treatment of partially edentulous patients. Part I: An up to 15-years clinical evaluation. Clin Oral Implants Res 2001;12:237–344.

52. Block MS, Lirette D, Gardiner D, Li L, Finger IM, Hochstedler J, et al. Prospective evaluation of implants connected to teeth. Int J Oral Maxillofac Implants 2002;17:473–487.

53. Lang NP, Pjetursson BE, Tan K, Brägger U, Egger M, Zwahlen M. A systematic review of the survival and complication rates of fixed dental prosthesis (FDPs) after an observation period of at least 5 years. II. Combined tooth–implant-supported FDPs. Clin Oral Implants Res 2004;15:643–653.

54. Srinivasan M, Padmanabhan TV. Intrusion in implant–tooth-supported fixed prosthesis: an in vitro photoelastic stress analysis. Indian J Dent Res 2008;19:6–11.

55. Blanes RJ, Bernard JP, Blanes ZM, Belser UC. A 10-year prospective study of ITI dental implants placed in the posterior region. II: Influence of the crown-to-implant ratio and different prosthetic treatment modalities on crestal bone loss. Clin Oral Implants Res 2007;18:707–714.

56. Rangert BR, Sullivan RM, Jemt TM. Load factor control for implants in the posterior partially edentulous segment. Int J Oral Maxillofac Implants 1997;12:360–370.

57. van den Bogaerde L, Pedretti G, Dellacasa P, Mozzati M, Rangert B, Wendelhag I. Early function of splinted implants in maxillas and posterior mandibles, using Brånemark System TiUnite implants: an 18-month prospective clinical multicenter study. Clin Implant Dent Relat Res 2004;6:121–129.

58. Misch CE, Steignga J, Barboza E, Misch-Dietsh F, Cianciola LJ, Kazor C. Short dental implants in posterior partial edentulism: a multicenter retrospective 6-year case series study. J Periodontol 2006;77:1340–1347.

59. Bergkvist G, Simonsson K, Rydberg K, Johansson F, Dérand T. A finite element analysis of stress distribution in bone tissue surroundinguncoupled or splinted dental implants. Clin Implant Dent Relat Res 2008;10:40–46.

60. Abboud M, Koeck B, Stark H, Wahl G, Paillon R. Immediate loading of single-tooth implants in the posterior region. Int J Oral Maxillofac Implants 2005;20:61–68.

61. Glauser R, Ruhstaller P, Windisch S, Zembic A, Lundgren A, Gottlow J, et al. Immediate occlusal loading of Brånemark System TiUnite implants placed predominantly in soft bone: 4-year results of a prospective clinical study. Clin Implant Dent Relat Res 2005;7(Suppl 1):S52–S59.

62. Renouard F, Nisand D. Short implants in the severely resorbed maxilla: a 2-year retrospective clinical study. Clin Implant Dent Relat Res 2005;7(Suppl 1):104–110.

63. Glauser R, Zembic A, Ruhstaller P, Windisch S. Five-year results of implants with an oxidized surface placed predominantly in soft quality bone and subjected to immediate occlusal loading. J Prosthet Dent 2007;97(Suppl 6):S59–S68.

64. Abrahamsson I, Berglundh T, Glantz PO, Lindhe J. The mucosal attachment at different abutments: An experimental study in dogs. J Clin Periodontol 1998;25:721–727.

65. Rasperini G, Maglione M, Cocconcelli P, Simion M. In vivo early plaque formation on pure titanium and ceramic abutments: a comparative microbiological and SEM analysis. Clin Oral Implants Res 1998;9:357–364.

66. Rimondini L, Cerroni L, Carrassi A, Torricelli P. Bacterial colonization of zirconia ceramic surfaces: an in vitro and in vivo study. Int J Oral Maxillofac Implants 2002;17:793–798.

67. Kucey BK, Fraser DC. The Procera abutment: the fifth generation abutment for dental implants. J Can Dent Assoc 2000;66:445–449.

68. Piconi C, Maccauro G. Zirconia as a ceramic biomaterial. Biomaterials 1999;20:1–25.

69. Cho HW, Dong JK, Jin TH, Oh SC, Lee HH, Lee JW. A study on the fracture strength of implant-supported restorations using milled ceramic abutments and all-ceramic crowns. Int J Prosthodont 2002;15:9–13.

70. Goodacre CJ, Bernal G, Rungcharassaeng K, Kan JY. Clinical complications with implants and implant prostheses. J Prosthet Dent 2003;90:121–132.

# The Complete Denture – Museum Object with a Future?

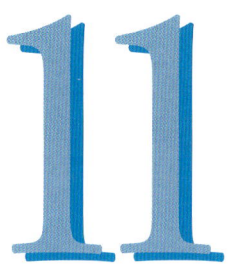

Sandro Palla and Ina Nitschke

*The complete denture is more than just 28 artificial teeth in an acrylic resin piece.*

## Introduction

There are a few well-established facts about edentulism and complete dentures. The first is that edentulism is generally decreasing in all industrialized countries. The second is that chewing efficiency, the objective measure of food comminution, is markedly decreased in the majority of complete denture wearers compared with dentate subjects and patients with dental or implant-supported overdentures. The third is that there is no correlation between chewing efficiency and chewing ability, where chewing efficiency refers to the food comminution degree while chewing ability refers to the subject's appraisal of his/her mastication. The fourth is that, in general, patients do not change their nutritional status even when they feel that chewing has been improved by renewing the old denture or by replacing it with an implant-supported overdenture. The fifth is that the majority of patients with a complete denture are satisfied with their denture no matter how good it is, and approximately 10–15% is dissatisfied even if their denture is perfectly constructed. The sixth and last fact is that the

quality of life of edentulous patients improves with mandibular-supported overdentures. These facts, in particular the first and sixth, seem to indicate that the time for complete dentures, at least in industrialized countries, will soon be over, thus supporting the title suggested by the book editor for this chapter. However, the question is whether this is a correct or a premature conclusion.

## Needs for Complete Dentures

In Switzerland, edentulism decreased from 5.7% to 3.1% within a 10-year period (1992 to 2002), with a two-fold reduction in every age group: from 1.1% to 0.4% in those aged 35–44 years, from 4.9% to 2.2% in those aged 45–54 years, from 12.6% to 5.5% in those aged 55–65 years, and from 26.8% to 13.8% in those aged 65–74 years. Edentulism was more pronounced in the maxilla than in the mandible and in subjects with lower educational and socioeconomic levels.[1,2] However, more than just educational and socioeconomic factors are associated with edentulism, and there is no consensus whether the most important risk factors are related

145

to dental/periodontal pathologies or to sociobehavioral and economics factors.[3]

A decrease in edentulism over the last few decades has been observed in most industrialized countries, although there are significant differences between countries and between geographical regions within countries, as well as between groups with differing background characteristics, such as education, urbanization, occupation, personal economic circumstances, attitudes to dental care, and lifestyle factors.[3]

In parallel with the prevalence decline, the incidence has also fallen significantly in the last few decades and there is a trend towards further decreases in the future. Comparison of the prevalence of edentulism between age cohorts a decade apart (i.e. those aged 45–54 years in 1992 compared with those aged 55–64 years in 2002) would suggest an estimated incidence of edentulism in the Swiss population of approximately 1.1% per decade,[2] a value similar to that reported for the Scandinavian countries (0–2% per year). However, it must be kept in mind that the incidence varies among different age groups, the prevalence increasing with the age (details about prevalence and incidence are given by Müller and coworkers[3] and Zitzmann and coworkers[2]).

The interpretation of epidemiological studies requires a careful evaluation of the study design and coverage rate. For instance, the highest age group is presented frequently as 70+ without any detail on the mean or median age or the upper age limit. Studies often include only community-dwelling persons while residents of long-term care facilities are excluded in order to reduce the effort required in data collection, but the prevalence of endentulousness is usually higher in long-term care facilities than in the general population. In the population-representative Berlin Aging Study, which included both those dwelling in the community and those in long-term care facilities, nearly 80% of those aged 85–90 years were edentulous.[4] The Fourth German Oral Health Study showed that in 2005 nearly 30% of 12-year-old Germans had caries; 20.5% of the middle age group (35–44 years) had a community periodontal index of 4, and 22% in the old age group (65–74 years) were edentulous. In addition, the rate of edentulousness had not changed since the third evaluation, which was performed in 1997. In all age groups, approximately 20% of the subjects had dental problems, indicating that these are likely socially related, that they follow some people during their whole life and that they are not easy to eradicate.[5]

The decrease in the prevalence and incidence of edentulousness gives rise to the question as to whether complete dentures will soon disappear in industrialized countries. Two phenomena could well counteract the prevalence decrease: the demographic changes, with the very rapid increase in the proportion of older people, who are more at risk for edentulousness; and the migration of peoples from countries with higher edentulism prevalence. Indeed, while even the most pessimistic projections do not predict an increase in the need for complete dentures, at least in Sweden, Finland and the UK,[6] projections from the USA are less optimistic and indicate that the prevalence decrease will not be sufficient to overcome the demographic population changes: the 79% increase in the population older than 55 years will largely offset the 10% decrease in edentulism that had been experienced in the last three decades. Consequently, the adult population in need of one or two complete dentures will increase from 33.6 million in 1991 to 37.9 million in 2020.[7] The view that complete dentures will disappear in the next three to four decades seems hazardous, premature and too optimistic, as stated also by Carlsson and Omar:[8] 'In spite of declines in edentulousness, there are still millions of edentulous people worldwide who need appropriate treatment, and the great majority of them will have to rely on complete dentures. Providing patients with complete dentures will, therefore, continue to be an important prosthodontic task for many more decades.'

Though edentulism eradication is one of the primary goals of dentistry, the fact that there are still individuals in need of complete dentures has serious teaching and clinical implications. The decline in edentulousness has already reduced the need for teaching complete denture prosthodontics, a fact that parallels the difficulty that several universities experience in recruiting sufficient and adequate edentulous subjects for undergraduate teaching. This phenomenon coincides with the fact that, in practice, clinicians are seeing fewer and fewer patients with complete dentures but these patients are getting more and more difficult to deal with, leading the clinicians to feel more and more uncomfortable in managing them. In addition, the rapid development of predictable dental implants has not only revolutionized prosthodontic treatment since the late 1980s but has also markedly decreased clinicians' interest and skill in complete dentures. The future challenge that universities and dental community are facing will be to educate enough specialists sufficiently interested in this area of prosthodontics to have the clinical expertise to manage these difficult cases. Indeed, there are still a number of patients who for health, anatomical, psychological, or financial reasons are not candidates for implant therapy.

Given the fact that complete dentures are not yet a museum object, the following sections will address a few problems related to the impact that complete dentures have on patients' health and quality of life.

# Chewing Efficiency and Nutrition

Final goals of treatment for the edentulous patient are to maintain/improve patient's nutrition, to provide him/her with a natural appearance, to maintain the ability to speak, and to maintain homeostasis in the masticatory system.

Chewing efficiency (the person's ability to comminute a test food) depends on two separate processes: selection of particles and breakage.[9–11] Tooth morphology, chewing force, and the direction of the closing path are factors influencing food breakage, while the selection process is influenced by the size of the occluding surface and the ability to maintain and position the food on it,

which are themselves functions of the tongue and perioral musculature (the degree of neuromuscular coordination). Chewing efficiency depends upon the number of occluding teeth: individuals with less than 20 teeth have far less chewing efficiency than those with more than 20 teeth (premolar occlusion)[12–15] (further details are given by Gotfredsen and Walls[16]). In addition, patients with a complete denture have markedly reduced chewing efficiency compared with dentate individuals and swallow fewer disrupted boli than dentate subjects,[12,17–21] a fact that is mainly determined by the instability of the mandibular denture. In effect, chewing efficiency increases by improving its stability by means of implants,[22-24] denture adhesive,[25] or preprosthetic surgery.[26] The better mechanical stability of the reconstruction allows the patient to produce higher chewing forces and to manipulate food more effectively using the tongue and perioral musculature, as the reconstruction does not need muscle stabilization.

For the patient's health, the subjective appraisal of chewing efficiency is actually more important than the objective evaluation as the former can lead to behavioral changes. With an objectively impaired masticatory function, people often start unconsciously avoiding certain foods or modifying the intake form. Consciously avoiding certain foods is usually a sign of grossly impaired function. Conscious or unconscious masticatory problems may lead to dietary restrictions; for example, individuals with 21 or more natural teeth eat more of the majority of nutrients than those with fewer.[15,27–31] The situation is even worse for wearers of complete dentures, who, indeed, are considered medically at risk because of restricted food selection. At the population level, wearers of complete dentures consume less food energy and significantly less protein, intrinsic and milk sugars, non-starch polysaccharide (fiber), calcium, non-heme iron, niacin and vitamin C than dentate people,[30] although the difference from dentate subjects is relatively small. They also consume less vegetables and fruits.[28,29,32,33] Insufficient intake of some nutrients that are hard to chew has been reported in several[15,30,33–37] but not all[38–41] studies.

Energy intake decreases physiologically with age owing to reduced activity. Geriatricians do not have problems with overweight, rather with malnutrition. This is a multifactorial problem and the loss in motivation to eat, the hunger decline, the decrease in taste and smell, and the loss of appetite are factors that may be even more important than the degree of chewing efficiency in itself.

The treatment of the edentulous patient should, therefore, aim to improve his/her nutritional status in case it has changed as a consequence of tooth loss. Unfortunately, the literature clearly shows that, in general, people do not change the way they eat even if they feel that they can chew better with the new reconstruction. Complete denture wearers did not change food intake when old dentures were replaced with better ones, with subjectively more efficient ones or with implant-supported removable reconstructions.[42–45] Only one study showed a significant improvement in the nutritional status with implant-supported overdentures.[46]

The general lack of dietary change post-therapy indicates that food selection, like any complex human behavior, is influenced by many inter-relating factors and is influenced to a far larger extent by non-prosthetic (e.g. attitude, self-identity, knowledge about healthy nutrition, education, tradition, culture), social, logistic (e.g. nursing home), and economic factors.[47,48] Indeed, perceived chewing ability could explain only 4% of the variance in fruit and vegetable intake in one study[48] and a community-based study indicated that Americans consumed diets of similar quality independently of their dental condition.[49,50]

In summary, to improve food selection it is not sufficient to provide the patient with a more stable reconstruction. A tailored dietary intervention is mandatory to change the diet, and regular reinforcements are essential to achieve a long-term adherence to the new dietary behavior.[51,52] A food history before and at the end of the prosthetic therapy, therefore, becomes an essential part of the management of the edentulous patient independent of whether the patient is to be provided with conventional, implant-supported, removable, or fixed reconstructions. The use of appropriate questionnaires may be of help. However, as questionnaires generally have broad questions, patients must be specifically interrogated as to whether or not they eat particular foods.

# Gastrointestinal Disorders

There is some evidence that complete denture wearers suffer from gastrointestinal disorders more often, and it is often hypothesized that this is the consequence of insufficient food comminution. A substantial improvement in digestive complaints was recorded in a group of female denture wearers 1 year after replacement of the poor-fitting mandibular complete dentures and improvement of the atrophic mandibular ridge by pre-prosthetic surgery. Before replacement therapy, 60% of the females had digestive complaints, such as abdominal pain (burning sensation, bloating, cramps), stool transit alteration (constipation or diarrhea), or both. The disorders decreased in 85% of the females after improving masticatory function. The authors concluded that the high incidence of digestive complaints and the symptom improvement after jaw reconstruction supported the hypothesis that poor mastication favors the development of digestive symptoms.[53] A higher risk of developing gastrointestinal problems in the presence of poor mastication has been reported also in other studies, and the risk for individuals with poor mastication to develop gastrointestinal problems was estimated to be approximately three times higher in a case–control investigation: odds ratio 2.62 (95% confidence interval, 1.02–6.95, after correction for age).[32,54]

There are several reasons why a poor chewing efficiency could increase the risk for gastrointestinal disorders. One possibility is that less-chewed food rests longer in the stomach. Unfortunately, the literature is not in agreement on this issue. A study performed on edentulous subjects who had to swallow cooked liver cubes either as a whole piece or after mastication did not report a difference in gastric emptying time.[55] By contrast, a second study performed on dentate young adults concluded that gastric emptying rate was significantly influenced by masticatory efficiency, as it was significantly shorter when the test meal was chewed during 50 instead of 25 cycles.[56] This finding may be supported by the delayed absorption of meat proteins in denture wearers compared with age-matched dentate subjects. The delayed protein absorption could be caused by a decrease in the gastric emptying rate.[57]

In the gastric-emptying studies, subjects ate easily masticable foods. It is, therefore, possible that the effect of mastication could be different when less-digestible foods are eaten. It could also be that good chewing efficiency is essential for patients with gastrointestinal problems. Indeed, patients with dyspepsia who had poor chewing efficiency had more pronounced gastric inflammatory alterations and *Helicobacter pylori* infections than those with dyspepsia who had good chewing efficiency.[58] This may be because the food lasted longer in the stomach in the former.

There are, of course, other factors that may explain a possible relationship between chewing efficiency and gastrointestinal disorders, and, indeed, it is certain that the relationship must be multifactorial as is often the case in a biological system. A factor that is often discussed in the literature in relation to gastrointestinal disorders is the fiber intake, and those wearing complete dentures in general eat fewer fiber nutrients. However, recent systematic reviews have questioned the protective effect of fiber intake against gastrointestinal disorders and pathologies.[59][62]

# Patient Satisfaction

Patient satisfaction with complete dentures is a very complex, multifactorial issue. The following are considered to be important: denture quality, quality of mandibular residual ridge, patient–clinician relationship, patient's attitude towards dentures, patient's personality, socioeconomic factors, psychological disorders (neuroticism, somatization, obsessivness, dysmorphism) and psychic disorders.[63–66] Although the literature is far from being concordant on the relevance of these factors, it is important to remember that the physical, mechanical aspect of a denture (its quality) plays only a minor role in patients' satisfaction, though it is the most extensively discussed. Indeed, this is likely related more to psychological/psychic factors than physical factors. For instance, the probability of dissatisfaction increases by an estimated 44% in persons with mild depression, and by 391% in persons with severe depression.[65] Patients with prosthesis incompatibility score higher in depressive distress level, global severity index, and positive symptom distress index.[67]

The role of psychological/psychic factors in denture dissatisfaction is too often overlooked by clinicians, who have the tendency to emphasize the physical, mechanical aspect of a denture and consequently to look for construction errors in dissatisfied patients. This approach is problematic as every new dental treatment may convince the dissatisfied patient that his/her problem is actually caused by denture errors, making it more and more difficult to convince him/her that in reality this is not the case. For instance, an association has been reported between the degree of somatization, obsessiveness, and tentativeness in social contact on the Symptoms Check List 90-R (SCL-90-R) scale[68] and the subjective dissatisfaction symptoms chewing and phonation ability in patients with psychological prosthesis incompatibility.[67]

Patients with psychological prosthesis incompatibility must be recognized right away; diagnostic criteria for distinguishing between a dental- and a psychological-related difficulty to wear dentures have been described elsewhere.[67] Often these misdiagnosed patients are provided with implant-supported reconstructions under the wrong assumption that a more stable or even a fixed reconstruction will solve the problem when, in fact, they need a tailored psychological/psychiatric diagnosis and therapy, with the decision whether a denture should be corrected or replaced, and if so when, being taken with-

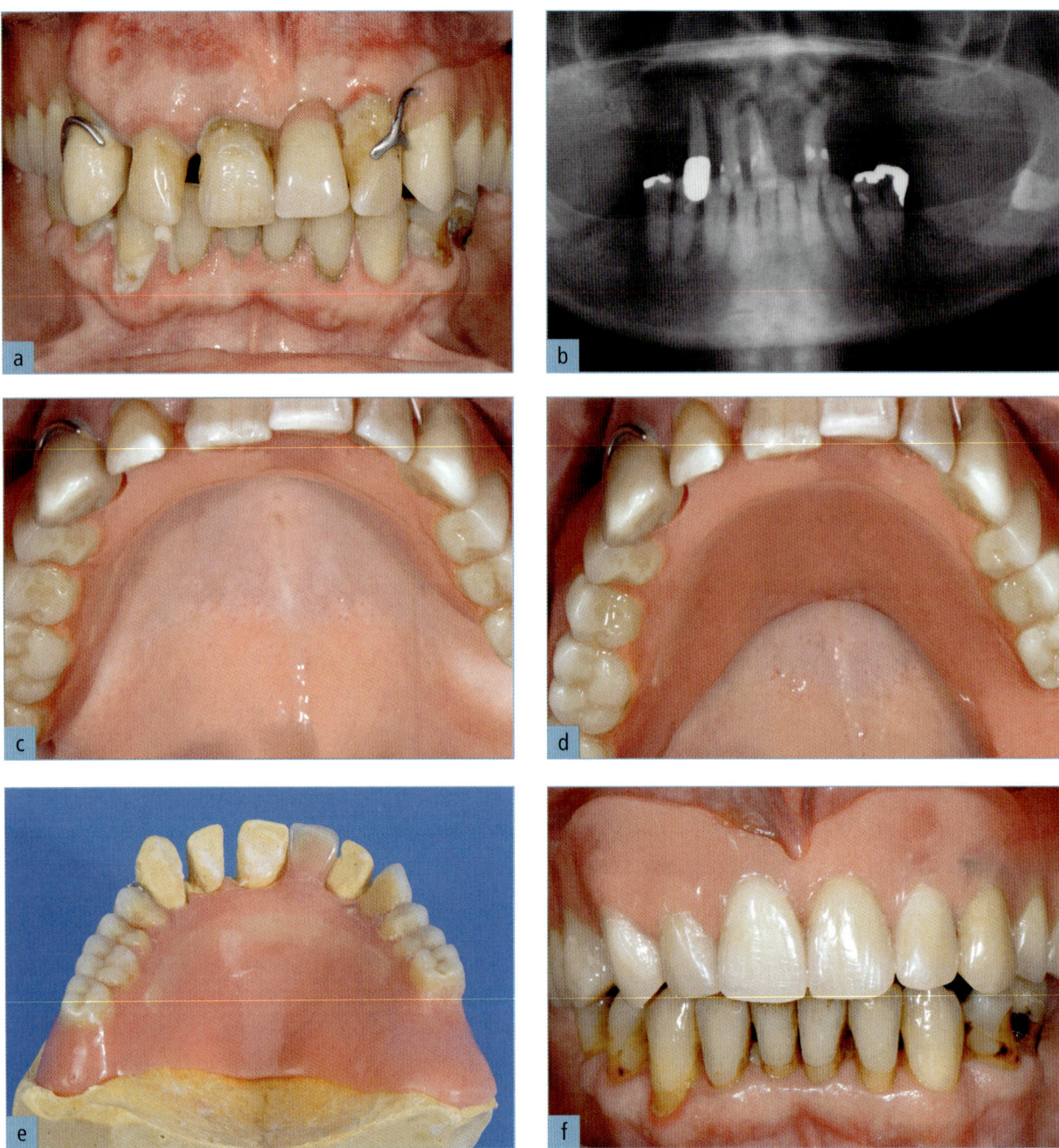

**Fig 11-1a–f** This patient was referred because of difficulty wearing the acrylic partial denture (a–c) as well as a burning mouth sensation. The orthopantomogram shows the unfavorable prognosis of the upper anterior teeth (b). The patient was sent to a psychologist for anxiety treatment. Thereafter, in a first step, the acrylic denture was extended palatinally in two steps (d,e). Finally, the anterior teeth were extracted and the acrylic partial denture converted into a complete denture with full coverage of the palate (f). The burning sensation was treated with clomazepam.

in the team. The challenge in these cases is how to explain to the patient that his/her dissatisfaction is not related to errors in the denture construction.

In the author's experience, a psychological prosthesis incompatibility is often triggered by a too-sudden transition from the dentate to the edentate condition. The insertion of an immediate denture after extraction of all remaining teeth is a practice that may have been well tolerated when edentulism was an integral part of the aging process, but today this procedure is highly risky. Wearing a denture becomes more and more an exception. Therefore, it becomes mandatory to plan the transition from the dentate to the edentulous condition correctly, as this is an event that can be highly traumatic for a patient. Getting dentures requires a lot of adaptation, about as much coping skill as is necessary to cope with major life events such as conflict with a partner, being unemployed for 1 month or more, getting married or retired, changing work, or partner stopping work.[69–71]

The transition from the dentate to the edentate condition should be scheduled in a most 'stress-free' life period and in patients at risk must be preceded and accompanied by a psychological support therapy. Furthermore, it has to happen in steps, and for the maxilla it may be suitable to start by inserting a palatal plate in order for the patient to get used to the palate coverage. In the absence of medical contraindications that requires immediate handling, tooth extraction will start in the posterior area, possibly one side after the other one, leaving the extraction of the anterior teeth to the end (Fig 11-1).

# Quality of Life

While patient satisfaction evaluates how pleased the patient is with the reconstruction, the appraisal of the oral health-related quality of life (OHRQoL) assesses how the reconstruction influences the subject's quality of life. According to Ingelhart and Bagramian, the OHRQoL refers to the part of quality of life that is affected by a person's oral health, or how oral health affects the person's ability to function (e.g. bite, chew, speak), psychological state (such as self-esteem and satisfaction with appearance), social factors, and pain/discomfort related to oral health.[72]

Complete denture wearers have, in general, a reduced OHRQoL in comparison with that of patients with natural dentition or fixed reconstructions, and the OHRQoL improves when conventional mandibular complete dentures are replaced by implant-supported overdentures. However, evidence is lacking to indicate that patients' satisfaction with implant-supported maxillary overdentures is better than with conventional maxillary dentures. Overall, the literature on OHRQoL supports the recommendation that mandibular two-implant overdentures should be the standard of care for the therapy of the edentulous mandible[73] but not for the maxilla (discussed in more detail by Thomason and coworkers[74] and Strassburger and coworkers[75]).

It is worth mentioning that not all wearers of complete dentures have a reduced OHRQoL[76] and that the OHRQoL also increases significantly when an old mandibular complete denture is replaced by a new one.[77,78] In this respect, two studies are worth mentioning. The first is by John and coworkers, who analyzed the changes in OHRQoL of patients treated in private offices with fixed or removable dentures.[78] They showed that the OHRQoL improved over a 1-year period in all groups and, more importantly, that the OHRQoL of the patients requiring treatment was worse than that of the general population,[78] an observation that is compatible with the fact that people seek medical and dental treatment when they feel that something is wrong rather than because of clinical signs and symptoms. This indicates that results obtained by studies performed only in patients seeking therapy can be biased through lacking external validity.

The second study analyzed the long-term improvement in OHRQoL in edentulous older adults receiving mandibular implant-supported overdentures or conventional complete dentures.[79] The OHRQoL was evaluated using the Oral Health Impact Profile (OHIP), which assesses five domains related to functional limitation, pain, psychological discomfort, physical disability, psychological disability, social disability, and handicap.[80] Patients were divided into three groups: a group comprising patients who required and obtained replacement of the mandibular complete denture with an implant-supported overdenture; a group desiring the same treatment but receiving a complete denture; and a group of those requesting replacement of their complete removable dentures by conventional means. Reasons for not providing implant therapy in the second group were that significant improvement was thought possible using conventional means, the patient was unwilling to undergo the proposed procedure, the patient was medically or psychiatrically unfit for this form of treatment, or the patient could not afford it. Results indicated that the pretreatment OHRQoL was poorer in subjects requesting implants than in those requesting conventional dentures. The OHRQoL improved more in the first and third groups, where patients essentially received the treatment they requested, than in the second group, where patients did not get the treatment with an implant-supported overdenture they had initially desired. Patients who received the implant-supported reconstruction (group 1) still had a lower OHRQoL than those who received the complete denture.

These results have clinical implications as they show that patients requiring implants have a lower OHRQoL than those asking for conventional denture replacement. Evaluation of the OHRQoL prior to therapy could help the clinician in filtering out those patients who will need an implant-supported reconstruction from those who will benefit from conventional dentures. Indeed, it has been shown that not all edentulous patients seek stabilization of the lower denture by means of implants: around one third of denture wearers refused an offer to stabilize the lower denture by means of one or two implants even though the therapy was free of charge. Those people who felt disturbed by a combination of chewing and speaking difficulties, pain, and dissatisfaction with appearance were most likely to choose implants, while the main reason for the non-acceptance of implant therapy was a concern about surgical risks.[81]

The fact that implant-supported mandibular overdentures lead, on average, to better patient satisfaction and OHRQoL does not warrant concluding that complete dentures are no longer indicated for the rehabilitation of the edentulous patient. As mentioned above, there are denture wearers who are satisfied with complete dentures, and a not irrelevant number of patients with an uncomfortable denture manage to eat most of the food available to them and are, therefore, medically not at risk. There are also individuals who cannot afford implant-supported dentures, who have medical contraindications, and who do not desire, even deny, them.

The advances in dental implantology has allowed a not insignificant part of the dental profession to think that all teeth need to be replaced by implants and that edentulous patients need to have reconstruction by means of implant-supported prostheses as these are more similar to the dentate condition. Moreover, implant-supported reconstructions are probably the kind of reconstruction that the vast majority of clinicians would like for themselves in case of tooth loss. However, the decision-making process on how tooth loss is managed should not be driven by the clinicians' feelings about their own preferences. The medical and dental literature since the mid-1990s clearly shows that the criteria on which patients base their decision often differ from those that guide the decisions taken by the medical/dental profession. For example, a cross-over study with fixed and removable implant-supported reconstructions showed that those subjects who felt that the removable reconstruction allowed a better hygiene than the fixed one chose the first reconstruction, despite the fact that those patients also rated stability and ability to chew with the fixed reconstruction as significantly better than with the removable prosthesis.[82]

The decision-making process, as an interaction between practitioner and patient, must be patient-centered; that is, patient-centered outcome measures should be used to find an individual, patient-tailored prosthetic solution that provides the best improvement of that particular patient's quality of life. This requires an in-depth psychosocial history, in particular an evalu-

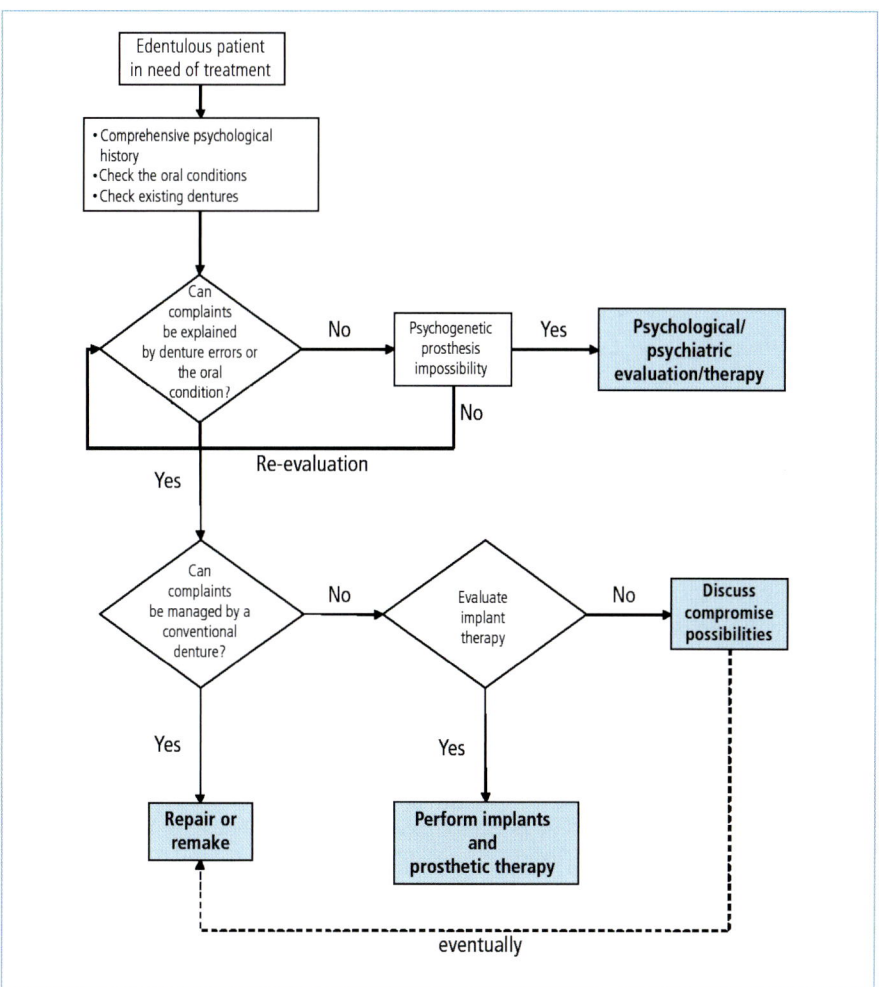

**Fig 11-2** Decision-making process for the treatment of the edentulous patient.

ation of how the edentulous condition and the complete dentures affect the patient in daily life. The decision-making process for the edentulous patient is depicted in Fig 11-2.

Unfortunately, the paternalistic model, underpinned by clinician-led decision making often prevails in dentistry and patients are excluded from treatment decision making.[83] Medicine, by comparison, is increasingly acknowledging that a 'patient centered approach' is necessary. This encourages patients to participate in and share control of treatment and management decisions and it takes into account individual preferences within social contexts. Delivering care in a manner that is meaningful for the individual is more likely to lead to long-term 'adherence'.[84] The growing number of treatment alternatives make it necessary to involve the

patient actively in the decision-making process. Indeed, the vast majority of patients interviewed in one study favored shared decision making in the choice among treatment alternatives.[85] Attention must, however, be drawn to the fact that the decision-making process differs with age. When patients were specifically asked who should have the final decision about the type of treatment, an opposite trend was seen: patients older than 60 years had the tendency to leave the final decision to the doctor, while the younger patients wanted to be in charge of the final decision. Differences in education level could explain, at least to some extent, this diversity. Indeed, among respondents with only a compulsory school background, a majority preferred shared decision making where the doctor has the final decision. Respondents with a university degree also preferred a shared decision making, but most of them wanted to have the final word themselves.[85] The literature on shared decision making in dentistry is scarce, but this also indicates that patients prefer this approach, though a passive role was more commonly perceived as the one attained.[83]

# Complete Dentures and Appearance

It is a fact that the demand for esthetic dentistry has increased tremendously since the mid-1990s. Almost parallel to this esthetic trend, we have experienced an increased demand for cosmetic dental procedures that has made cosmetic dentistry a significant part of dental practice and boosted interests and understanding for procedures such as tooth bleaching, bonding, and adhesive ceramic restorative procedures in order to improve tooth appearance. However, the esthetic trend is still limited to restorative dentistry, and esthetics in removable reconstructions remains aleatory. This is somehow

strange as dentistry is faced with a population that is getting older and that keeps more of its natural teeth. Consequently, wearing an unnaturally looking removable reconstruction is no longer the age-related phenomenon it once was. In our cosmetic and youth-oriented societies, wearing an unnaturally looking reconstruction may, therefore, be a cause of severe psychological distress.

Too often it is said that the goal in restoring a mutilated anterior dentition is to improve the patient's smile. The benefits of smiling have been accepted throughout human history. Smiling facilitates problem solving both interpersonally and in a group setting, and it puts people at ease, promoting expression and the exchange of ideas. Smiling, and especially laughing, reduces stress, anxiety, worry, and frustration and increases sociability. However, patients disclose the anterior teeth and the dental arches more often during talking than smiling. Therefore, the goal in reconstructing a dental arch cannot be reduced simply to smile improvement. On the contrary, the ultimate goal of the treatment of the edentulous patient is to provide the subject with a natural appearance during all aspects of facial expression: to give the illusion that the subject has

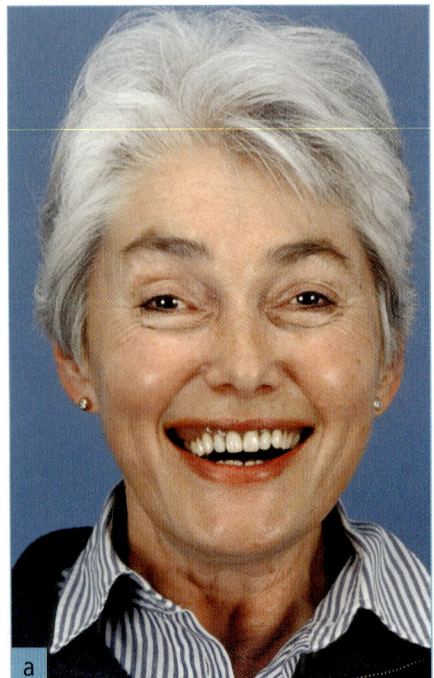 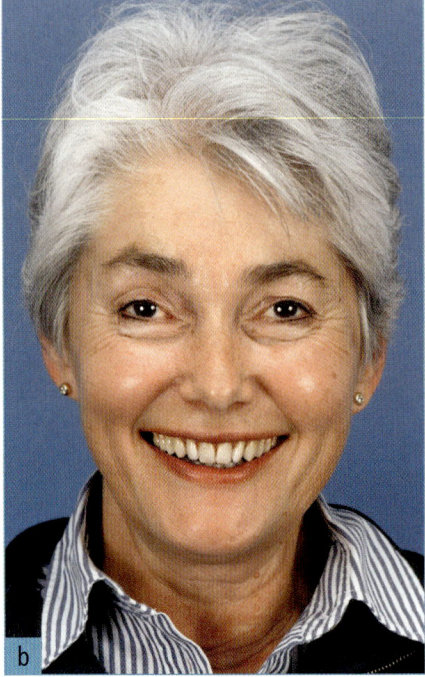

**Fig 11-3a–b** (a) The dental arch of the old denture is too small, too caudal, too narrow, and too tilted dorsocaudally; the posterior teeth are too short. As a consequence, the patient is disclosing the artificial 'gum' too much and has an unnatural buccal corridor. (b) The correct orientation of the dental arch and the selection of larger teeth allowed the artificial dentition to blend in the patient's face, providing the illusion of a natural dentition. To avoid incorrect orientation of the occlusal plane, the denture try-in needs to be done with the patient standing in front of the clinician at 1 m distance. *(Denture by Dr Bruna Ernst)*

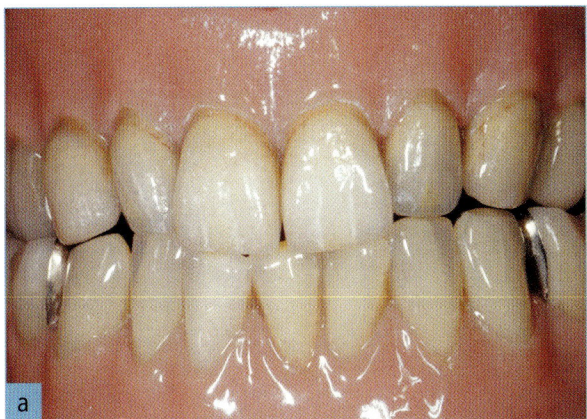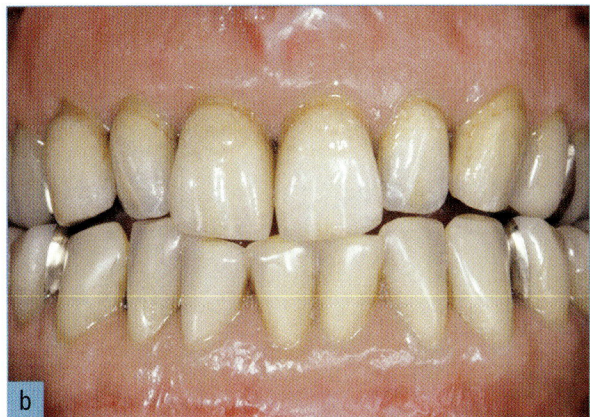

**Fig 11-4a–b**  Unnatural (a) and natural (b) shape of the artificial gingiva. (a) The gingival contour is correct but the interdental papillae gives the appearance of artificiality as they all have an interdental groove. (b) The full and convex papillae plus the individual coloring of the artificial gingiva provide a much more natural look. *(from Palla S 86, with permission)*

his/her own teeth. 'Esthetic' is, therefore, not what looks nice but what looks natural – what provide the illusion of a natural appearance.

There are several points that need to be addressed in order to reach this goal, the most important being correct sustaining of the soft tissues, adequate vertical dimension, proper dental arch shape and orientation, incisal margin shape, modeling of the gingiva, and indi-

vidual coloring of the artificial gingiva in patients who display it. These points have been described elsewhere, and a detailed description is outside of the scope of this chapter.[86,87] Figures 11-3 to 11-8 are typical examples of errors and solutions in attempting to provide the illusion of a natural dentition. The demand for a naturally appearing dentition may, however, cause difficulties. Healthy and fit older people may like to have a young

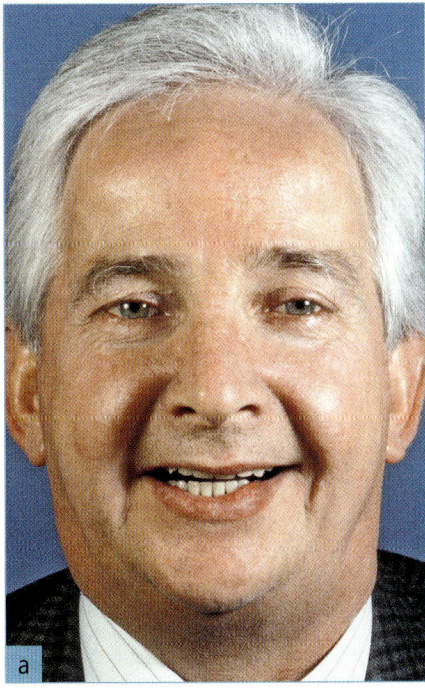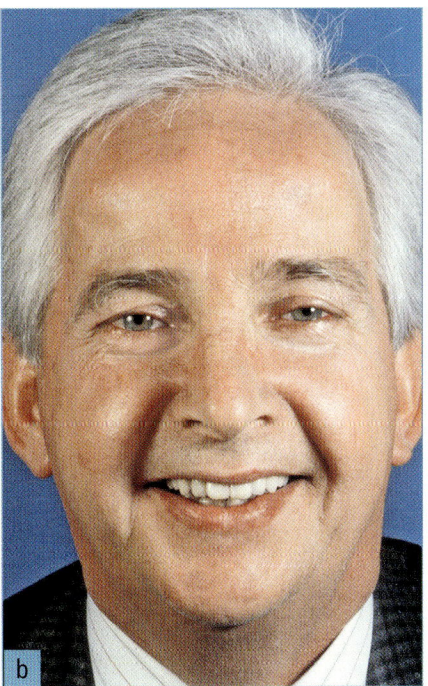

**Fig 11-5a–b**  (a) The dental arch of the old denture is positioned too cranially and the teeth are too small. Consequently, the dental arch is too narrow. In addition, the lower anterior teeth are too long and too regular, and the incisal margins are too convex, as if the teeth had not worn. (b) The width and position of the dental arch of the new denture fit harmoniously in the patient's face, providing the illusion of a natural dentition.

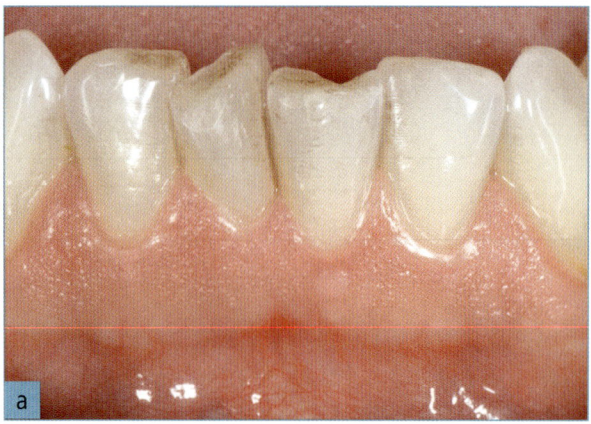

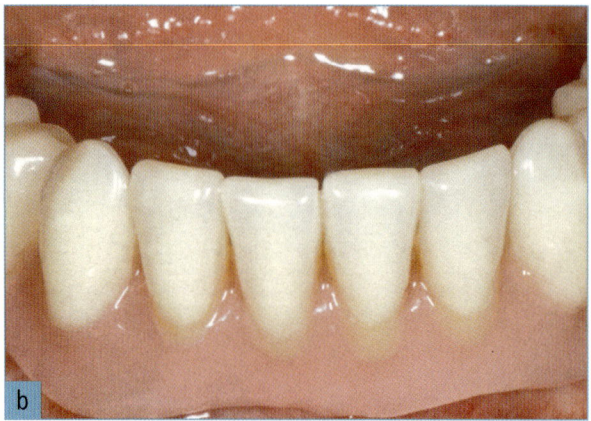

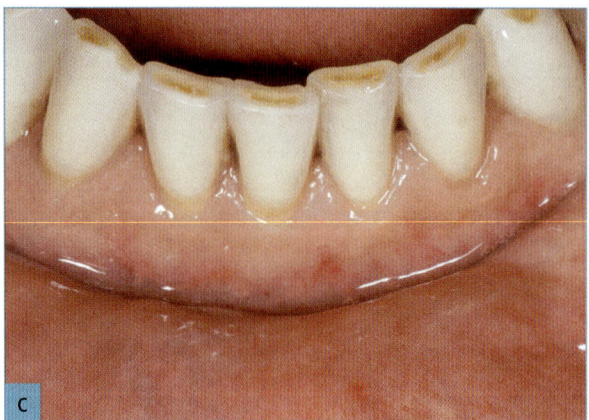

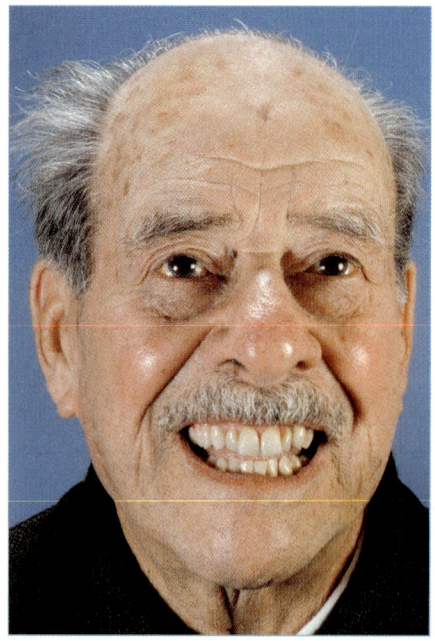

**Fig 11-7**   Final try-in. Though the patient also discloses the artificial gingiva, the illusion of a natural dentition is provided by the appropriate length of the anterior and posterior teeth, the natural modeling of the gingival margin, and the crowding of the upper and lower anterior teeth. *(Denture by Dr Bruna Ernst)*

**Fig 11-6a–c**   Most elderly whites have crowded lower anterior teeth (a). Unfortunately, a very symmetrical lower front is the 'rule' in complete denture (b). Imitation of the crowding in the lower front, the correct modeling of the incisal margins, and of the artificial gingiva as well as the coloring of the artificial soft tissues provides the impression of a natural dentition (c).

dentition, as promoted by the media in our youth-oriented society. The request to utilize too light a shade, a shade that is similar to that of primary teeth or to arrange the teeth in a too regular and symmetric manner is well known to all clinicians. In these cases, it is the clinician's duty to educate the patient.

In recent years, some authors have started to challenge the use of the classic technique to construct complete dentures. Kawai and coworkers showed that dentures constructed with a simplified technique were as good as those constructed with the classic approach in that patients were equally satisfied.[88] The difference in fabrication techniques had minimal impact on patient satisfaction or on how difficult it was to chew with the new dentures, suggesting that the time-consuming procedures of the traditional method, such as final impressions using border molding and secondary impression materials, face bow transfer, semi-adjustable articulator and re-mount procedures, have little influence on out-

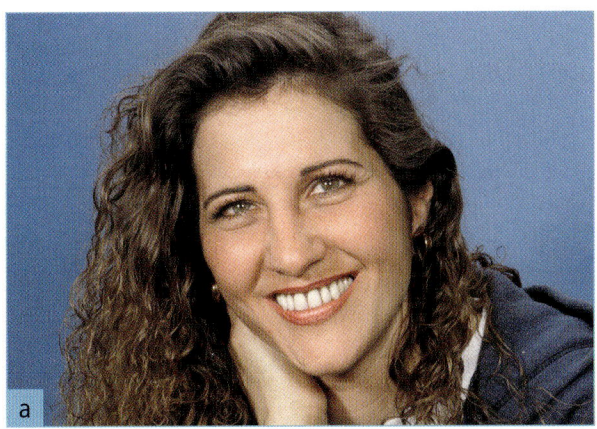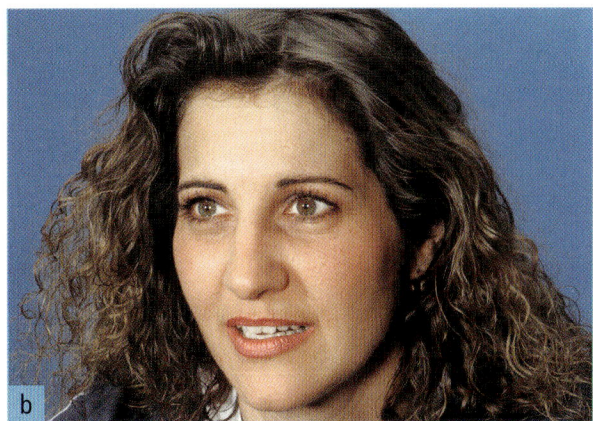

**Fig 11-8a–b** While the old denture disfigures the face of this young woman (a), the new denture beautifies her face (b). *(from Palla S[86], with permission)*

come. Actually this is not surprising, as patient's satisfaction is explained only to a small degree by denture quality. While one can understand the need to simplify denture construction in order to decrease the fabrication costs in a 'time' in which society is pressured by feelings of getting poorer and states are becoming more and more indebted, it is to hope that this approach will not decrease further the value of complete dentures. While the study of Kawai and coworkers indicates that a simplified technique is sufficient to provide adequate masticatory function,[88] it is unlikely that it will allow dentures to be constructed that provide the illusion of a natural dentition.

## Conclusions

Though the prevalence of edentulous patients has greatly decreased in industrialized countries, edentulousness is not eradicated and complete dentures are not yet confined to the museum. Unfortunately, there are still a number of patients who need them, and the dental profession is very far from having reached in industrialized countries the goal set by the World Health Organization in 1992, namely that the retention throughout life of at least 20 teeth should be the treatment goal for oral health.[89]

The improvement in implantology and the introduction of the mandibular implant-supported overdenture have greatly facilitated the clinician's task and have improved the quality of life for many edentulous patients. Nevertheless, it is not correct to assume that all edentulous patients are unsatisfied with complete dentures and have a poor OHRQoL, or that complete dentures are a second line of treatment. It is the duty of the engaged clinician to treat the patient as a human being, considering the prosthetic treatment within the patient's psychosocial frame, and finalizing the treatment with nutritional counseling. The treatment of the edentulous patient cannot happen according to an inflexible treatment plan and in a unique standardized treatment course. In the foreground must always be the individual patient, who is one of a heterogeneous group of edentulous individuals. Though all may require a denture, the therapeutic approach may differ widely among patients: that of an edentulous middle-aged healthy person may be completely different from that for an aged person living at home, for whom life is already a misery, or from that of a geriatric patient who receives, in addition to other medical comorbidities, also the diagnosis of an 'insufficient masticatory apparatus.'

Lastly, it is important to consider complete dentures as a valuable treatment modality for the edentulous patient and not just as a piece of acrylic resin with artificial teeth or a cheap 'social' treatment modality for the edentulous patient. Only a change in this thinking will allow the construction of dentures, with or without implants, that restore the patient's integrity and dignity.

# References

1. Zitzmann NU, Marinello CP, Zemp E, Kessler P, Ackermann-Liebrich U. Zahnverlust, prothetische Versorgung und zahnärztliche Inanspruchnahme in der Schweiz [Tooth loss, dental restorations and dental attendance in Switzerland.] Schweiz Monatsschr Zahnmed 2001;111:1288–1294.

2. Zitzmann NU, Staehelin K, Walls AW, Menghini G, Weiger R, Zemp SE. Changes in oral health over a 10-yr period in Switzerland. Eur J Oral Sci 2008;116:52–59.

3. Müller F, Naharro M, Carlsson GE. What are the prevalence and incidence of tooth loss in the adult and elderly population in Europe? Clin Oral Implants Res 2007;18(Suppl 3):2–14.

4. Nitschke I, Hopfenmüller W. Die zahnmedizinische Versorgung älterer Menschen. [The dental therapy of elderly people.] In: Mayer KU, Baltes PB (eds). Die Berliner Altersstudie. Berlin: Akademie Verlag, 1996:429–448.

5. Micheelis W, Schiffner U (eds).Vierte Deutsche Mundgesundheitsstudie (DMS IV). Köln: Institut der Deutschen Zahnärzte, 2006.

6. Mojon P, Thomason JM, Walls AW. The impact of falling rates of edentulism. Int J Prosthodont 2004;17:434–440.

7. Douglass CW, Shih A, Ostry L. Will there be a need for complete dentures in the United States in 2020? J Prosthet Dent 2002;87:5–8.

8. Carlsson GE, Omar R. Trends in prosthodontics. Med Princ Pract 2006;15:167–179.

9. Lucas PW, Luke DA. Computer simulation of the breakdown of carrot particles during human mastication. Arch Oral Biol 1983;28:821–826.

10. Lucas PW, Luke DA, Voon FC, Chew CL, Ow R. Food breakdown patterns produced by human subjects possessing artificial and natural teeth. J Oral Rehabil 1986;13:205–214.

11. van der Bilt A, Olthoff LW, van der Glas HW, van der Weelen K, Bosman F. A mathematical description of the comminution of food during mastication in man. Arch Oral Biol 1987;32:579–586.

12. Helkimo E, Carlsson GE, Helkimo M. Chewing efficiency and state of dentition. A methodologic study. Acta Odontol Scand 1978;36:33–41.

13. Leake JL. An index of chewing ability. J Public Health Dent 1990;50:262–267.

14. Leake JL, Hawkins R, Locker D. Social and functional impact of reduced posterior dental units in older adults. J Oral Rehabil 1994;21:1–10.

15. Sheiham A, Steele JG, Marcenes W, Finch S, Walls AW. The impact of oral health on stated ability to eat certain foods; findings from the National Diet and Nutrition Survey of Older People in Great Britain. Gerodontology 1999;16:11–20.

16. Gotfredsen K, Walls AW. What dentition assures oral function? Clin Oral Implants Res 2007;18(Suppl 3):34–45.

17. Slagter AP, Olthoff LW, Steen WH, Bosman F. Comminution of food by complete-denture wearers. J Dent Res 1992;71:380–386.

18. Gunne HS. Masticatory efficiency and dental state. A comparison between two methods. Acta Odontol Scand 1985;43:139–146.

19. Kapur KK, Soman SD. Masticatory performance and efficiency in denture wearers. J Prosthet Dent 1964;687–694.

20. Liedberg B, Stoltze K, Owall B. The masticatory handicap of wearing removable dentures in elderly men. Gerodontology 2005;22:10–16.

21. Yven C, Bonnet L, Cormier D, Monier S, Mioche L. Impaired mastication modifies the dynamics of bolus formation. Eur J Oral Sci 2006;114:184–190.

22. Geertman ME, Slagter AP, van Waas MA, Kalk W. Comminution of food with mandibular implant-retained overdentures. J Dent Res 1994;73:1858–1864.

23. Geertman ME, Slagter AP, van 't Hof MA, van Waas MA, Kalk W. Masticatory performance and chewing experience with implant-retained mandibular overdentures. J Oral Rehabil 1999;26:7–13.

24. Fueki K, Kimoto K, Ogawa T, Garrett NR. Effect of implant-supported or retained dentures on masticatory performance: a systematic review. J Prosthet Dent 2007;98:470–477.

25. Fujimori T, Hirano S, Hayakawa I. Effects of a denture adhesive on masticatory functions for complete denture wearers. Consideration for the condition of denture-bearing tissues. J Med Dent Sci 2002;49: 151–156.

26. Watson CJ. Masticatory performance before and after mandibular vestibuloplasty. Br Dent J 1987;162:417–422.

27. Sarita PT, Witter DJ, Kreulen CM, van't Hof MA, Creugers NH. Chewing ability of subjects with shortened dental arches. Community Dent Oral Epidemiol 2003;31:328–334.

28. Hung HC, Willett W, Ascherio A, Rosner BA, Rimm E, Joshipura KJ. Tooth loss and dietary intake. J Am Dent Assoc 2003;134:1185–1192.

29. Hung HC, Colditz G, Joshipura KJ. The association between tooth loss and the self-reported intake of selected CVD-related nutrients and foods among US women. Community Dent Oral Epidemiol 2005;33:167–173.

30. Sheiham A, Steele JG, Marcenes W, Lowe C, Finch S, Bates CJ, et al. The relationship among dental status, nutrient intake, and nutritional status in older people. J Dent Res 2001;80:408–413.

31. Sheiham A, Steele J. Does the condition of the mouth and teeth affect the ability to eat certain foods, nutrient and dietary intake and nutritional status amongst older people? Public Health Nutr 2001;4:797–803.

32. Brodeur JM, Laurin D, Vallee R, Lachapelle D. Nutrient intake and gastrointestinal disorders related to masticatory performance in the edentulous elderly. J Prosthet Dent 1993;70:468–473.

33. Sahyoun NR, Lin CL, Krall E. Nutritional status of the older adult is associated with dentition status. J Am Diet Assoc 2003;103:61–66.

34. Österberg T, Steen B. Relationship between dental state and dietary intake in 70-year-old males and females in Göteborg, Sweden: a population study. J Oral Rehabil 1982;9:509–521.

35. Joshipura KJ, Willett WC, Douglass CW. The impact of edentulousness on food and nutrient intake. J Am Dent Assoc 1996;127:459–467.

36. Krall E, Hayes C, Garcia R. How dentition status and masticatory function affect nutrient intake. J Am Dent Assoc 1998;129:1261–1269.

37. Papas AS, Palmer CA, Rounds MC, Russell RM. The effects of denture status on nutrition. Spec Care Dentist 1998;18:17–25.

38. Greksa LP, Parraga IM, Clark CA. The dietary adequacy of edentulous older adults. J Prosthet Dent 1995;73:142–145.

39. Griep MI, Verleye G, Franck AH, Collys K, Mets TF, Massart DL. Variation in nutrient intake with dental status, age and odour perception. Eur J Clin Nutr 1996;50:816–825.

40. Österberg T, Tsuga K, Rothenberg E, Carlsson GE, Steen B. Masticatory ability in 80-year-old subjects and its relation to intake of energy, nutrients and food items. Gerodontology 2002;19:95–101.

41. Liedberg B, Stoltze K, Norlen P, Öwall B. 'Inadequate' dietary habits and mastication in elderly men. Gerodontology 2007;24:41–46.

42. Allen F, McMillan A. Food selection and perceptions of chewing ability following provision of implant and conventional prostheses in complete denture wearers. Clin Oral Implants Res 2002;13:320–326.

43. Ellis JS, Thomason JM, Jepson NJ, Nohl F, Smith DG, Allen PF. A randomized-controlled trial of food choices made by edentulous adults. Clin Oral Implants Res 2008;19:356–361.

44. Müller F, Nitschke I. Mundgesundheit, Zahnstatus und Ernährung im Alter [Oral health, dental state and nutrition in older adults.] Z Gerontol Geriatr 2005;38:334–341.

45. Hamada MO, Garrett NR, Roumanas ED, Kapur KK, Freymiller E, Han T, et al. A randomized clinical trial comparing the efficacy of mandibular implant-supported overdentures and conventional dentures in diabetic patients. Part IV: comparisons of dietary intake. J Prosthet Dent 2001;85:53–60.

46. Morais JA, Heydecke G, Pawliuk J, Lund JP, Feine JS. The effects of mandibular two-implant overdentures on nutrition in elderly edentulous individuals. J Dent Res 2003;82:53–58.

47. Shepherd R. Influences on food choice and dietary behavior. Forum Nutr 2005;57:36–43.

48. Bradbury J, Thomason JM, Jepson NJA, Walls AWG, Mulvaney CE, Allen PF, et al. Perceived chewing ability and intake of fruit and vegetables. J Dent Res 2008;87:720–725.

49. Shinkai RS, Hatch JP, Sakai S, Mobley CC, Saunders MJ, Rugh JD. Oral function and diet quality in a community-based sample. J Dent Res 2001;80:1625–1630.

50. Shinkai RS, Hatch JP, Rugh JD, Sakai S, Mobley CC, Saunders MJ. Dietary intake in edentulous subjects with good and poor quality complete dentures. J Prosthet Dent 2002;87:490–498.

51. Bradbury J, Thomason JM, Jepson NJ, Walls AW, Allen PF, Moynihan PJ. Nutrition counseling increases fruit and vegetable intake in the edentulous. J Dent Res 2006;85:463–468.

52. Pierce JP, Newman VA, Natarajan L, Flatt SW, Al-Delaimy WK, Caan BJ, et al. Telephone counseling helps maintain long-term adherence to a high-vegetable dietary pattern. J Nutr 2007;137:2291–2296.

53. Mercier P, Poitras P. Alimentary tract and pancreas. Gastrointestinal symptoms and masticatory dysfunction. J Gastroenterol Hepatol 1992;7:61–65.

54. Tosello A, Foti B, Sedarat C, Brodeur JM, Ferrigno JM, Tavitian P, et al. Oral functional characteristics and gastrointestinal pathology: an epidemiological approach. J Oral Rehabil 2001;28:668–672.

55. Poitras P, Bolvin M, Morais J, Picard M, Mercier P. Gastric emptying of solid food in edentulous patients. Digestion 1995;56:483–487.

56. Pera P, Bassi F, Schierano G, Appendino P, Preti G. Implant anchored complete mandibular denture: evaluation of masticatory efficiency, oral function and degree of satisfaction. J Oral Rehabil 1998;25:462–467.

57. Rémond D, Machebeuf M, Yven C, Buffiere C, Mioche L, Mosoni L, et al. Postprandial whole-body protein metabolism after a meat meal is influenced by chewing efficiency in elderly subjects. Am J Clin Nutr 2007;85:1286–1292.

58. Sierpinska T, Golebiewska M, Dlugosz J, Kemona A, Laszewicz W. Connection between masticatory efficiency and pathomorphologic changes in gastric mucosa. Quintessence Int 2007;38:31–37.

59. Leung FW. Etiologic factors of chronic constipation: review of the scientific evidence. Dig Dis Sci 2007;52:313–316.

60. Müller-Lissner SA, Kamm MA, Scarpignato C, Wald A. Myths and misconceptions about chronic constipation. Am J Gastroenterol 2005;100:232–242.

61. Tan KY, Seow-Choen F. Fiber and colorectal diseases: separating fact from fiction. World J Gastroenterol 2007;13:4161–4167.

62. Zuckerman MJ. The role of fiber in the treatment of irritable bowel syndrome: therapeutic recommendations. J Clin Gastroenterol 2006;40:104–108.

63. Fenlon MR, Sherriff M. An investigation of factors influencing patients' satisfaction with new complete dentures using structural equation modelling. J Dent 2008;36:427–434.

64. Fenlon MR, Sherriff M, Newton JT. The influence of personality on patients' satisfaction with existing and new complete dentures. J Dent 2007;35:744–748.

65. John MT, Micheelis W, Steele JG. Depression as a risk factor for denture dissatisfaction. J Dent Res 2007;86:852–856.

66. Klages U, Esch M, Wehrbein H. Oral health impact in patients wearing removable prostheses: relations to somatization, pain sensitivity, and body consciousness. Int J Prosthodont 2005;18:106–111.

67. Eitner S, Wichmann M, Heckmann J, Holst S. Pilot study on the psychologic evaluation of prosthesis incompatibility using the SCL-90-R scale and the CES-D scale. Int J Prosthodont 2006;19:482–490.

68. Derogatis L. The SCL-90R Manual II: Administration, Scoring and Procedures. Baltimore, MD: Clinical Psychometric Research, 1983.

69. Bergendal B. The relative importance of tooth loss and denture wearing in Swedish adults. Community Dent Health 1989;6:103–111.

70. Haugejorden O, Rise J, Klock KS. Norwegian adults' perceived need for coping skills to adjust to dental and non-dental life events. Community Dent Oral Epidemiol 1993;21:57–61.

71. Klock KS, Haugejorden O. Measurement and predictors of young adults' perceived ability to cope with dental life events. Acta Odontol Scand 2002;60:129–135.

72. Ingelhart M, Bagramian R. Oral health related quality of life: an introduction. In: Ingelhart M, Bagramian R (eds). Oral Health Related Quality of Life. Chicago, IL: Quintessence, 2002:1–6.

73. Feine JS, Carlsson GE, Awad MA, Chehade A, Duncan WJ, Gizani S, et al. The McGill Consensus Statement on Overdentures. Mandibular two implant overdentures as first choice standard of care for edentulous patients. Gerodontology 2002;19:3–4.

74. Thomason JM, Heydecke G, Feine JS, Ellis JS. How do patients perceive the benefit of reconstructive dentistry with regard to oral health-related quality of life and patient satisfaction? A systematic review. Clin Oral Implants Res 2007;18(Suppl 3): 168–188.

75. Strassburger C, Heydecke G, Kerschbaum T. Influence of prosthetic and implant therapy on satisfaction and quality of life: a systematic literature review. Part 1 Characteristics of the studies. Int J Prosthodont 2004;17:83–93.

76. Forgie AH, Scott BJ, Davis DM. A study to compare the oral health impact profile and satisfaction before and after having replacement complete dentures in England and Scotland. Gerodontology 2005;22:137–142.

77. Allen PF, Thomason JM, Jepson NJ, Nohl F, Smith DG, Ellis J. A randomized controlled trial of implant-retained mandibular overdentures. J Dent Res 2006;85:547–551.

78. John MT, Slade GD, Szentpetery A, Setz JM. Oral health-related quality of life in patients treated with fixed, removable, and complete dentures 1 month and 6 to 12 months after treatment. Int J Prosthodont 2004;17:503–511.

79. Allen PF, McMillan AS. A longitudinal study of quality of life outcomes in older adults requesting implant prostheses and complete removable dentures. Clin Oral Implants Res 2003;14:173–179.

80. Slade GD, Spencer AJ. Development and evaluation of the Oral Health Impact Profile. Community Dent Health 1994;11:3–11.

81. Walton JN, MacEntee MI. Choosing or refusing oral implants: a prospective study of edentulous volunteers for a clinical trial. Int J Prosthodont 2005;18:483–488.

82. Feine JS, de Grandmont P, Boudrias P, Brien N, LaMarche C, Tache R, et al. Within-subject comparisons of implant-supported mandibular prostheses: choice of prosthesis. J Dent Res 1994;73:1105–1111.

83. Redford M, Gift HC. Dentist–patient interactions in treatment decision-making: a qualitative study. J Dent Educ 1997;61:16–21.

84. Holliday RC, Cano S, Freeman JA, Playford ED. Should patients participate in clinical decision making? An optimised balance block design controlled study of goal setting in a rehabilitation unit. J Neurol Neurosurg Psychiatry 2007;78:576–580.

85. Rosén P, Anell A, Hjortsberg C. Patient views on choice and participation in primary health care. Health Policy 2001;55:121–128.

86. Palla S. L'ésthétique en prothèse amovible totale. [Esthetics in removable prosthodontics.] Cahiers Prothèse 1999;108:109

87. Palla S. Aesthetik in der Totalprothetik. [Esthetics in complete dentures.] Quintessenz 2000;51:905–919.

88. Kawai Y, Murakami H, Shariati B, Klemetti E, Blomfield JV, Billette L, et al. Do traditional techniques produce better conventional complete dentures than simplified techniques? J Dent 2005;33:659–668.

89. World Health Organization. Recent Advances in Oral Health. WHO Technical Report Series. No. 826. Geneva: World Health Organization,1992:16–17.

# Invisible Orthodontics

**12**

Hans-Peter Bantleon, Bernhard Christian Psneiner and Josef Freudenthaler

## Introduction

Physician intervention and plastic surgery aiming at better esthetics and good looks have increased substantially since the late 1980s, in terms of both investment and public interest. Consequently, the number of adult patients asking for orthodontic treatment has greatly increased.

The main concern for most of these patients is improvement in the esthetics related to the front teeth rather than an improvement in their oral function. The latter is the primary objective in interdisciplinary treatment planning and oral restoration among the specialties of dentistry. However, the patient's wish to have nicely aligned and esthetically pleasing teeth drives the demand for invisible orthodontic devices. This is the reason why orthodontists are striving for a treatment with invisible brackets, bands, and wires. Many patients did not have the possibility of orthodontic treatment in their childhood, and now that modern orthodontics can provide improved appliances that are 'more invisible', this group of patients is showing interest in the correction of malpositioned teeth.

This chapter will scrutinize the claim for invisible orthodontic devices. In addition, other orthodontic items that may be considered to be 'minimally visible' are introduced:

♦ Invisalign and similar aligners
♦ lingual therapy
♦ ceramic brackets
♦ fiber-reinforced composites (FRCs)
♦ skeletal anchorage.

## Invisalign and Similar Aligners

In 1945, Kesling used a positioner made on the casts of an idealized set-up as retention device after debanding, which enabled minor tooth movement for a final correction.[1] Based on this concept, the Essix aligner was introduced in 1993. Approximal enamel reduction enabled tooth movement using a series of these aligners. Align Technology used computer-aided design and manufacture (CAD/CAM) techniques to produce the aligners and developed Kesling's idea to clinical practice in 1997. Using the CAD technology, the orthodontist can create a virtual treatment outcome using the internet and can present and discuss the planned therapy with the patient. The orthodontist then sends the usual patient's records plus the treatment plan to the commercial center in California, USA.

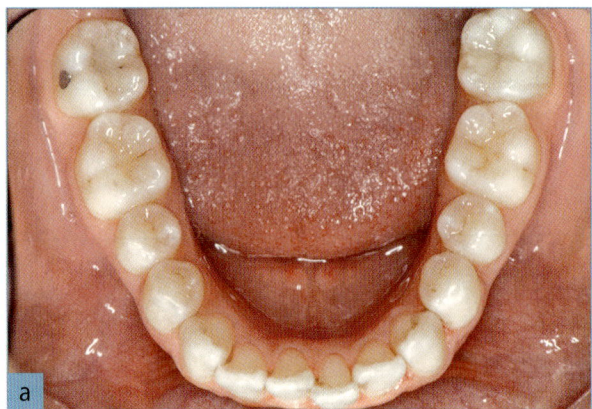

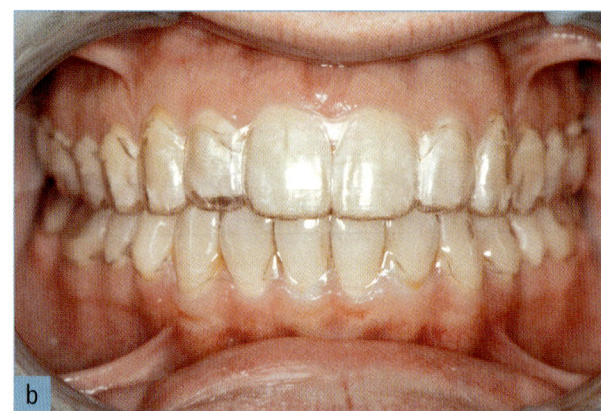

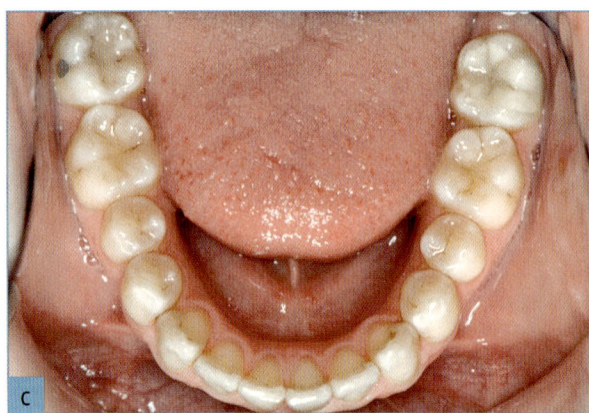

**Fig 12-1a–c** Use of an aligner was the chosen approach to deal with minor to moderate crowding in the mandible. **(a)** After enamel reduction at the contact points, the first aligner was inserted. **(b)** Every 2 weeks, a new pair of splints was inserted. **(c)** The use of the aligners over a period of 3 months resulted in perfectly aligned teeth.

Up to this point, changes in planning are possible. Once this is completed, the aligners are produced based on the designated therapeutical set-up. An aligner is a 1 mm thick splint made of clear plastic. Within 2 weeks of use of the aligner, teeth will have moved between 0.25 and 0.3 mm (Fig 12-1). Cooperation and compliance of the patient in using the aligner 20–22 hours a day is essential for its success. Over 200 000 patients worldwide have used this technology for correction of minor malocclusions such as crowding or spacing (1–5 mm), relapses after fixed therapy, and correction of tooth discrepancies in the arches (Fig 12-2). Contraindications for this treatment modality include skeletal dysgnathia, rotations of teeth more than 20 degrees, open-bite malocclusions, extrusions of teeth, moving severely tipped teeth towards upright, a reduced clinical coronal height, and patients with tooth agenesis.[2] A review of the literature since the early 1990s revealed only four clinical studies dealing with Invisalign technology.[3–6] Despite use of the technology over a 12-year period, no consensus concerning the possibilities and limitations of this technology can be seen in the orthodontic community.[7]

In the early 1980s, Burstone showed that to ensure tooth movement a certain moment-to-force-ratio had to be created.[8] It is not clear if the removable aligner is fullfilling this essential requirement as even the single acting force on the tooth by the aligner is unknown. Hence, the main indication for aligners is with enamel reduction for resolving a minor crowding in the mandible (Fig12-3). This is not surprising as a tendency to spontaneous space closure is seen after the loss of a single front tooth in the mandible. In the peer-reviewed literature, no case with bicuspid extraction

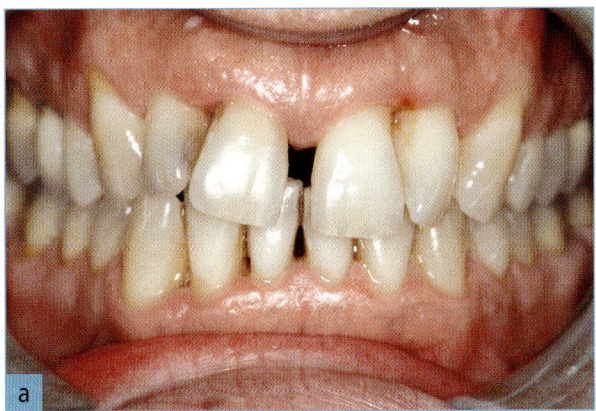

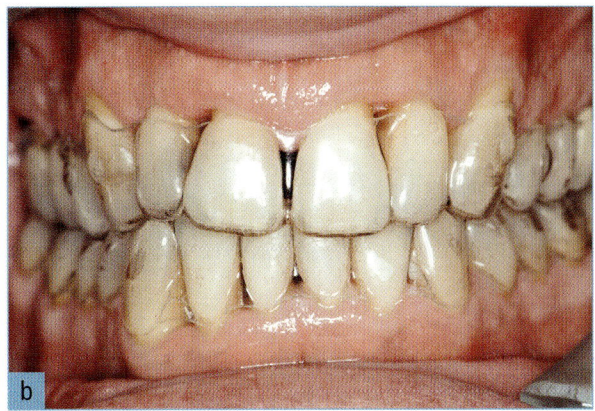

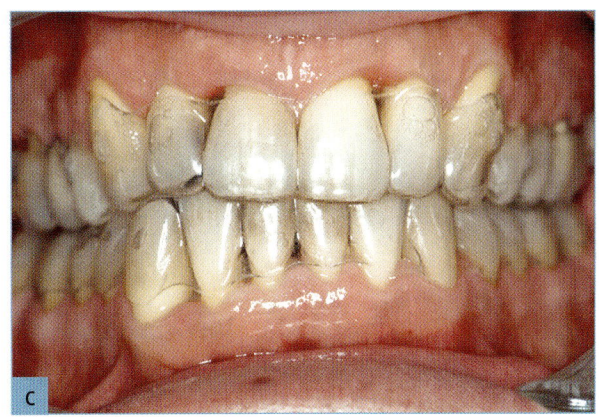

Fig 12-2a–c  Space closure of a central diastema in the maxilla using Invisalign technology as chosen by the patient. (a) View before therapy. (b) The aligners were changed every 2 weeks. (c) The result achieved during 4 months must be maintained forever.

was described that would match the Objective Grading System of the American Board of Orthodontics.[9] This would suggest that aligners are unable to exert a translatory tooth movement after bicuspid extraction. In addition, they are unable to meet the requirements for anchorage preparation. Christensen has reported recently that 48 000 dentists have passed Invisalign instruction courses since the market launch in 1999; this is a rather small proportion of the participating orthodontists (36%).[10] The survey reported the findings of 43 evaluators with 1–9 years of experience (mean, 4.2 years) with the Invisalign process. Within this group, 24 (56%) found the learning curve moderately difficult and less than 20% rated achieving treatment goals and time to reach treatment objectives as excellent. Patient satisfaction was 'excellent' for 54% compared with 45% good for dentists' satisfaction.

Selection of this treatment mode seems to be driven by the insistence of patients for esthetical orthodontic devices. Easy handling and facilitated oral hygiene are not the main reasons. In term of adverse effects of Invisalign therapy, evaluators noted lack of patient compliance and difficulties in moving teeth in 24% of the observed cases. Typical average fees from the company to the dentist are US$1425, with an overall average clinical fee of US$4750 for a comprehensive treatment in both dental arches. The survey concluded: 'The Invisalign concept has made a positive impact on orthodontic therapy by providing esthetically acceptable orthodontic treatment for minor to moderate orthodontic need situations. Patients for treatment of crowded teeth are served best'.[10]

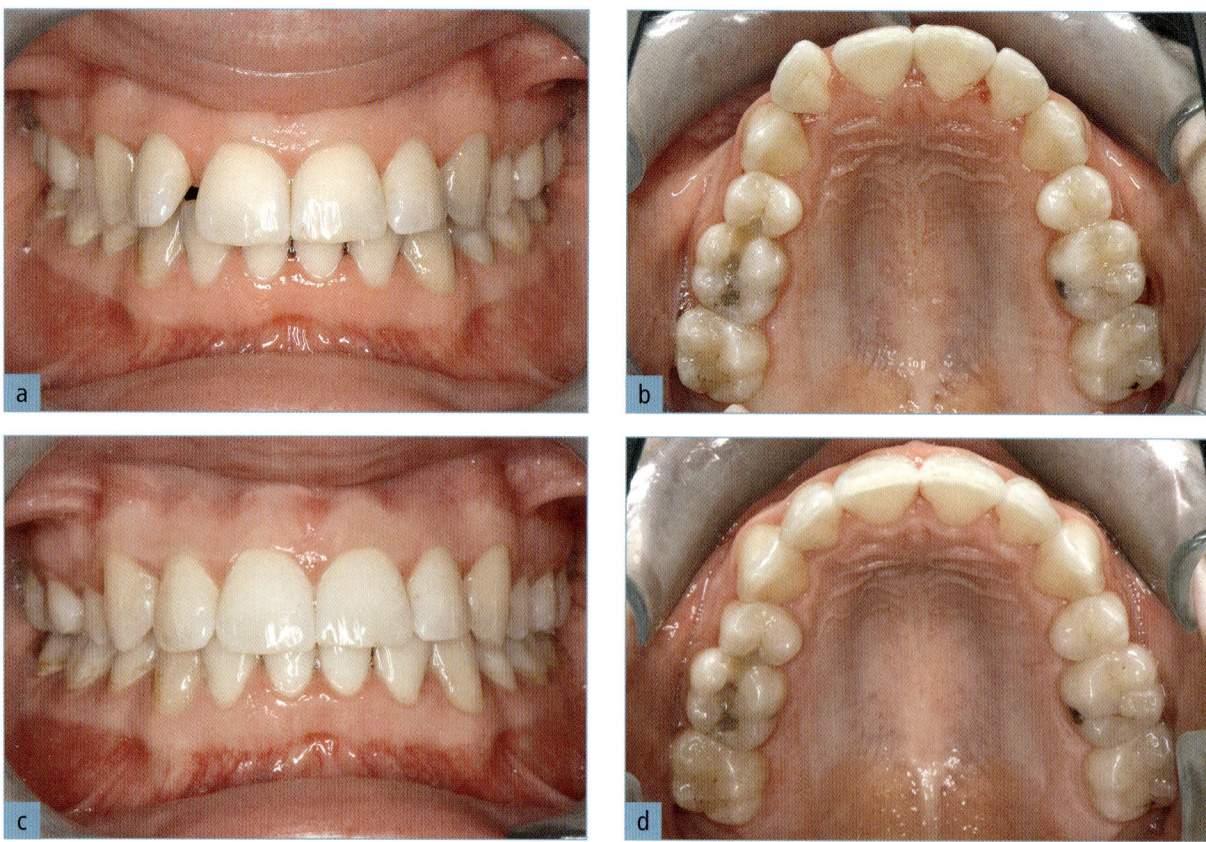

**Fig12-3a–d** The chief complaint of the patient was the buccally positioned right lateral incisor. **(a)** Frontal view. **(b)** Occlusal view of the rotated tooth, which was moved with the help an Essix aligner produced in the clinic laboratory. **(c)** Treatment phase, which lasted for 2 months. **(d)** Occlusal view after treatment, with the corrected right lateral incisor.

# Lingual Therapy

Fixed lingual bracket systems are an alternative to aligners for invisible comprehensive correction of complex malocclusion. The mechanics involved are equivalent to those in conventional techniques. This method was invented contemporaneously in Japan and the USA in the 1970s.

The demands concerning site and accessibility are complicated and, furthermore, the lingual surfaces of the teeth have considerable anatomical variability. This necessitates individual design for the bracket base and indirect bracket placement in the laboratory. The technician positions the plaster teeth in a wax set-up according to the requirements of the treatment plan. The brackets are repositioned on the malocclusion casts and thermoplastic splints are prepared for indirect bonding.

A revolutionary advance in this approach is seen in the Incognito-bracket, which is produced in Germany (TOP-Labor, Bad Essen) (Fig 12-4).[11,12] This technique uses three-dimensional CAD/CAM processes for moulding and positioning the individualized brackets. Carrying out two steps at once allows high specificity and individual shaping. Using CAD/CAM, the brackets are designed in the computer and placed on a set-up model, which is then scanned in three dimensions. The virtual brackets are converted to wax-like brackets in a prototyping machine prior to gold moulding. A bending machine is primed with the necessary information for the creation of the wire sequences (Fig 12-4f).

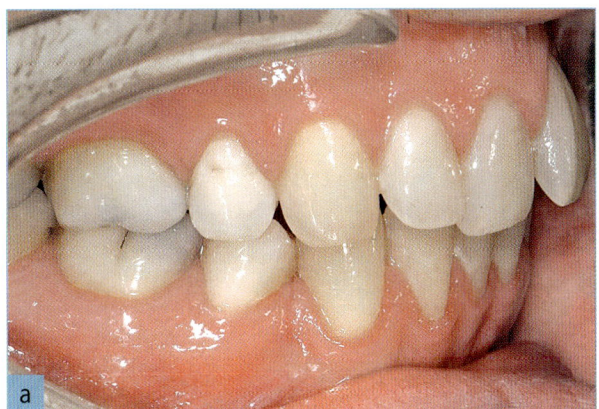

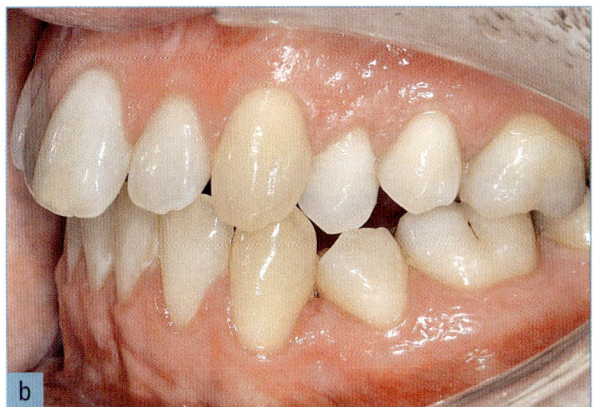

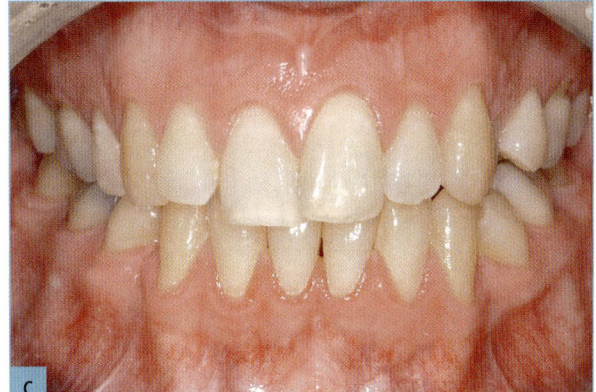

**Fig 12-4a–n** Correction of an Angle Class II malocclusion and harmonizing the midlines in both arches using lingually placed brackets (Incognito, TOP-Service, Bad Essen, Germany). **Fig 12-4f** shows the archwires produced by a computer-controlled bending machine.

**Fig.12-4g** Frontal view after insertion of the custom made archwires with a minimum bite opening effect.

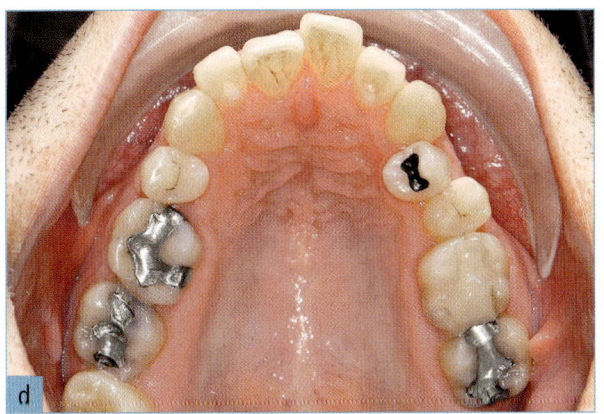

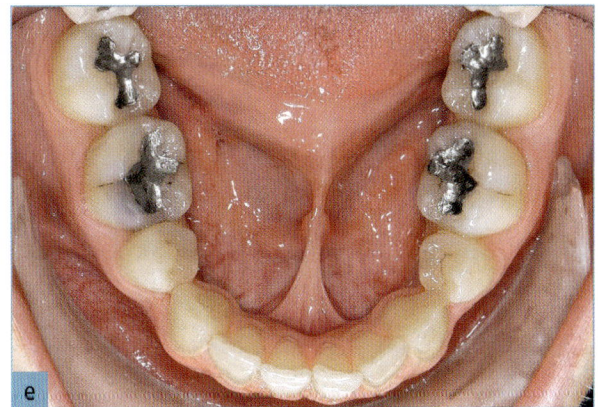

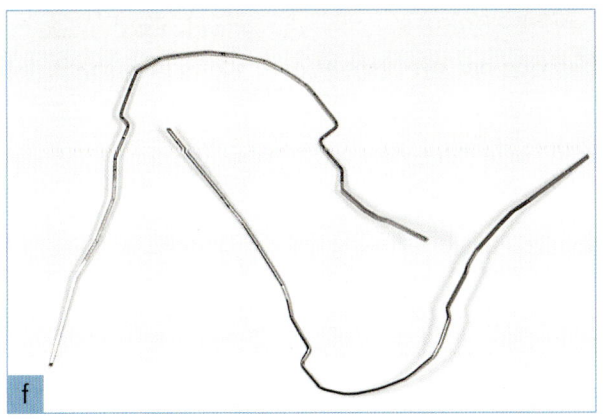

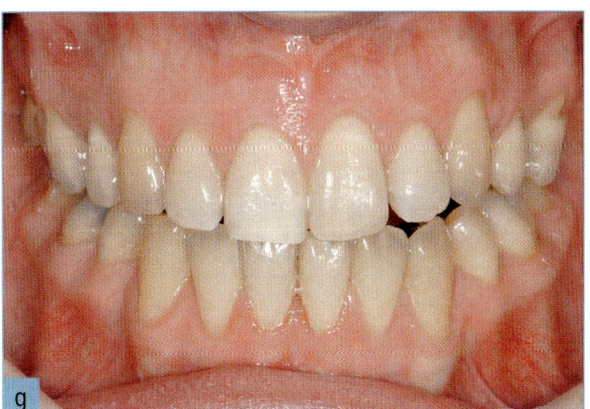

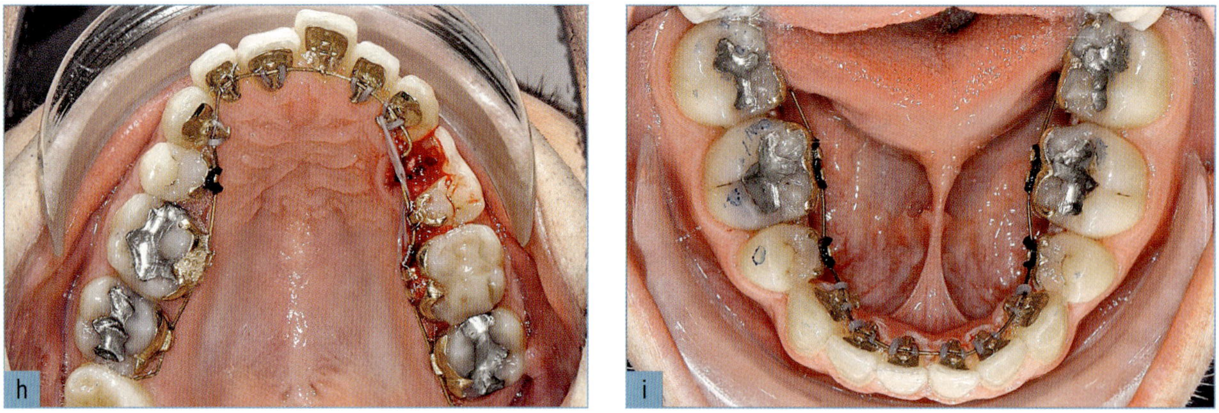

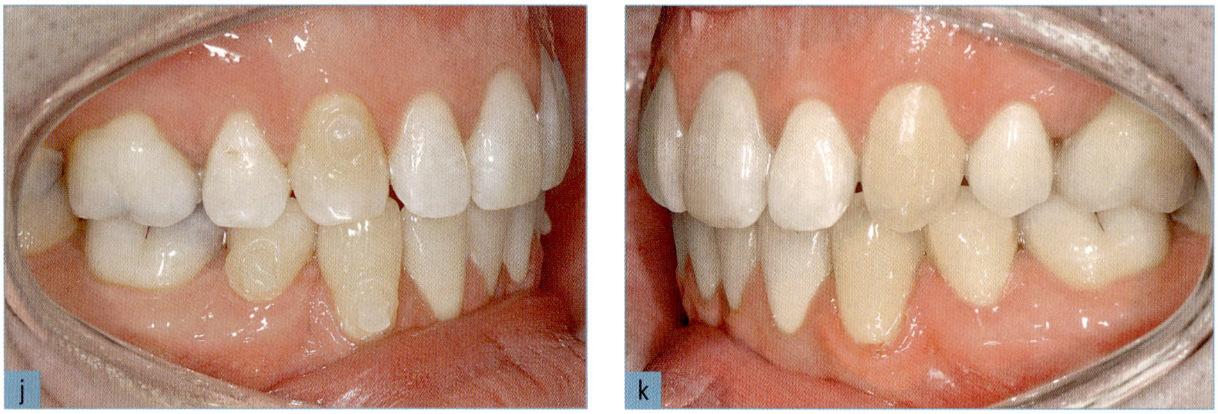

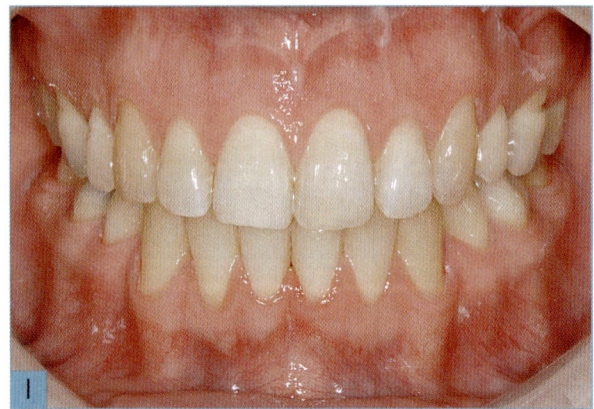

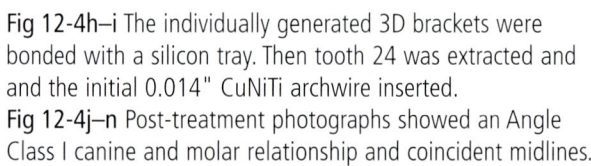

Fig 12-4h–i The individually generated 3D brackets were bonded with a silicon tray. Then tooth 24 was extracted and and the initial 0.014" CuNiTi archwire inserted.

Fig 12-4j–n Post-treatment photographs showed an Angle Class I canine and molar relationship and coincident midlines.

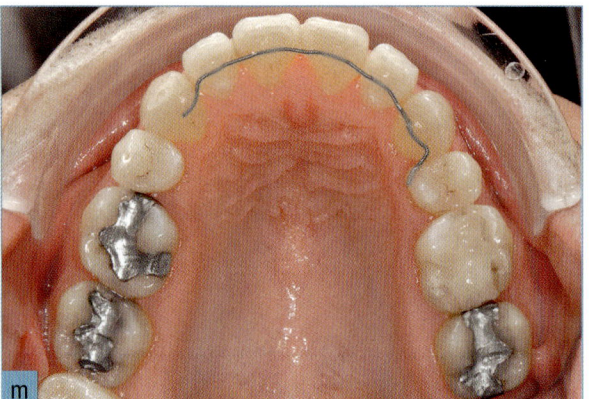

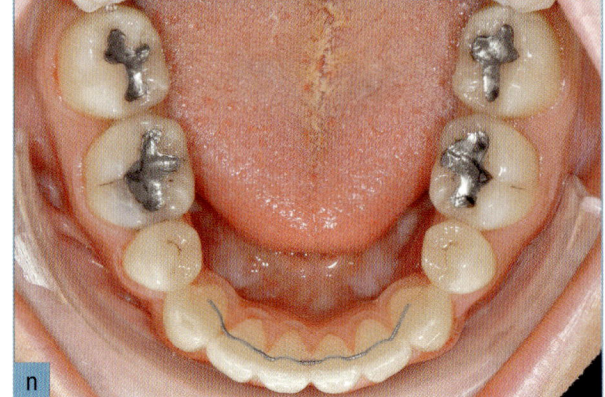

Fig 12-5a–p Use of lingual brackets for a patient with a negative anterior overjet. (a) View before treatment. (b) The maxillary right first premolar and the mandibular right first molar were missing, showing an Angle Class II angle molar relationship and an Angle Class I canine relationship. (c) The maxillary left first premolar and the mandibular left first molar were missing, showing an Angle Class II molar relationship and an Angle Class III canine relationship. (d) Maxillary arch with a buccally outblocked canine and crowded right lateral incisor. The midline was shifted to the right. (e) Spaces in the lower arch after extraction of the first lower molars.

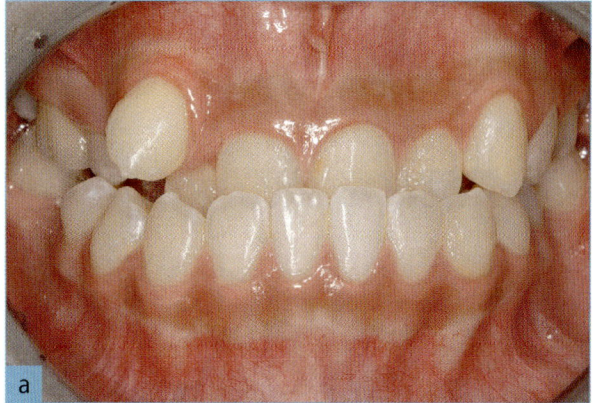

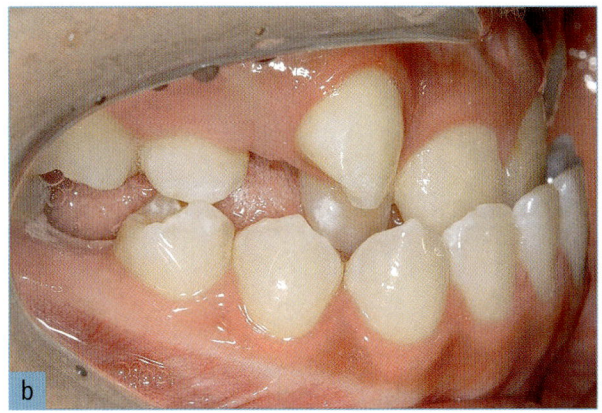

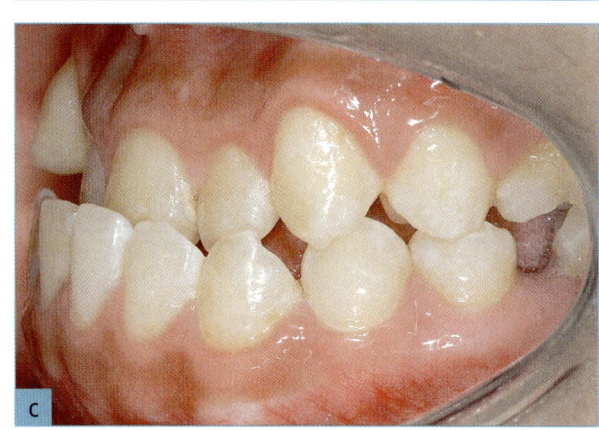

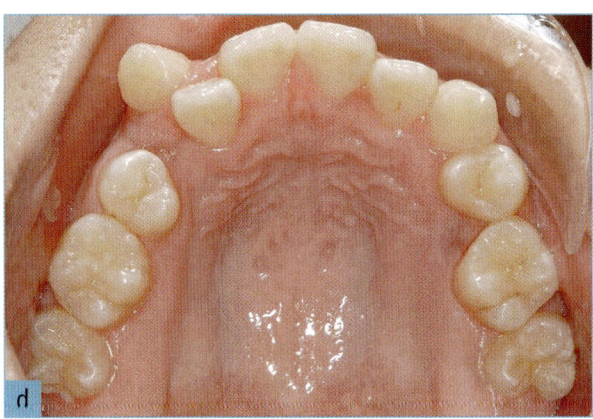

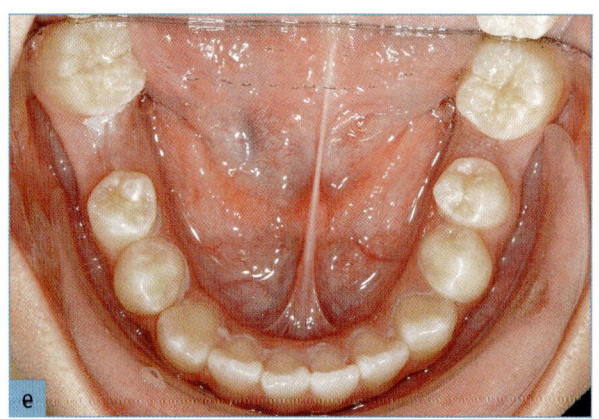

The main problems in lingual therapy are patient discomfort during the adaptation phase and reduced space for tongue function, which may lead to phonetical restriction and irritation. Tongue function is also reduced by the very low profile of the moulded bracket (Fig12-5). According to the manufacturer's specification (www.lingualtechnik.de), brackets can also be directly precision bonded because of their large base.

Finishing problems may occur with conventional laboratory processes as a result of inaccurate laboratory work and varying torque play between archwire and bracket slot. The precise bracket slot of the moulded bracket minimizes torque problems.[13]

Patient's advantages include amelioration of tooth position in the invisible approach.

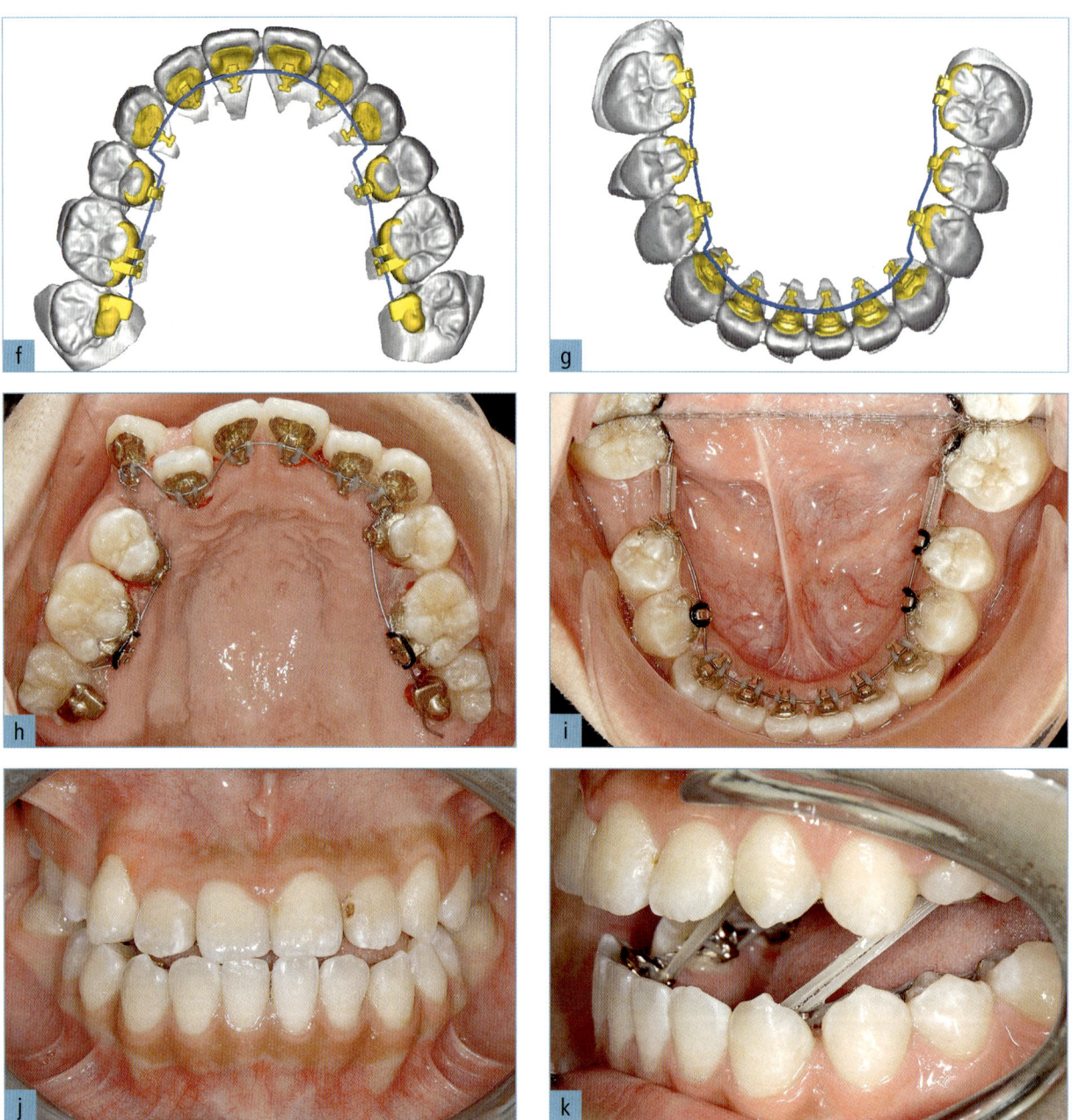

**Fig 12-5a–p** (f,g) Scanned set-up models with brackets manufactured with prototyping machines and archwires using bending robots. (h) First Ni-Ti archwire inserted in the maxillary arch. (i) Ni-Ti archwire with plastic tubes placed in the lower arch. (j) Sagittal expansion of the maxillary arch using preformed archwires and Class III elastics. (k) Class III elastics were applied from the lower canines to the maxillary first molars.

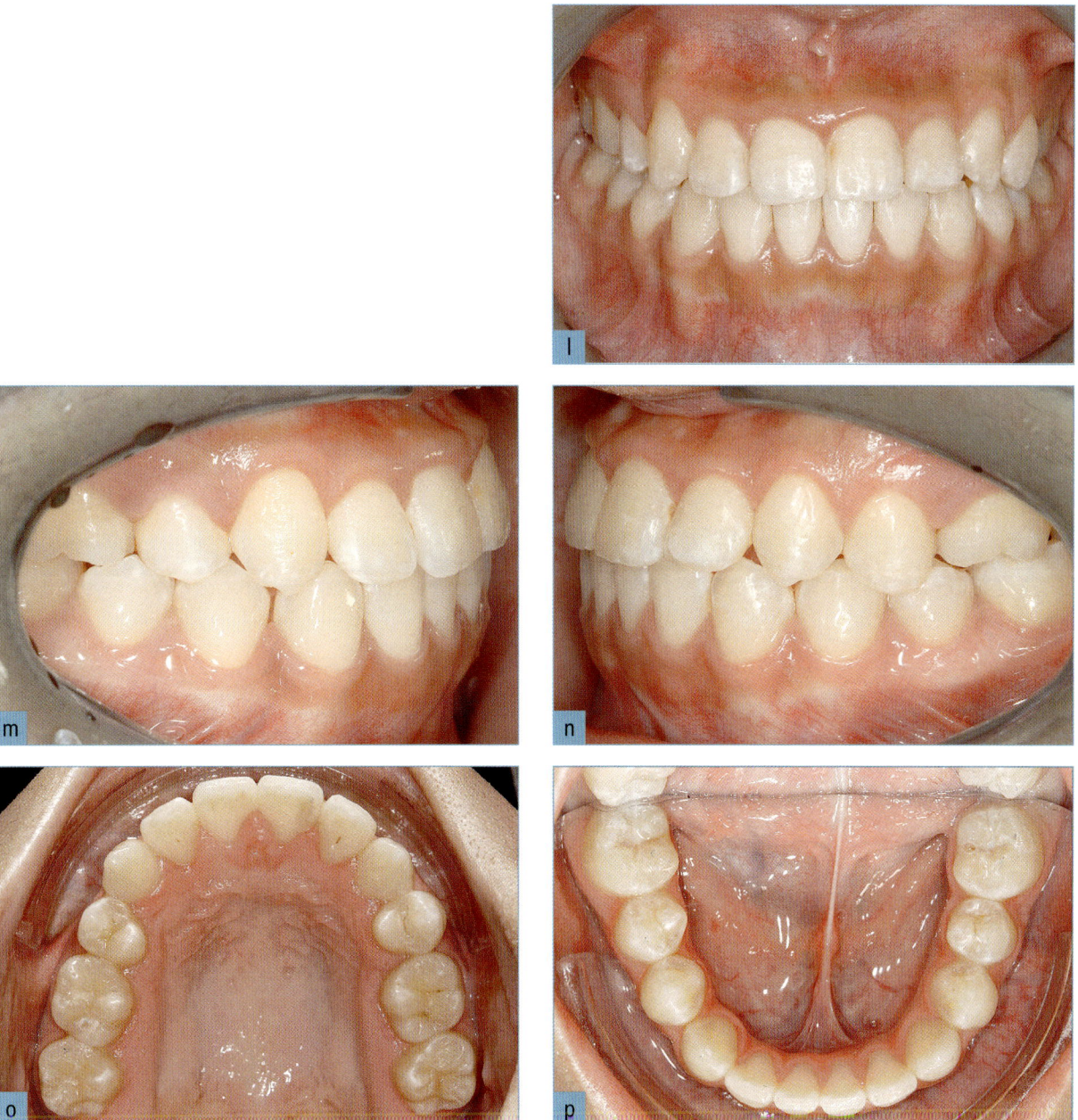

Fig 12-5a–p (l–p) Post-treatment intraoral photographs showed an Angle Class I canine and Class II molar relationship and coincident midlines. The negative overjet was corrected and the overbite considerably improved.

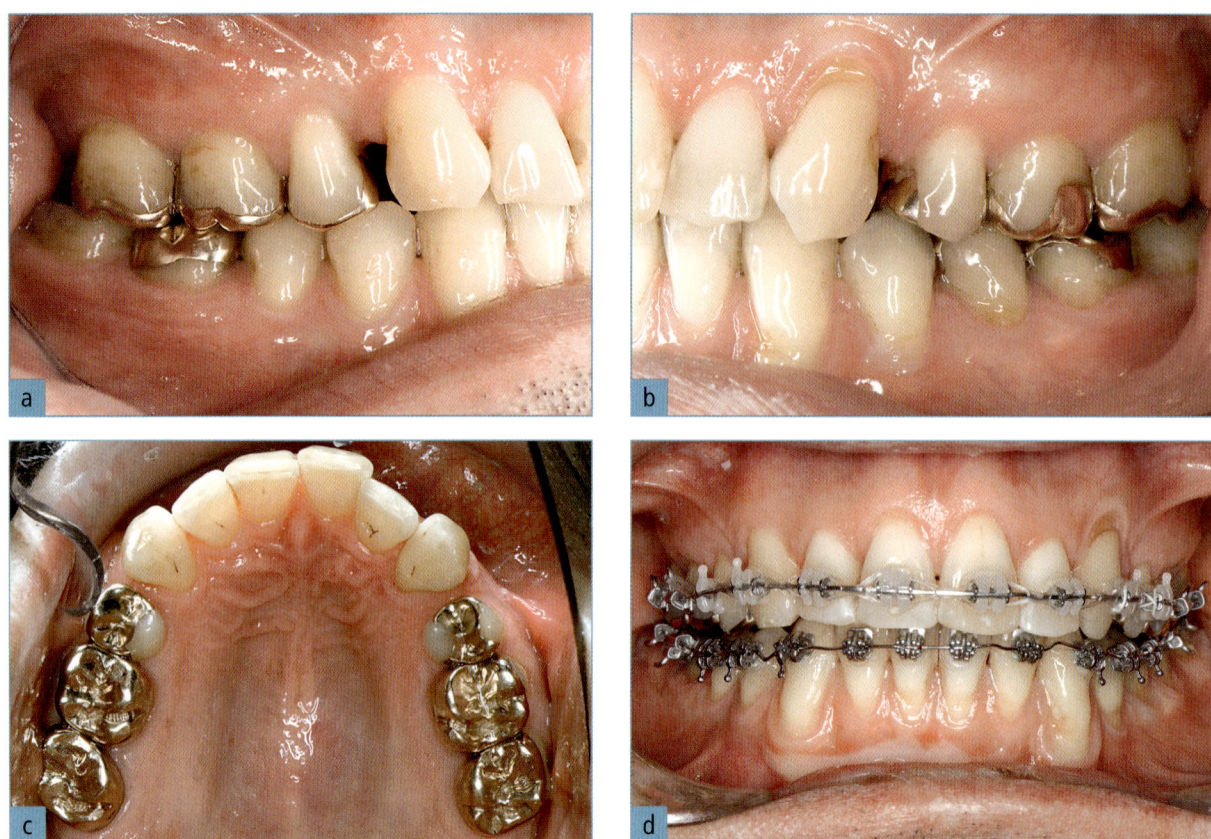

**Fig 12-6a–h** Use of ceramic brackets. **(a–c)** Views after extraction of the maxillary first premolar and opening of the necessary space for the subsequent orthodontic treatment. **(d)** The maxillary arch is bonded with self-ligating ceramic brackets. Self-ligating steel brackets were bonded in the mandibular arch.

# Ceramic Brackets

Ceramic brackets bonded to the buccal surface of the teeth are an esthetic alternative to conventional brackets. They are visible of course, especially when the metallic arch wire reflects light.

The main shortcoming of ceramic brackets is their brittleness.[14] While ceramic is resistant against high pressure, shear forces can cause fractures of the fragile wings of the bracket, so caution is needed when applying torquing forces.[15] In contrast to plastic brackets, ceramic brackets do not change color with the type of food eaten. Another advantage lies in the stability of the bracket slot dimension.[16] Recently, self-ligating ceramic brackets have been introduced to the market (Fig 12-6). The removal of ceramic brackets must be done extremely carefully to avoid enamel fractures.

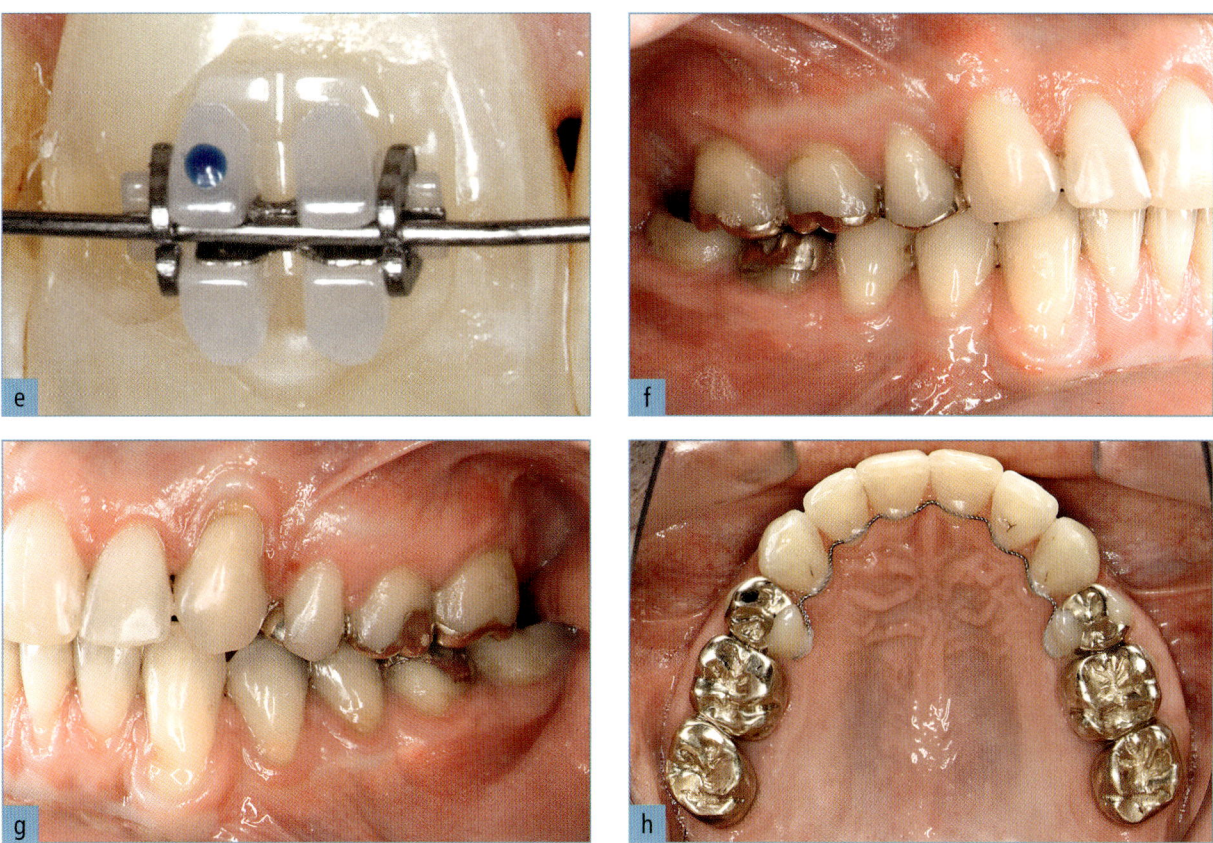

**Fig 12-6a-h** (e) Fitting of a self-ligating ceramic bracket (Clarity SL, 3M Unitek, Monrovia, CA, USA). (f–h) Post-treatment intraoral photographs showed an Angle Class I canine and an Angle Class II molar relationship, plus coincident midlines and normal overjet and overbite. The gaps between the maxillary canines and second premolars were closed and retained with a wire extended to the maxillary second premolars.

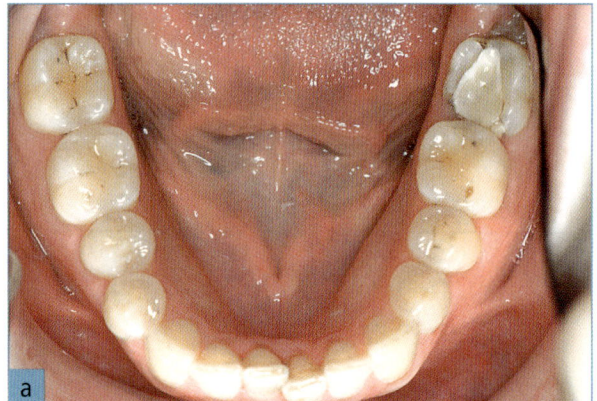
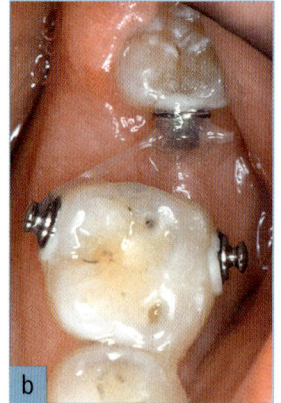
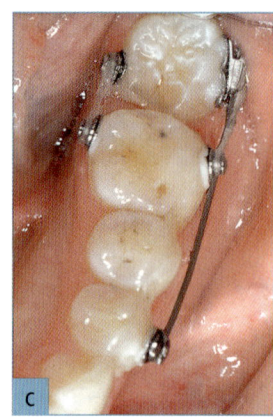
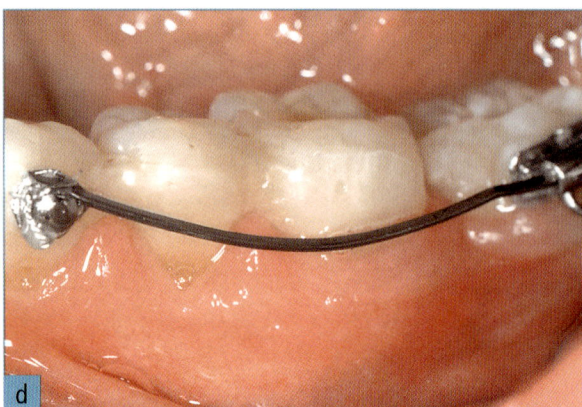

**Fig 12-7a–d** The use of fiber-reinforced composites (FRCs) to adjust spacing after tooth extraction. **(a)** Tooth 37 in a patient with a Class I occlusion had to be extracted because of chronic inflammation. **(b)** The FRC was used to establish a tooth-borne anchorage unit between teeth 34 and 36. Tooth 38 was moved mesially by elastics placed buccally and lingually. **(c,d)** The third left lower molar was moved to a more upright position with a lever arm made from 0.43 mm x 0.64 mm (0.017 inch by 0.025 inch) TMA-wire and hooked with a single point to the bonded bottom. The space closure was achieved within 7 months.

# Fiber-Reinforced Composites

The FRCs are additional orthodontic tools used in certain, well-defined situations. The FRC consists of prefabricated strips that need to be adjusted prior to the final polymerization. The strips are attached to the enamel with a flowable bonding agent. Originally, FRCs were used in prosthodontic dentistry as retainers, resin-bonded fixed dental protheses, and splints. In orthodontics, they serve as parts of the passive unit or as a base for attachments (Fig 12-7). The FRCs are not invisible but they are far less compromising for dental appearance than conventional metallic brackets (Fig 12-8). They clearly are easy to handle and a safe and firm fit is achieved with the conditioned enamel.[17–20]

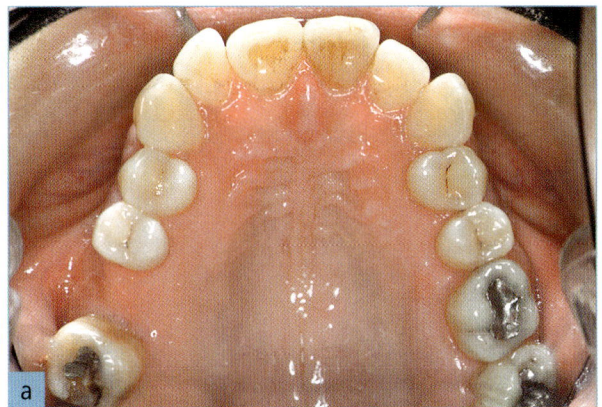
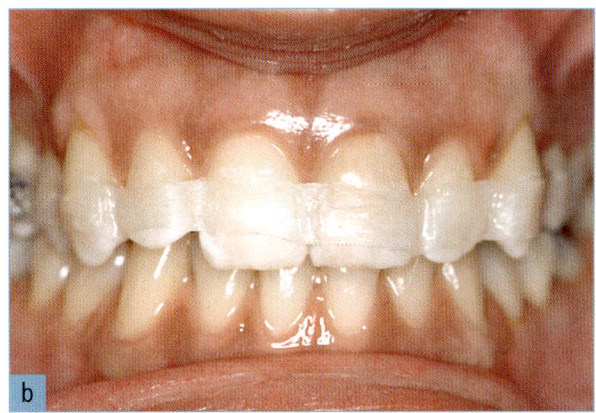
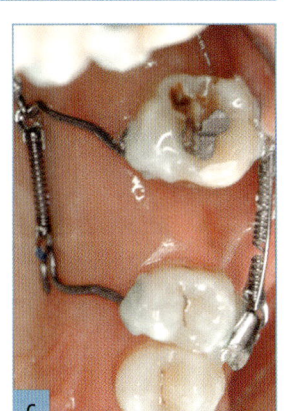
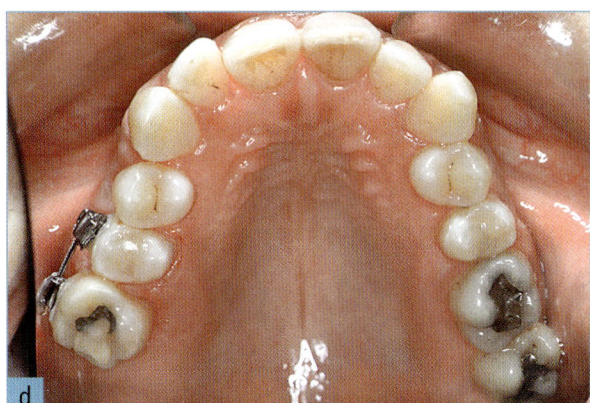

**Fig 12-8a–d** The use of fiber-reinforced composites (FRCs) to adjust spacing after tooth extraction. (a) Following the extraction of tooth 16, space closure was planned prior to prosthodontic restoration. (b) A FRC was bonded between teeth 15 and 25 in the maxillary arch for retention. (c) Lever arms were bonded to teeth 17 and 15 and loaded with superelastic coil springs buccally and lingually. This enabled a translatory tooth movement. (d) Result after completing treatment at 1 year.

# Skeletal Anchorage

In the early 1990s, Albino Triaca made the first palatial placements of implants.[21] Skeletal anchorage devices have been used since that initial development, particularly in Europe and Asia. Palatal implants were the initial preferred option, but, nowadays, there is a strong trend for the use of so-called miniscrews, alone or in combination with miniplates.[22] A temporary skeletal anchorage can achieve maximum anchorage control in situations where a tooth-borne anchorage is not compatible with treatment requirements.[23] No healing period for osseointegration is necessary as the correct positioning of the screws leads to a primary stability. The success rate of miniscrews is as high as 90%, that of palatal implants over 90%.[24] Skeletal anchorage systems are replacing the esthetically displeasing extraoral devices such as headgear and Delaire, or Grummons facemasks (Fig12-9). These were not acceptable by adults and so these patients were unable to take advantage of a comprehensive orthodontic treatment.

The main indications for skeletal anchorage systems are space closure with mesial tooth movement and distal shifting of molars (Fig12-10).[25] Among the patients who are profiting from this novel technique prior to prosthodontic treatment are those with reduced dental arches (multiple agenesis and a mutilated dentition).[26]

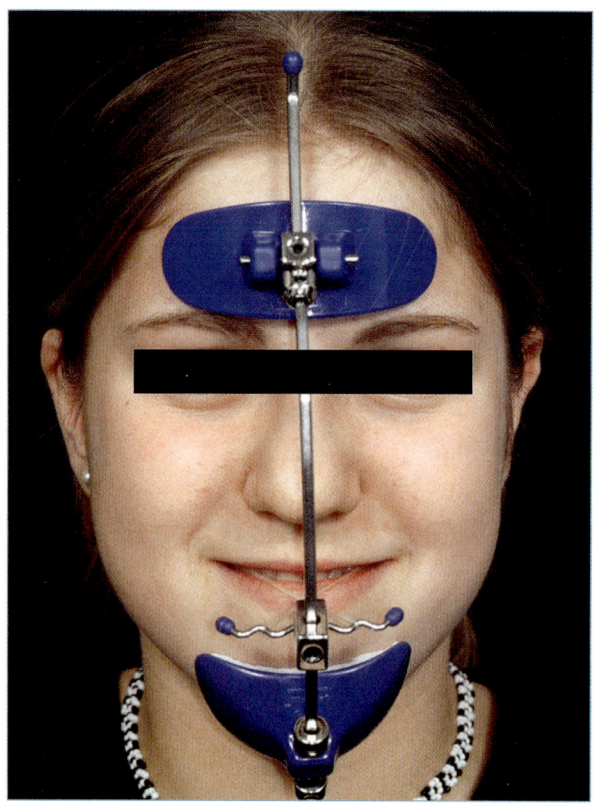

**Fig 12-9** Before skeletal anchorage elements became available, extraoral devices had to be used for anchorage preparation. In this case, a Delaire facemask was used for molar protraction.

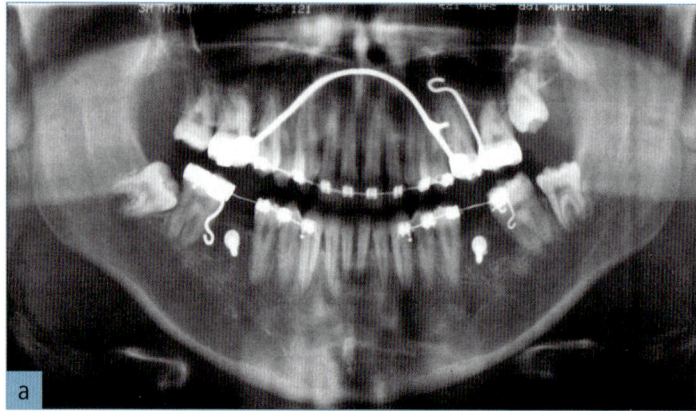

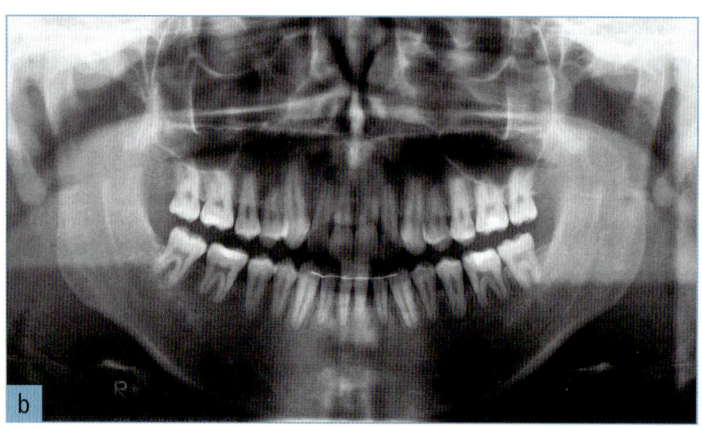

**Fig 12-10a–b** **(a)** The use of a skeletal anchorage system in a patient who had lost all first molars through juvenile aggressive periodontitis. Bicortical screws were placed in the mesial socket of the extraction site. **(b)** Situation after treatment: Elastic traction moved the posterior teeth mesially, maintaining a Class I occlusion.

# Retention

At the end of therapy with a fixed appliance, the position of the teeth should be ideal. However, this needs to be maintained under the natural pressures of the modelling and remodelling that occurs in the dentoalveolar apparatus. According to Reitan, the periodontal fibers need almost a year for stabilization of the treatment result.[27] This explains why there is a tendency for relapse after orthodontic therapy; this is particularly a problem in males and during prolonged growth periods.[28] To avoid this relapse from the treated positions, several devices, all called retainers, have been developed to hold the teeth in place. Removable plates such as the Hawley-Retainer can be used or fixed wires can be bonded to the lingual surface of the teeth. As mentioned above, FRC or plastic splints can also be used as retainers.

Long-term studies have examined the stability of achieved treatment results over a period of 10 years. Almost 50% of the relapses occur in the first 2 years after the retention period.[28,29] After that time, the treatment position stabilizes, apart from in the mandibular intercanine segment. Discouraging results were published by Little, who showed that after 10 years the position of the mandibular front teeth was as bad as prior to the orthodontic treatment.[30] Therefore, realignment of crowded teeth cannot be regarded as stable. The distance between the lower canines decreases throughout life. Growth increments are seen in adults as well as in children and they may be accompanied by compensatory changes in the dentition. It is obvious that the orthodontist is unable to influence such processes. However, relapse is not as severe in adults as in children.[31]

There is no consensus in the orthodontic community as to the length of time that retention should continue as scientific evidence is lacking. The use of retention for 5 to 10 years is a good prerequisite for stable results. However, based on the data provided by Little[30] and Zachrisson,[32] only long-term retention should be recommended to the patient.

# References

1. Elsasser WA. Some observations on the history and uses of the Kesling positioner. Am J Orthod 1950;36:568–574.
2. Phan X, Ling PH. Clinical limitations of Invisalign. J Can Dent Assoc 2007;73:363–366.
3. Vlaskalic V, Boyd RL. Clinical evolution of the Invisalign appliance. J Calif Dent Assoc 2002;30:1069–1076.
4. Bollen AM, Huang G, King G, Hujoel P, Ma T. Activation time and material stiffness of sequential removable orthodontic appliances. Part 1: ability to complete treatment. Am J Orthod Dentofacial Orthop 2003;124:496–501.
5. Clements KM, Bollen AM, Huang G, King G, Hujoel P, Ma T. Activation time and material stiffness of sequential removable orthodontic appliances. Part 2: dental improvements. Am J Orthod Dentofacial Orthop 2003;124:502–508.
6. Djeu G, Shelton C, Maganzini A. Outcome assessment of Invisalign and traditional orthodontic treatment compared with the American Board of Orthodontics objective grading system. Am J Orthod Dentofacial Orthop 2005;128:392–398.
7. Turpin DL. Clinical trials needed to answer questions about Invisalign. Am J Orthod Dentofacial Orthop 2005;127:257–258.
8. Koenig HA, Vanderby R, Solonche DJ, Burstone CJ. Force systems from orthodontic appliances: an analytical and experimental comparison. J Biomech Eng 1980;102:494–300.
9. Lagravère MO, Flores-Mir C. The treatment effects of Invisalign orthodontic aligners: a systematic review. J Am Dent Assoc 2005;136:12724–12729.
10. Christensen GC. Evaluator Survey on Non-Conventional Movement of Teeth, Part 1. Clinicians Report, CR Foundation; Provo.2008 Volume1
11. Wiechmann D. A new bracket system for lingual orthodontic treatment. Part 1: theoretical background and development. J Orofac Orthop 2002;63:334–345.
12. Wiechmann D, Rummel V, Thalheim A, Simon JS, Wiechmann L. Customized brackets and archwires for lingual orthodontic treatment. Am J Orthod Dentofacial Orthop 2003;124:593–599.
13. Ye L, Kula KS. Status of lingual orthodontics. World J Orthod 2006;7:461–468.
14. Bishara SE, Fehr DE. Ceramic brackets: something old, something new, a review. Semin Orthod 1997;3:378–388.
15. Russell JS. Aesthetic orthodontic brackets. J Orthod 2005;32:246–263.
16. Karamouzos A, Athanasiou AE, Papadopoulos MA. Clinical characteristics and properties of ceramic brackets: a comprehensive review. Am J Orthod Dentofacial Orthop 1997;112:14–40.
17. Freudenthaler JW, Tischler GK, Burstone CJ. Bond strength of fiber-reinforced composite bars for orthodontic attachment. Am J Orthod Dentofacial Orthop 2001;120:648–653.
18. Cacciafesta V, Sfondrini MF, Lena A, Scribante A, Vallittu PK, Lassila LV. Flexural strengths of fiber-reinforced composites polymerized with conventional light-curing and additional postcuring. Am J Orthod Dentofac Orthop 2007;132:424–427.
19. Cacciafesta V, Sfondrini MF, Lena A, Scribante A, Vallittu PK, Lassila LV. Force levels of fiber-reinforced composites and orthodontic stainless steel wires: a 3-point bending test. Am J Orthod Dentofacial Orthop 2008;133:310–313.
20. Kirzioglu Z, Ertürk MS. Success of reinforced fiber material space maintainers. J Dent Child 2004;71:258–2562.

21. Wehrbein H, Merz BR, Diedrich P, Glatzmaier J. The use of palatal implants for orthodontic anchorage. Design and clinical application of the orthosystem. Clin Oral Implants Res 1996;7:410–416.

22. Leung MT, Lee TC, Rabie AB, Wong RW. Use of miniscrews and miniplates in orthodontics. J Oral Maxillofac Surg 2008;66:7461–7466.

23. Wehrbein H, Göllner P. Skeletal anchorage in orthodontics: basics and clinical application. J Orofac Orthop 2007;68:643–661.

24. Papadopoulos MA, Tarawneh F. The use of miniscrew implants for temporary skeletal anchorage in orthodontics: a comprehensive review. Oral Surg Oral Med Oral Pathol Oral Radiol Endod 2007;103:e6–e15.

25. Fishel DL, Vanarsdall RL Jr. The use of miniscrews for orthodontic anchorage. Compend Contin Educ Dent 2007;28:1238–1242.

26. Heymann GC, Tulloch JF. Implantable devices as orthodontic anchorage: a review of current treatment modalities. J Esthet Restor Dent 2006;18:28–79; discussion 80.

27. Reitan K. Clinical and histologic observations on tooth movement during and after orthodontic treatment. Am J Orthod 1967;53:1021–1045.

28. Al Yami EA, Kuijpers-Jagtman AM, van 't Hof MA. Stability of orthodontic treatment outcome: follow-up until 10 years postretention. Am J Orthod Dentofac Orthop 1999;115:300–304.

29. Binda SK, Kuijpers-Jagtman AM, Maertens JK, van 't Hof MA. A long-term cephalometric evaluation of treated Class II division 2 malocclusions. Eur J Orthod 1994;16:401–408.

30. Little RM. Stability and relapse of dental arch alignment. Br J Orthod 1990;17:335–341.

31. Littlewood SJ, Millett DT, Doubleday B, Bearn DR, Worthington HV. Orthodontic retention: a systematic review. J Orthod 2006;33:305–312.

32. Zachrisson BU. Long term experience with direct bonded retainers: update and clinical advice. J Clin Orthod 2007;41:728–737

# Principles for Selection of Metal-Ceramic and All-Ceramic Prostheses

13

Kenneth J. Anusavice and Josephine F. Esquivel-Upshaw

## Introduction

Fixed dental prostheses (FDPs) represent one of the most costly options that a dental patient can face. The cost of a single ceramic crown ranges from US$500 to $3000 depending on materials, complexity of oral conditions (disease, occlusion, bone quality, and tissue health), location in the dental arch, and the clinician's training and experience.

The recent increased demand for esthetics and the development of stronger and tougher core ceramics and associated processing technologies have led to the introduction of ceramic products for crowns and FDPs well before the limitations of these products have been fully explored. Furthermore, the increased acceptance by the profession of minimally invasive dentistry concepts has resulted in the development of thinner metal substrates (0.1–0.3 mm) such as burnished metal foil, e.g., Captek, or electroformed metal copings for metal–ceramic crowns. Ceramic core substrates for total ceramic crowns have a minimal thickness of 0.4 mm although thicknesses of up to 0.7 mm are recommended. For FDPs, the connector shape and size as well as the crown design control survival probability.

Unfortunately, dental patients unwittingly serve as test subjects for many new all-ceramic products and prosthesis designs, which have been introduced with limited long-term study data that demonstrate their effectiveness and durability. Furthermore, like metal–ceramics, they also have an external veneering ceramic, which is the weak link in the system. The outermost ceramic veneers used today exhibit the lowest flexural strength and fracture toughness of any ceramic product used for FDP applications. These veneering ceramic formulations have not improved significantly since metal–ceramic restorations were introduced in the early 1960s. This part of the structure, which is composed predominantly of a glass phase, has been and still remains the Achilles heel of FDP restorations.

We have been able to improve the fracture resistance of veneering glasses and feldspathic-based porcelains by supporting them with relatively stiff cast metal substrates. However, the elastic moduli of alumina (418 GPa) and zirconia (210 GPa) core ceramics exceed those of palladium-silver alloy (92 GPa), type III gold alloy (100 GPa), tooth enamel (130 GPa), and nickel-chromium alloy (145 GPa). This suggests that a certain proportion of tensile stress generated under occlusal forces or as a result of thermal incompatibility will be transferred to the stiffer core material and away from the more fragile veneering ceramic. In principle, the survival probability of all-ceramic prostheses generally should increase as the elastic modulus of the core increases, as the fracture toughness of structural components increases, as the thicknesses of the components and design areas increase, and as the population density of critical flaws decreases.

Recent introductions of ultrathin burnished metal foil, e.g., Captek, or electroformed metal copings, which are made by electrodeposition of metal on a die, have led to premature failures of crowns and FDPs in certain cases, especially when adequate tooth reduction is not possible or when the teeth have not been adequately reduced to the optimal dimensions needed for maximum survival. The fact is that the designs of FDPs[1] have been based primarily on empirical evidence and minimal science. There are many reasons for this, not the least of which is the lack of funding for well-designed clinical trials that are free of bias. Review of the scientific literature reveals relatively few studies of the biomechanics-based designs that are required to ensure high-survival times and probabilities for all-ceramic restorations. However, a few excellent studies have been published and these provide some initial insights into the variables that are most likely to control the resistance of the prostheses to fracture. Fracture origins have been observed primarily at the gingival embrasure of the connectors in fractured and retrieved Cercon four-unit FDPs made from a zirconia core ceramic.[1] The importance of connector design has been demonstrated in several studies.[2–4]

Failures of dental prostheses can be caused by patient factors, clinician errors, laboratory technician errors, and material deficiencies. Patient factors, such as biting, chewing, clenching, and bruxing habits, cannot be controlled by the clinician, although oral hygiene and other disease-controlling regimens can be promoted through education. The last three variables can be corrected to a potentially greater extent through biomechanics, translational, and clinical translational research.

# Requirements of Ceramic-Based Restorations

One of the primary functions of ceramic-based restorations is their ability to mimic sound tooth structure and blend with what is natural. Esthetics is defined as the branch of philosophy dealing with beauty and beautification. The development of ceramic-based restorations has primarily been driven by the need to satisfy the demand for tooth-colored restorations; for most of the population, this reflects the desire to be beautiful or physically attractive. Our esthetically aware society is constantly demanding more life-like restorations, and this generates the need to develop ceramic based products with a wide range of chroma, hue, value, fluorescence, and translucency to match natural tooth structures. The increased strength and toughness of alumina and zirconia core ceramics do not necessarily mean success since these ceramics reflect a significant level of opacity that must be compensated for by increasing the veneer/core thickness ratio.

Marginal integrity, defined as the proper adaptation of the margin of the restoration to the cavosurface angle or margin of the tooth, is another requirement for ceramic-based restorations, as with any type of restoration. The marginal gap of any restoration is defined as the 'weak link' since it often provides ingress of bacteria for recurrent caries, for periodontal deterioration, or for dissolution of cement if the adaptation is inadequate.[5] There has been much debate as to the maximum amount of marginal opening allowable before failure of the restoration occurs. With properly prepared margins and an experienced technician, cast and porcelain margins can be as low as 10 and 50 μm, respectively. At the time of writing, there is still no agreement on what degree of opening is considered acceptable. Marginal adaptations can range anywhere from 30 to 100 μm and still yield acceptable clinical results.[6]

Fracture resistance is defined as the ability to resist fracture. One of the main factors in a crown's ability to resist fracture is the design of the preparation itself, which allows for adequate thickness of the restorative material, proper occlusion, adequate height, and good marginal adaptation. The physical properties of the restorative materials are secondary to the fracture resistance of a restoration. These include hardness, elastic modulus, fracture toughness, flexural strength of the ceramic, and thermal compatibility. However, excessive wear of enamel by ceramics can be a cause of failure.

Wear is defined as the 'progressive loss of substance from the surface of a solid caused by mechanical action'.[7] Ceramics are known to cause abrasive wear of opposing enamel or to develop excessive wear on the ceramic surface. One of the major requirements of ceramic-based materials is that they are wear resistant and show minimal wear through years of mastication, but they must not induce excessive wear on opposing enamel or abrasive resistance. Microfracture is the dominant mechanism responsible for surface breakdown of ceramics and the subsequent damage that a roughened ceramic surface can cause within tooth enamel surfaces. Enamel is also susceptible to microfracture abrasion through one or more mechanisms: asperities extending from the ceramic surface, which produce high localized stresses and microfracture; gouging, which results from high stresses and large hardness differences between two surfaces or particles extending from these surfaces; impact or erosion, which occurs through the action of abrasive particles carried in a flowing liquid such as saliva; and contact stress microfracture, which increases localized tensile stress and also enhances the damage caused by asperities, gouging, and impact or erosion. Periodic polishing of the ceramic surface is often required because of these microfracture mechanisms. Of major concern is the potential catastrophic damage that can be incurred by enamel in contact with polycrystalline asperities having high fracture toughness values, such as alumina (3.5–4.0 MPa·m$^{1/2}$), Mg-stabilized zirconia (9–12 MPa·m$^{1/2}$), yttria-stabilized zirconia (6–9 MPa·m$^{1/2}$), or ceria-stabilized zirconia (10–16 MPa·m$^{1/2}$). In contrast, glass has a fracture toughness of only 0.75 MPa·m$^{1/2}$ and should cause less gouging, contact stress, and impact damage within contacting enamel surfaces.

The abrasiveness of ceramics against enamel is affected by numerous factors that include hardness of both surfaces, shape and size of the crystalline phase particles of a ceramic, tensile strength, fracture toughness of each material, fatigue resistance, particle–glass bond, particle–glass interface integrity, chemical durability, exposure frequency to corrosive chemical agents (acidulated phosphate fluoride, carbonated beverages, citric acid), abrasiveness of foods, residual stress state, subsurface quality such as voids or imperfections, surface roughness, chemical durability of the ceramic, residual stress type (tension, compression or shear), magnitude and orientation of applied forces, chewing and bruxing frequency, lubricant properties, contact area, and wear debris. It is important to understand why the hardness of the ceramic is not a good predictor of potential wear of enamel surfaces by a ceramic. Comparative analysis of wear of different restorative materials has been ranked along with their hardness values[8] and no correlation was found between wear performance and material hardness. However, hardness does contribute to the wear process, since larger hardness differences between two sliding surfaces are associated with greater degrees of gouging.

# Metal-Ceramic Systems

In 2003 the American Dental Association reclassified casting metals from the 1984 classification according to their titanium content and their noble metal content (gold, iridium, osmium, palladium, platinum, rhodium, and ruthenium). Typically, the noble metals that are used primarily for cast dental alloys are gold and two platinum group metals, palladium and platinum. The four casting metal classes are as follows:

1. High Noble: ≥ 40 wt% gold and ≥ 60 wt% noble metal
2. Titanium and Titanium Alloys: ≥ 85 wt% titanium
3. Noble Metal: ≥ 25 wt% noble metal (no gold requirement)

4. Predominantly Base Metal: < 25 wt% noble metal (no gold requirement).

High noble metal alloys contain a minimum of 60% by weight of noble metal (gold, platinum, palladium and/or other noble elements) and at least 40% by weight of gold. Historically, formulations have been based on gold-platinum-palladium (Au-Pt-Pd), gold-palladium-silver (Au-Pd-Ag) and gold-palladium (Au-Pd) alloys. Noble metal alloys require a minimum of 25% by weight of noble metals with no requirement for gold content. Formulations of noble metal alloys are based on a majority of palladium. Typical alloys include palladium-silver (Pd-Ag), palladium-copper-gallium (Pd-Cu-Ga), and palladium-silver-gold (Pd-Ag-Au). Predominantly base metal alloys contain less than 25% by weight of noble metals and may or may not have any gold content. Formulations include nickel-chromium (Ni-Cr), nickel-chromium-beryllium (Ni-Cr-Be), and cobalt-chromium (Co-Cr).

There are different types of margin available for a metal-ceramic restoration.[6] The most commonly used are:
- chamfer, which provides obtuse internal and external line angle
- heavy chamfer, which exhibits obtuse internal line angle but provides a 90 degree angle at the cavosurface margin
- shoulder, which provides a 90 degree internal line angle and is desirable for all-ceramic restorations as it provides the most esthetic result, the major disadvantage being the requirement for a maximum amount of tooth reduction
- radial shoulder, a modified version of the shoulder but with a rounded internal line angle; this design also exhibits a 90 degree cavosurface margin and stress concentration is minimized with the rounded line angle
- shoulder with a bevel, which can be utilized in situations where esthetics is not of as much concern and provides for added retention for short axial walls
- knife-edge, which is usually used for full-metallic restorations, although poor laboratory work can result in

overcontoured restorations; it provides the advantage of minimizing tooth reduction.

Marginal designs have been examined to determine which ones are more likely to distribute stress to ceramic and which are more apt to distort. Chamfer preparations have been shown to exhibit greater distortion than the shoulder or shoulder-bevel designs, although there was no significant difference noted between the last two.[9] Others have reported greater marginal distortion with a base metal alloy compared with a Au-Pt-Pd alloy when fired with porcelain.[10] They further concluded that the greatest marginal gap change occurred with the oxidation cycle (70 μm for the base metal alloy and 7 μm for the gold alloy). A subsequent study revealed that grinding and sandblasting are more likely causes of marginal distortion than the thermal contraction mismatch.[11] A metal coping thickness of 0.1 mm or less and the asymmetrical marginal extremities are more susceptible to localized or generalized distortion.[12]

A study of the effects of margin design (rounded shoulder, rounded shoulder with a bevel, and a chamfer) on the tensile stress distribution revealed no significant effects at the cement-dentin or metal-cement interfaces for all designs.[13] However, the mean tensile stress along the porcelain-metal interface was higher for the rounded shoulder than for the chamfer. There is no conclusive evidence from the study to promote the superiority of one margin design over the other. Margin design should be based on other factors, including adequate tooth reduction for ceramic, esthetic demands of the restoration, accuracy of fabrication, and the need to conserve tooth structure.

In another study of the effect of marginal distortion as a function of varying axial height versus uniform axial height, it was found that marginal distortion of an incompatible metal-ceramic system decreased as the axial length of the tooth preparation margins became more uniform.[14] The largest gap widths for the nonuniform copings were detected after either the grinding or the porcelain firing cycles.

The choice of metal alloys for use in FDPs is dependent on the physical properties of the alloys, cost, biocompatibility, and esthetics. High noble metal alloys are the preferred metal of choice for crowns and FDPs of up to three units because of their favorable bond strength to ceramic. Some base metal alloys without beryllium form thick or nonadherent oxides on the surface, creating difficulties in chemical bonding with ceramic.[15] However, base metal alloys offer several advantages, including low cost since they do not contain gold, which is expensive; a higher modulus of elasticity,[16-18] which makes them more suitable for long-span prostheses; and a higher melting temperature range and creep (sag) resistance, which makes them more resistant to framework distortion during porcelain firing.[19]

An area of concern for metal–ceramic restorations is the risk of allergic reactions with both the noble metal alloys and the base metal alloys.[20-23] There have been widespread reports on allergic reactions to nickel and concerns over the potential toxic effects of beryllium as well as reports on the release of metal ions in saliva, which could compromise health.[24] There have even been implications of burning mouth syndrome being associated with the presence of some of these metals in the mouth[25-27] and the potential for long-term debilitating effects.

Despite these challenges, metal–ceramic restorations have been the preference of clinicians because of their predictability and survivability. Prostheses can span from as little as three units, replacing one missing tooth, to full arch units ('round-house' FDPs), replacing several missing teeth. However, the more units involved in the prostheses, the more complex is the casting of the metal substructure and the more challenging are the achievement of excellent fit and marginal adaptability. A retrospective study of the survival of short-span versus long-span FDPs revealed survival rates of 70.8% and 52.8%, respectively, after 20 years of use.[28] Failure of the short-span restorations was primarily associated with biological factors (caries, periodontal disease, root fracture, etc.) in 55.6–66.7% of the restorations, while failures in the long-span restorations were attributed to

technical factors (fracture of connector through metal fatigue, fracture of porcelain, etc.) in 56–84% of the cases. Interestingly, there was a significant difference reported in the survival of short-span FDPs depending on their location. Maxillary prostheses had a survival rate of 70.2% compared with 96.3% for mandibular restorations.[29] These survival statistics for metal–ceramic prostheses are consistent with the reports from other studies, which reported survival rates of 93% at 10 years and 79% between 18 and 23 years.[30] The average lifespan of these FDPs is 10 years, after which survival decreases significantly. Causes for failure include loss of retention of the prosthesis, caries, metal fracture, or a combination of biological and technical factors.[31-34]

The thermal mismatch of alloy–porcelain systems can be one of the causes of technical failure of metal–ceramic restorations. One study analyzed the influence of framework design, contraction mismatch, and thermal history on the fracture resistance of the ceramic.[35] Thermally compatible and incompatible metal–ceramic three-unit FDPs were studied using three experimental designs (Fig 13-1) and four heating and cooling conditions. These included fast heating and fast cooling, fast heating and slow cooling, slow heating and fast cooling, and slow heating and slow cooling. All specimens were subjected to nine firing cycles, which included opaque, body, and glaze firings. Fluorescent light illumination, fiberoptic transillumination, and penetrant dye inspection with ultraviolet light illumination were used to determine the presence of cracks in the porcelain. The results indicated that multiple firings were a primary cause for the failure of both metal-ceramic systems. It can be surmised that the design exhibiting a high ceramic-to-metal thickness ratio may contribute to larger temperature gradients, thereby producing high tensile stresses in these areas. The investigators also concluded that rapid cooling tended to minimize the negative thermal mismatch of thermal expansion or contraction coefficients ($\Delta_\alpha = \alpha_m - \alpha_c$, where $\alpha$ is the contraction coefficient, m is metal and c is ceramic) because of the faster transfer of heat from the metal, thereby producing greater compressive stress in the ceramic.

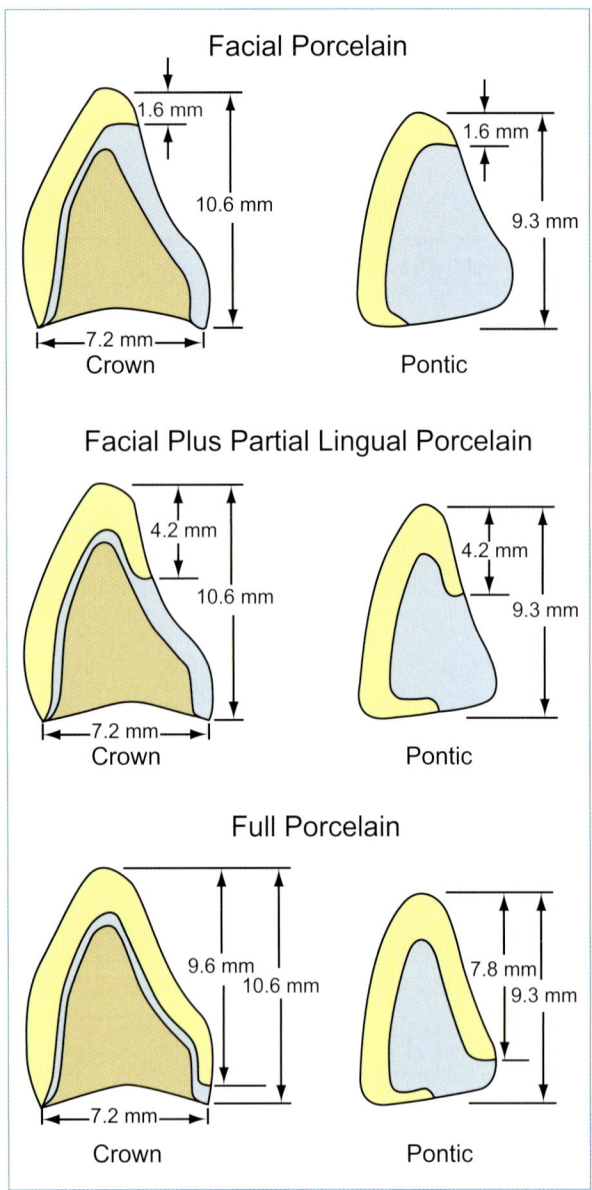

Fig 13-1  Three crown and pontic designs for metal-ceramic FDPs.[35] (with permission from Elsevier)

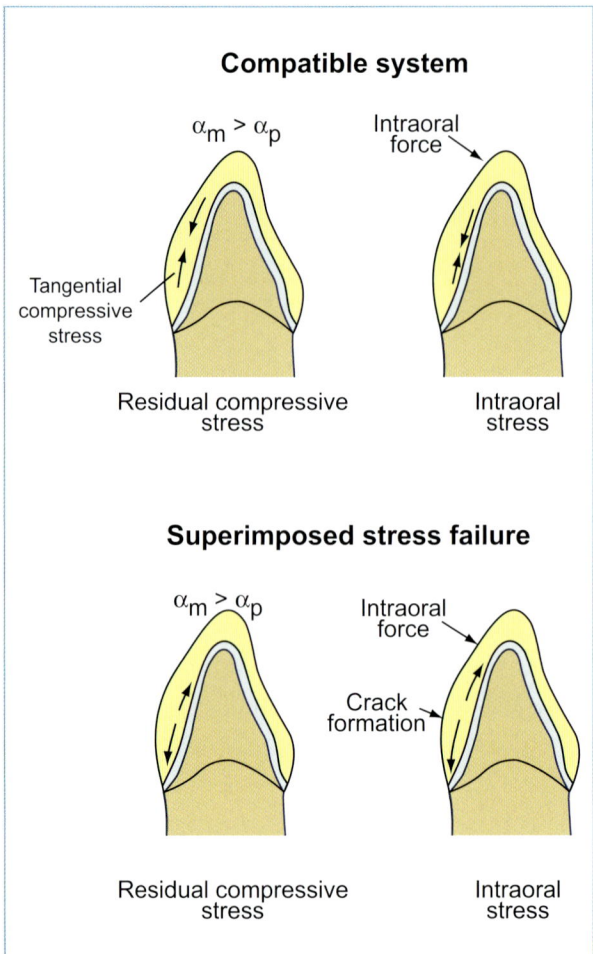

Fig 13-2 (Top)  Combined effect of residual compressive stress and tensile stress induced by load P in a metal (m) – porcelain (p) crown, which is less likely to fail prematurely. (Bottom) The residual tensile stress caused by a greater thermal contraction of the porcelain than the metal is more likely to cause premature failure when combined with the tensile stress induced by load P.[37] (with permission from Quintessence Publishing)

The relatively low intraoral tensile stresses that develop from applied forces can contribute to metal-ceramic system failure when combined with residual thermal incompatibility tensile stress.[36] Figure 13-2 is an illustration of the effect of superimposing tensile stresses from intraoral forces on the residual tensile stresses associated with a thermally incompatible system.[37] Unfortunately, there are no reported clinical studies that document the effect of these combined stresses on premature failure of metal–ceramic restorations.

# All-Ceramic Restorations

The evolution of all-ceramic prostheses for use as anterior or posterior FDPs began in 1967 with the development of a ceramic with high alumina content for FDP pontics. Through the years, several new high-strength ceramic materials have been developed for use in all-ceramic prostheses.

## Glass-Infiltrated Ceramics

The glass-infiltrated alumina ceramic was one of the first systems introduced for the fabrication of anterior FDPs. Commercially known as In-Ceram Alumina, its flexural strength ranges from 236 to 600 MPa and the fracture toughness ranges from 3.1 to 4.6 $MPa·m^{1/2}$. This ceramic must be veneered with Vita ceramic to produce sufficient esthetics. Another product, In-Ceram Spinell, is a more translucent core ceramic made from a combination of magnesia and alumina. However, its lower strength and toughness restricts its use to anterior crowns. For maximum fracture resistance, In-Ceram Zirkonia is available as a core ceramic.[38-40] Prosthetic frameworks can be fabricated with the core ceramic using the slip-casting technique or milled from prefabricated ceramic blanks. The recommended connector thicknesses are 4 mm occlusogingivally and 3 mm buccolingually. This ceramic core material is quite opaque in appearance. A more translucent core ceramic, In-Ceram Spinell, which is structure composed of alumina and magnesia, was introduced to improve the appearance of anterior ceramic crowns. It is not recommended for posterior crowns and anterior or posterior FDPs.

## Glass-Ceramics Based on Lithia Disilicate

Commercially known as IPS Empress 2 or e.max Press, the lithia-disilicate-based glass-ceramic core material is indicated for anterior or posterior FDPs, with the second premolar being the most posterior terminal abutment. It can be fabricated using either the lost-wax and hot-pressing technique or milled from prefabricated blanks. Mechanical properties include a flexural strength ranging from 300 to 400 MPa[22] and a fracture toughness of 2.8–3.5 $MPa·m^{1/2}$.[41,42] This material exhibits excellent esthetics with relatively high translucency, although cementation requires the use of an adhesive resin cement to enhance the fracture resistance of cemented prostheses. The minimal critical dimensions that are recommended by the manufacturer are 4–5 mm occlusogingivally and 3–4 mm buccolingually.[43] Clinical data reveal that lithia-disilicate-based posterior FDPs have a clinical success rate of 86% after 4 years.[44] Both of the e.max lithia-disilicate-based core ceramic products (e.maxPress and e.max CAD) can be veneered with the e.max Ceram 'nanofluorapatite' glass-ceramic veneer.

## Densely Sintered High-Purity Procera Alumina and Zirconia

Procera Crown Alumina (1991), Procera Bridge Alumina (1999), Procera Crown Zirconia (2001) and Procera Bridge Zirconia (2004) are based on densely sintered core ceramics that are processed from oversized dies to compensate for sintering shrinkage. The zirconia core ceramics are more fracture resistant than the alumina ceramics. The recommended NobelRondo veneering ceramic can be used for either core ceramic. The Procera zirconia products exhibit a flexural strength ranging from 487 to 699 MPa[45] and a fracture toughness ranging from 4.5 to 6.0 $MPa·m^{1/2}$.[46] The core materials are made of densely sintered high-purity zirconium oxide and they are more opaque than their alumina ceramic counterparts. The recommended connector height and width for anterior FDPs are 3 mm and 2 mm, respectively. The strongest and toughest of this family of materials is In-Ceram Zirconia. However, it is, like In-Ceram Alumina, quite opaque. and it is best suited for posterior crowns and FDPs.

## Glass-Infiltrated Alumina and Partially Stabilized Zirconia

A hybrid core material commercially marketed as the In-Ceram Zirconia system contains approximately 69 vol% alumina and a balance of yttria stabilized zirconia

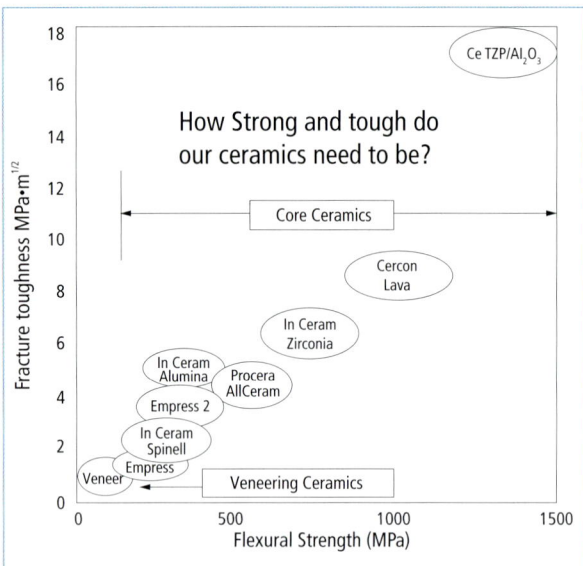

**Fig 13-3** Fracture toughness versus flexural strenght plot for framework (core) ceramics and glassphase veneering ceramics. The Ce/TZP/Al$_2$O$_3$ ceramic core material has not been introduced in the dental market. Note that the value of fracture toughness for this material is based on a test that tends to overestimate the true fractue toughness.

whose partially sintered structure is infiltrated with 20-25 vol% of glass. Flexural strength ranges from 421 to 800 MPa,[38,40,47] with fracture toughness of 6 to 8 MPa·m$^{1/2}$.[48] The recommended connector dimensions are 4–5 mm in height and 3–4 mm in width.[48] Because of the high opacity of the core material, it is not recommended for anterior prostheses.

## Yttria-Stabilized Tetragonal Zirconia Polycrystal Ceramic

The yttria-stabilized tetragon zirconia polycrystal (Y-TZP) ceramics are the most recent addition to the core materials for all-ceramic FDPs. These materials exhibit the highest flexural strength and fracture toughness in the ceramic market so far. The clinical success rate for all-ceramic FDPs ranges from 86% to 93%[44,48-51] within a 5-year time frame. This relatively good success rate is a result of the unique mechanical properties of the ceramics, which make them brittle and less resistant to fracture. The long-term failure probability and loading capacity of all-ceramic FDPs using Empress 1, Empress 2, In-Ceram Alumina and yttria-stabilized zirconia were assessed using lifetime prediction analysis based on the NASA post-processor Ceramic Analysis and Reliability Evaluation of Structure Life Prediction (CARES/LIFE) analysis.[52] Results indicated that FDPs made of zirconia had very high mechanical long-term reliability. A zero failure probability was predicted for zirconia FDPs even after 10 years of static loading. Other results indicate that Empress 1 and In-Ceram Alumina were not suitable for use as posterior FDP materials and that Empress 2 was more suitable to be used in the molar region, with the failure rate being three times smaller than that for In-Ceram Alumina. Another study examined strength probability–time diagrams for porcelain, alumina, and Y-TZP ceramics.[53] The results suggested that Y-TZP has a higher fracture strength with a resistance to subcritical crack growth compared with the other two ceramics. Although these lifetime predictions must be validated with clinical data, it is clear evidence that zirconia ceramics should be far superior to other ceramics used for all-ceramic FDPs.

Zirconia ceramics exist in the monoclinic, tetragonal, and cubic phases. The monoclinic phase is the low-temperature phase and remains stable up to 1170°C, above which it transforms into the tetragonal phase.[54] The stability of the tetragonal phase is dependent on the amount of the stabilizing oxide present as well as the grain size of the zirconia particles. At a temperature over 2370°C, zirconia transforms into the cubic phase, which only remains stable at very high temperatures. Pure zirconia ceramics, without stabilizing oxides, can undergo a reverse tetragonal to monoclinic transformation, which occurs at 1070°C.[53] This can result in a 1–5% volume expansion, during which tensile stresses can develop that can cause pure zirconia ceramics to fracture at room temperature.

Based on the strength and biocompatibility demonstrated by zirconia in the medical field, the dental industry has been attracted to a pure Y-TZP for posterior prosthesis construction. Yttria (Y$_2$O$_3$) as a stabilizing agent allows the zirconium ceramic to exist in complete small metastable tetragonal grains. The sintered Y-

TZP has a flexural strength ranging from 900 to 1500 MPa.[46,55] This type of core ceramic is marketed under several brand names (Cercon by Dentsply, DCS-Precident by Bien-Air Group/DCS Dental AG, DC-Zirkon by Denstply, Lava by 3M ESPE, and e.max ZirCAD by Ivoclar Vivadent). It has gained popularity in the dental community because of its strength, fracture toughness, fatigue resistance, and flexibility for use in longer spans in the posterior areas of the mouth. Compared with other ceramic materials used for all-ceramic prostheses, such as lithia-disilicate-based glass-ceramics and zirconia-reinforced glass-infiltrated alumina, Y-TZP has demonstrated the highest flexural strength and fracture toughness (Fig 13-3).[46,56,57] The fracture toughness of Y-TZP ranges from 9 to 10 MPa/m$^2$, which is twice the value for alumina-based materials and three times the value for lithium disilicate-based glass-ceramics. Because of its increased strength, Y-TZP also allows for a smaller connector dimension, 7.6 mm$^2$ (2.8 mm occlusogingival height and 2.7 mm buccolingual width) for a posterior three-unit FDP, compared with other materials on the market.[58]

Y-TZP ceramics do not contain a glass phase and they are sintered with minimal voids, flaws, and cracks, thereby increasing their strength and fracture toughness. The absence of a glass phase also makes it resistant to subcritical crack propagation and stress corrosion susceptibility, which is caused by water in saliva reacting with the glass. The phenomenon known as transformation toughening (Fig 13-4)[59] occurs during a tetragonal to monoclinic crystal structure transformation. It is considered beneficial in that the material can actually 'heal' itself. When tensile stresses are generated at the tip of a crack, the reverse tetragonal to monoclinic transformation occurs. This phase change at the tip of the crack is accompanied by a volumetric expansion and subsequent compressive stresses around the crack tip. The volumetric expansion can result in partial closure of the crack and prevents its propagation through the entire structure.[60] Another phenomenon, known as low-temperature degradation, is controversial in that it can actually cause loss of strength and has adverse

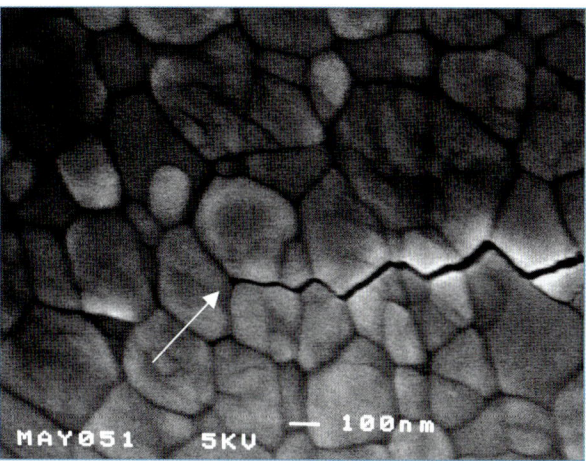

**Fig 13-4** Crack arrest associated with tetragonal to monoclinic crystal phase change (transformation toughening). *(From Guazzato M, Albkry M, Ringer SP, Swain MV. Strength, fracture toughness and microstructure of a selection of all-ceramic materials. Part II. Zirconia-based dental ceramics. Dent Mater 2004;20:449–456,59 with permission from Elsevier)*

effects on other mechanical properties. The low-temperature degradation phenomenon induces the tetragonal to monoclinic transformation at the surface of the specimen in the presence of moisture at 250°C.[61] Characteristics of low-temperature degradation include: tetragonal to monoclinic transformation occurring from the external surface of the material and proceeding internally; transformation occurring in water or in a humid environment; the transformation process being modified by the amount of stabilizer and the zirconia grain size; and degradation occurring over time at temperatures ranging from 65°C to 500°C but mostly at 250°C. Theories formulated to explain the possible cause of low-temperature degradation include a depletion of the stabilizer as a result of formation of yttrium hydroxide from water and yttria and the formation of this zirconium hydroxide on the surface from water chemisorption.[62,63] A study was conducted to analyze the effect of low-temperature degradation on the flexural strength and structural stability of Y-TZP by boiling Y-TZP samples for up to 7 days or storing them in humidified air at 250°C. These treatments did not significantly degrade the strength of the ceramic material.[60]

Other reports showed that finishing procedures, air abrasion, and polishing did not affect the strength of the ceramic but sandblasting increased the strength to some extent.[59,64]

Y-TZP frameworks can be fabricated using either conventional waxing techniques or computer-assisted design (CAD) technology. Once the frameworks have been designed, they can either be scanned from the waxed patterns or the data can be transferred to computer-assisted manufacturing (CAM) units. These CAM units can mill either partially sintered Y-TZP blanks or fully sintered blocks according to the system used and the design specifications of the framework. If partially sintered blanks are used, the size is usually increased by 20–25% to compensate for the firing shrinkage that will occur. There are benefits and drawbacks with using either partially sintered or fully sintered blanks. Proponents of partially sintered blanks claim that the process is faster and easier on the wear and tear of the hardware since the blanks are 'softer'. Advocates of the fully sintered blanks claim that the marginal adaptation is superior because there is no firing shrinkage. However, there are concerns regarding the introduction of microcracks in the surface during the processing of fully sintered Y-TZP.[65]

*In vitro* tests have shown that Y-TZP ceramics have the highest fracture toughness and flexural strength of all available all-ceramic materials in the market today. Since all-ceramic prostheses have been shown to have a slightly lower clinical success rate compared with metal–ceramic prostheses, the present and future goals are to develop a material that is close in strength and superior in structural reliability yet offers the same esthetic advantages. Many of the clinical fractures of all-ceramic FDPs have occurred by chipping of the veneer ceramic and fracture within the connector areas. Placement of an all-ceramic prosthesis in the posterior regions of the mouth is sometimes difficult because the connector dimensions are often compromised by the limited space available in the posterior region. In a clinical study, fractures occurred in FDPs that had lower than prescribed connector values.[44] The connector sizes

were dictated by other factors such as tooth height, occlusion, and esthetics. Although low-temperature degradation may be an issue with Y-TZP, *in vitro* studies have shown that it does not affect the strength or mechanical properties of this type of ceramic.[60] The temperature at which low-temperature degradation most rapidly occurs is at 250°C, with a temperature range of 65 to 500°C. Studies have shown that the temperature extremes under dental restorations range from 9 to 52°C,[65] with oral temperatures ranging from 15.4 to 68°C.60,[66–70] Another study has shown that soft tissues in the mouth would incur damage above 40°C and that the adaptive mechanism involved in ingesting hot fluids such as coffee (up to 64.4°C) is that the hot fluid does not stay in contact with any one area for more than 0.4 s.[71] In light of these data, there is only a very small possibility that the restorations will come into contact for more than a fraction of a second with fluid temperatures above 65°C, which is the temperature at which low-temperature degradation occurs. Further clinical research is needed to determine the effect, if any, of low-temperature degradation on Y-TZP restorations.

The driving force for the development of all-ceramic materials has been the demand for more esthetically pleasing and natural-looking restorative materials. The use of ceramic as a primary material in FDPs to replace missing teeth has gained popularity since the 1980s. With the advent of an esthetically conscious society, the total ceramic prosthesis has gained momentum and use in the dental community because of increased patient demand. However, the physical properties of ceramics confer major limitations for their use and account for a lower success rate compared with metal–ceramic prostheses. Meta analyses of clinical data for metal–ceramic fixed dental protheses have shown survival levels of 96–98%, 90–92%, and 74–75% at 5, 10, and 15 years, respectively.[71–73] Since the all-ceramic materials are relatively new, there have been few clinical studies to evaluate their success. Studies so far have shown survival rate for all-ceramic FDPs ranging from 86 to 93% within a 5-year observation period.[44,49–51] Almost all of these studies identified that the failures occurred by a fracture of

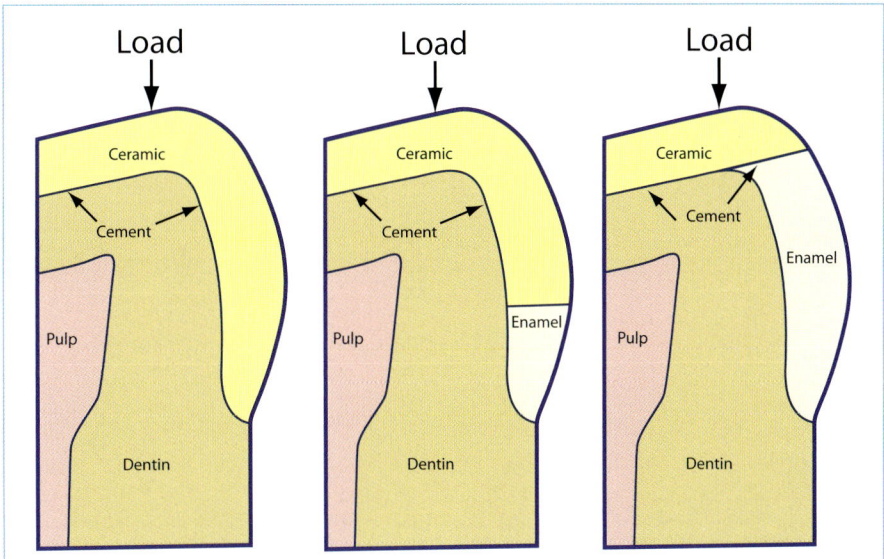

**Fig 13-5** Schematic of full crown (left), half crown (middle), and occlusal onlay (right).[77] *(with permission from IEEE Service Center)*

the connector through the framework or core material.

Several variables could affect survival of all-ceramic prostheses. These multfactorial variables were investigated in an *in vitro* study that considered variables that influenced stress in all-ceramic crowns.[74] These included the physical properties of the ceramic crown material, crown thickness, cement modulus, cement thickness, physical properties and design of the supporting core material, and position of the load on the prosthesis.

Proper design of the prosthesis is also a critical element in minimizing fracture and extending the survival time. The requirements for the fabrication of an all-ceramic crown are an axial reduction of 1.2–1.4 mm towards the gingival portion of the tooth. The tooth is also reduced 1.5–2.0 mm incisally or occlusally. The shoulder width should be a minimum of 1.0 mm all around the labial and lingual surfaces and should be a smooth transition between the two areas. All sharp angles should be smooth and rounded and a 90 degree angle should exist at the cavosurface margin.

An increase in the length of an all-ceramic crown has been shown to increase the fracture load.[75] Finite element analysis[76] has also been used to analyze the potential fracture resistance of full-length crowns, half-length crowns, and occlusal plates, each with a thickness of 1.5 mm (Fig 13-5).[77] Each design was given the same value for Young's modulus and Poisson's ratio for the ceramic crown, enamel, dentin, and pulp chamber with five combinations available for each design. A pressure load of 200 MPa was applied to an area of 2 mm$^2$ at four different occlusal sites, as shown in Fig 13-5. It was found that the maximum stress within the ceramic occlusal plate was 6–30% higher than those of the full-length or half-length crowns and increased as the loading site moved away from the center. The maximum stresses differed by less than 2% between the full-length and half-length crowns. This study also determined that the maximum stress decreased from 343 to 101 MPa as the thickness of the ceramic crowns increased from 0.5 to 1.5 mm. When the thickness was increased from 1.5 to 2 mm, the stress remained relatively constant. As mentioned above, the most common site for failure with these all-ceramic prostheses is located along the connector area. The longer the span or the more posterior the location of the prosthesis, the greater the connector dimensions should be. Occlusogingival dimension is more critical in determining longevity of the restoration than the buccolingual dimension of the connector.

| Prosthesis unit size | Cyclic fatigue 250 N | | Static load 800 N | | Recommendations | |
|---|---|---|---|---|---|---|
| FDPs | Diameter (mm) | Area (mm²) | Diameter (mm) | Area (mm²) | Diameter (mm) | Area (mm²) |
| 3 | 2.5 | 4.9 | 2.7 | 5.7 | >2.7 | 5.7 |
| 4 | 4.0 | 12.6 | 3.5 | 9.6 | >4.0 | 12.6 |
| 5 | 4.9 | 18.8 | 4.1 | 13.2 | >4.9 | 18.8 |

**Table 13-1** Minimum connector dimensions recommended for zirconia-based fixed dental prostheses.

From Studart et al. (2007)[78,79]

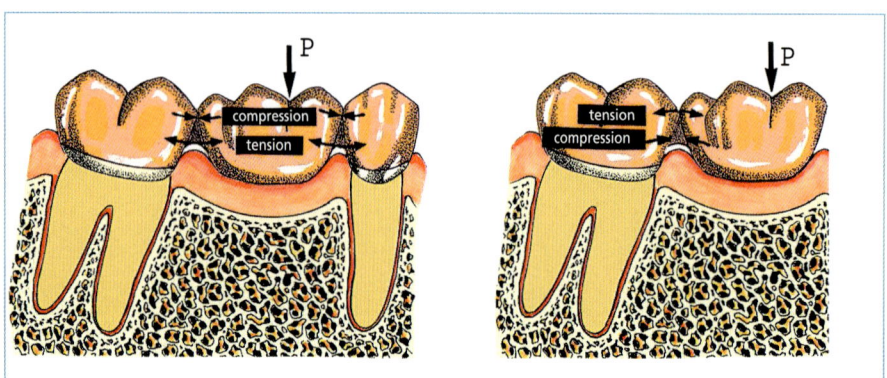

**Fig 13-6** Tensile and compressive stresses in metal-ceramic prostheses during loading of **(a)** a three-unit fixed dental prosthesis (FDP); and **(b)** a two-unit cantilever metal-ceramic FDP.

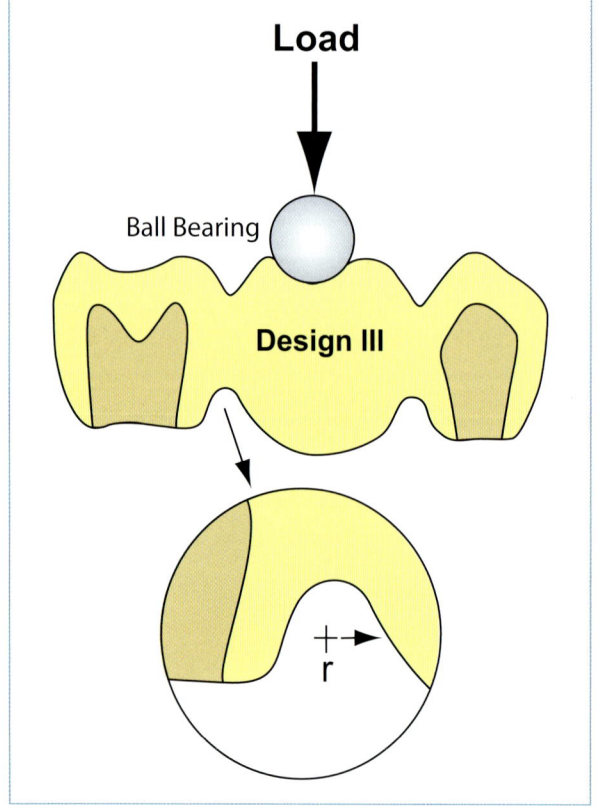

**Fig 13-7** Radius (r) of curvature at the gingival embrasure.[3] *(with permission from IADR)*

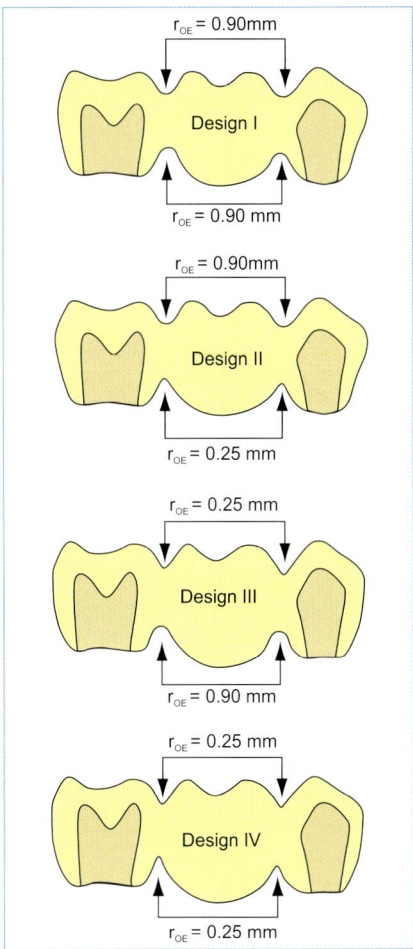

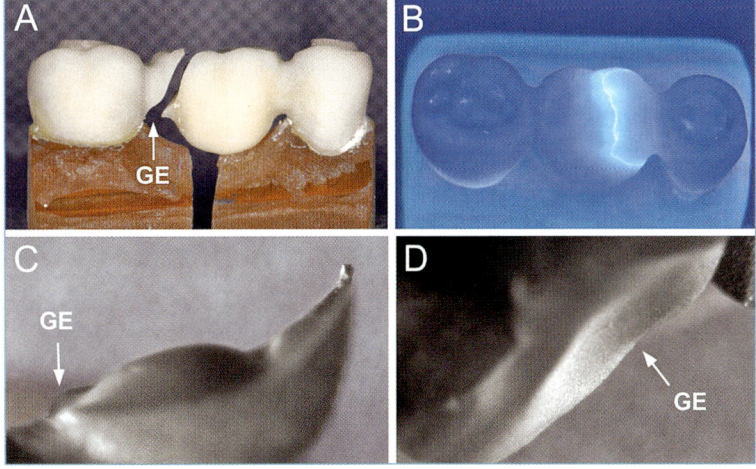

**Fig 13-8** Fixed dental prosthesis designs on gingival embrasure with variations on occlusal embrasure (OE) and gingival embrasure (GE) radii (r). Design IV had a maximum tensile stress of 156 MPa at a failure load of 740 N.[4] *(with permission from Elsevier)*

**Fig 13-9** Oblique orientation of fracture path **(a)** extending from the gingival embrasure (GE) to the occlusal contact area **(b)**. The sites of crack initiation are shown in **c** and **d**.[4] *(with permission from Elsevier)*

*In vitro* analyses were performed to examine the influence of fatigue loading and the connector diameter and cross-sectional area of three-, four-, and five-unit Y-TZP FDPs at a maximum fatigue load of 250 N and a control static load of 800 N, assuming a fracture rate of 5% over 20 years.[78,79] Based on these studies, the recommended connector diameter and cross-sectional area dimensions are as summarized in Table 13-1.[78,79] These studies suggest that the strength of FDPs containing a weak framework (fracture toughness $< 3$ MPa·m$^{1/2}$) is controlled by the low fracture resistance of the veneer ceramic, since crack arresting does not occur at the veneer–framework interface. Instead, ceramics of higher toughness (5 MPa·m$^{1/2}$) are recommended for core frameworks of posterior all-ceramic FDPs.

Another factor to consider in connector dimensions is the radius of curvature along the gingival embrasure. The curvature at the gingival embrasure must be broad when tension dominates. The occlusal embrasure must be broad for cantilever prostheses.[3] Figure 13-6 illustrates the principal compressive and tensile stresses within the connector areas for a three-unit FDP.[80] Finite element analyses and mechanical loading tests were performed[3,4] to determine the effect of the embrasure radius of curvature on the fracture potential (Figs 13-7 and 13-8). The results of these studies suggest that increasing the gingival embrasure radius from 0.25 to 0.90 mm more than doubles the connector strength (increase of 135%). These results also indicate that the occlusal embrasure radius has a negligible effect on the strength of three-unit FDPs (Fig 13-9).

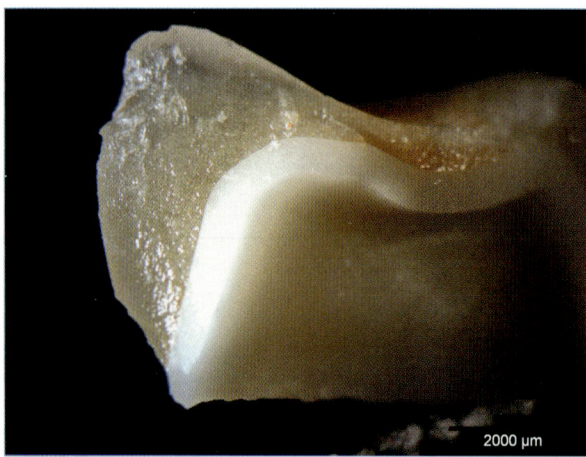

**Fig 13-10**   Lack of core support for ceramic veneer. *(Courtesy of Susanne Scherrer)*

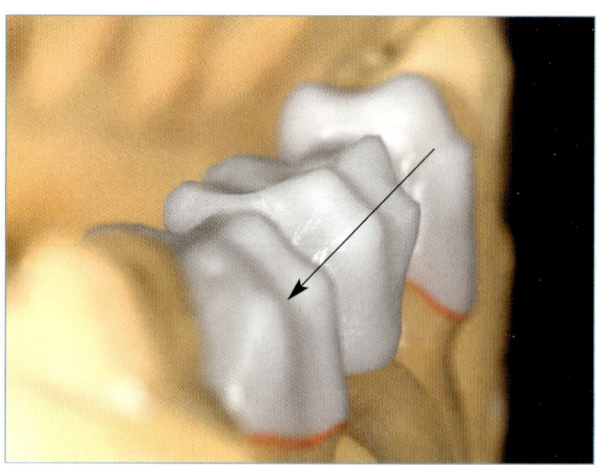

**Fig 13-11**   Cusp reinforcement (arrow) in framework design for veneer support.[81] *(with permission from Deutscher Ärzte-Verlag GmbH)*

Design of the core ceramic is also a factor in improving the longevity of all-ceramic prostheses. As indicated above for metal–ceramic core designs, there should be adequate support of the veneer ceramic. Figure 13-10 is a fracture surface of a failed all-ceramic crown for which fractography analysis shows the origin of the fracture within the veneer ceramic as a result of inadequate support by the core ceramic. A more supportive core design (Fig. 13-11) has been proposed[81] to reduce the risk of veneer ceramic fracture. The veneer ceramic is better supported especially in line with the forces that may be applied at the cuspal areas.

ment teeth to ensure proper connector dimensions and adequate occlusal clearance for provision of a proper thickness of the ceramic. The clinician and the laboratory technician need to ensure that the proper design for the margins are followed to allow for adequate thickness of the ceramic along the gingival area and that there is proper connector and embrasure design, which includes the gingival embrasure radius, to ensure longevity of the prosthesis. Although all-ceramic prostheses are superior in appearance to metal–ceramic restorations, the latter offers a stronger, more predictable, and proven option, especially for multiple unit fixed dental prostheses.

## Survival Statistics

In summary, all-ceramic prostheses are indicated for highly esthetic areas, for patients who have very high esthetic demands, or for those who have specific metal allergies. They are not indicated for everyone and there needs to be adequate treatment planning to include examination of factors such as the height of the abut-

## Conclusions

It is clear that all-ceramic restorations will be used more extensively because of their esthetic capability. However, for younger patients or those with a significant level of translucency and vitality in their anterior natural teeth, material systems with the highest core

Table 13-2 Decision matrix for selection of metal-ceramic versus all-ceramic prostheses.

| | Anterior and premolar crowns | Anterior and premolar FDPs | Posterior crowns | Posterior FDPs |
|---|---|---|---|---|
| Translucency | Glass-ceramic | Glass-ceramic | Not applicable | Not applicable |
| Strength (bite force > 250 N) | Ceramic core strength ≥ 250 MPa | $Al_2O_3$ and $ZrO_2$ core ceramics | PFM (excluding foil and galvanometal) | PFM (excluding foil and galvanometal) |
| Tooth conservation | Ceramic veneer, glass-ceramic, Thin-metal PFM | Implant-supported, $Al_2O_3$ and $ZrO_2$ core ceramics, thin-metal PFM | $Al_2O_3$ and $ZrO_2$ core ceramics, thin-metal PFM | Implant-supported, $Al_2O_3$ and $ZrO_2$ core ceramics, thin-metal PFM |
| Non-allergenic | All-ceramic or CP Ti core PFM | All-ceramic or CP Ti core PFM | $Al_2O_3$ and $ZrO_2$ core ceramics | $ZrO_2$ core ceramics |
| Survival probability for 95% ≥ 7 years | Glass-ceramic, $Al_2O_3$, and $ZrO_2$ core, PFM | $Al_2O_3$, and $ZrO_2$ core, PFM | PFM | PFM |
| Survival probability for 95% ≥ 10 years | PFM | PFM | PFM | PFM |

FDP, fixed dental prostheses; PFM, porcelain fused to metal.

ceramic strength and toughness will not be able to match this esthetic appearance routinely because of the core-ceramic core opacity. Instead, the hot-pressed core ceramics or glass-infiltrated ceramics of moderate strength and moderate toughness will be required. Concerns still exist regarding the incidence of chipping of all-ceramic crowns and FDPs; chipping indicates significant transient incompatibility tensile stress. which induces microcracks, and/or residual tensile stress, which may also lead to delayed cracking and subsequent localized fracture.

Metal–ceramic restorations can also be made with reasonably good anterior esthetics, especially when thin copings and butt-joint porcelain margin designs are used. There is little question of their excellence when used for FDPs involving molar crowns or abutments.

The main use of metal–ceramics will be for long-span FDPs, the so-called roundhouse designs, and in areas where partial denture clasp arms and occlusal rests are involved. The metal–ceramics will also be useful for patients who exhibit bruxism or high wear rates of enamel from opposing ceramic surfaces. However, in these cases, occlusal metal coverage will be required. Although posterior all-ceramic crowns appear to be relatively successful for some products for periods of up to 5 years, the survival probabilities of four-unit and longer FDPs is uncertain at this time because only limited clinical data are available. The connector design in these cases will play a much greater role than it does for metal–ceramic FDPs.

Patients who are allergic to certain common metals used for fixed prostheses and who insist on non-metallic restorations should be informed of the anticipated reduced survival probabilities of long-span all-ceramic prostheses in posterior areas. Even though commercially pure titanium is believed to be a more biocompatible substructure for metal–ceramic prostheses, this metal is highly technique sensitive and the survival probabilities of metal–ceramic prostheses are expected to be much lower than those made with high noble or noble substructures, even if the thermal compatibility between the metal and matching ceramic is well established.

In summary, it is apparent that, while all-ceramic prostheses will gain further acceptance by the dental profession because of their biocompatibility and esthetic capabilities, metal–ceramics will continue to be used, especially when long spans are required, bruxing is likely, or when partial removable dental protheses will be associated with the prostheses. Table 13-2 provides a decision matrix that could be used for consideration of future treatment needs.

# References

1. Taskonak B, Yan J, Mecholsky JJ, Jr, Sertgoz A, Kocak A. Fractographic analyses of zirconia-based fixed dental protheses. Gen Dent 2007;55:657–662.

2. Larsson C, Holm L, Lovgren N, Kokubo Y, Vult von Steyern P. Fracture strength of four-unit Y-TZP FPD cores designed with varying connector diameter. An in-vitro study. J Oral Rehabil 2007;34:702–709.

3. Oh W, Gotzen N, Anusavice KJ. Influence of connector design on fracture probability of ceramic fixed partial dentures. J Dent Res 2002;81:623–627.

4. Oh WS, Anusavice KJ. Effect of connector design on the fracture resistance of all-ceramic fixed partial dentures. J Prosthet Dent 2002;87:536–542.

5. Bronson MR, Lindquist TJ, Dawson DV. Clinical acceptability of crown margins versus marginal gaps as determined by pre-doctoral students and prosthodontists. J Prosthodont 2005;14:226–232.

6. Shillingburg HT, Hobo S, Whitsett LD, Jacobi R, Brackett SE. Fundamentals of Fixed Prosthodontics. Chicago, IL: Quintessence Publishing, 1997:139–154.

7. Sulong MZ, Aziz RA. Wear of materials used in dentistry: a review of the literature. J Prosthet Dent 1990;63:342–349.

8. Yap AU, Ong LF, Teoh SH, Hastings GW. Comparative wear ranking of dental restoratives with the BIOMAT wear simulator. J Oral Rehabil 1999;26:228–235.

9. Faucher RR, Nicholls JI. Distortion related to margin design in porcelain-fused-to-metal restorations. J Prosthet Dent 1980;43:149–155.

10. Buchanan WT, Svare CW, Turner KA. The effect of repeated firings and strength on marginal distortion in two ceramometal systems. J Prosthet Dent 1981;45:502–506.

11. Anusavice KJ, Carroll JE. Effect of incompatibility stress on the fit of metal-ceramic crowns. J Dent Res 1987;66:1341–1345.

12. Anusavice KJ, Hojjatie B. Stress distribution in metal-ceramic crowns with a facial porcelain margin. J Dent Res 1987;66:1493–1498.

13. Chai JY, Steege JW. Effects of labial margin design on stress distribution of a porcelain-fused-to-metal crown. J Prosthodont 1992;1:18–23.

14. Nakamura Y, Anusavice KJ. Marginal distortion of thermally incompatible metal ceramic crowns with overextended margins. Int J Prosthodont 1998;11:325–332.

15. Baran GR. Selection criteria for base metals for use with porcelain. Dent Clin North Am 1985;27:733–746.

16. Moffa JP. Alternative dental casting alloys. Dent Clin North Am 1983;27:733–746.

17. Wataha JC. Alloys for prosthodontic restorations. J Prosthet Dent 2002;87:351–363.

18. Wataha JC, Messer RL. Casting alloys. Dent Clin North Am 2004;48:vii-viii, 499–512.

19. Watanabe I, Benson AP, Nguyen K. Effect of heat treatment on joint properties of laser-welded Ag-Au-Cu-Pd and Co-Cr alloys. J Prosthodont 2005;14:170–174.

20. Hensten-Pettersen A. Casting alloys: side-effects. Adv Dent Res 1992;6:38–43.

21. Hensten-Pettersen A, Jacobsen N, Gjerdet NR. Adverse reaction to dental materials. In: Karlsson S, Nilner C, Dahl BL (eds). A Textbook of Fixed Prosthodontics: The Scandinavian Approach. Stockholm: Gothia,2000:131–134.

22. Mjör IA, Christensen GJ. Assessment of local side effects of casting alloys. Quintessence Int 1993;24:343–351.

23. Schmalz G, Garhammer P. Biological interactions of dental cast alloys with oral tissues. Dent Mater 2002;18:396–406.

24. Kalicanin B, Ajdukovic Z. Influence of saliva medium on freeing heavy metal ion from fixed dentures. Sci Total Environ 2008;397:41–45.

25. Maltsman-Tseikhin A, Moricca P, Niv D. Burning mouth syndrome: will better understanding yield better management? Pain Pract 2007;7:151–162.

26. Patton LL, Siegel MA, Benoliel R, De Laat A. Management of burning mouth syndrome: systematic review and management recommendations. Oral Surg Oral Med Oral Pathol Oral Radiol Endod 2007;103(Suppl S39):e31–e13.

27. Ship JA, Grushka M, Lipton JA, Mott AE, Sessle BJ, Dionne RA. Burning mouth syndrome: an update. J Am Dent Assoc 1995;126:842–853.

28. de Backer H, van Maele G, de Moor N, van den Berghe L. An up to 20-year retrospective study of 4-unit fixed dental prostheses for the replacement of 2 missing adjacent teeth. Int J Prosthodont 2008;21:259–266.

29. de Backer H, van Maele G, de Moor N, van den Berghe L. Single-tooth replacement: is a 3-unit fixed partial dentures still an option? A 20-year retrospective study. Int J Prosthodont 2006;19:567–573.

30. Palmqvist S, Swartz B. Artificial crowns and fixed partial dentures 18 to 23 years after placement. Int J Prosthodont 1993;6:279–285.

31. Eliasson A, Arnelund CF, Johansson A. A clinical evaluation of cobalt–chromium metal–ceramic fixed dental protheses and crowns: a three- to seven-year retrospective study. J Prosthet Dent 2007;98:6–16.

32. Lindquist E, Karlsson S. Success rate and failures for fixed dental protheses after 20 years of service: Part I. Int J Prosthodont 1998;11:133–138.

33. Motta AB, Pereira LC, da Cunha AR, Duda FP. The influence of the loading mode on the stress distribution on the connector region of metal–ceramic and all-ceramic fixed partial denture. Artif Organs 2008;32:283–291.

34. Randow K, Glantz PO, Zoger B. Technical failures and some related clinical complications in extensive fixed prosthodontics. An epidemiological study of long-term clinical quality. Acta Odontol Scand 1986;44:241–255.

35. Anusavice KJ, Gray AE. Influence of framework design, contraction mismatch, and thermal history on porcelain checking in fixed dental protheses. Dent Mater 1989;5:58–63.

36. Coffey JP, Anusavice KJ, DeHoff PH, Lee RB, Hojjatie B. Influence of contraction mismatch and cooling rate on flexural failure of PFM systems. J Dent Res 1988;67:61–65.

37. Anusavice KJ. Stress distribution in atypical crown design. Perspectives in dental ceramics. In: JD Preston (ed). Proceedings of the Fourth International Symposium on Ceramics. Chicago, IL: Quintessence Publishing, 1988:175–191.

38. Seghi RR, Denry IL, Rosenstiel SF. Relative fracture toughness and hardness of new dental ceramics. J Prosthet Dent 1995;74:145–150.

39. Seghi RR, Sorensen JA. Relative flexural strength of six new ceramic materials. Int J Prosthodont 1995;8:239–246.

40. Wagner WC, Chu TM. Biaxial flexural strength and indentation fracture toughness of three new dental core ceramics. J Prosthet Dent 1996;76:140–144.

41. Quinn JB, Sundar V, Lloyd IK. Influence of microstructure and chemistry on the fracture toughness of dental ceramics. Dent Mater 2003;19:603–611.

42. Schweiger M, Holand W, Frank M, Drescher H, Rheinberger V. IPS Empress 2: a new pressable high-strength glass-ceramic for esthetic all-ceramic restorations. Quintessence Dent Technol 1999;22:143–151.

43. Sorensen JA, Cruz M, Mito WT, Raffeiner O, Meredith HR, Foser HP. A clinical investigation on three-unit fixed partial dentures fabricated with a lithium disilicate glass-ceramic. Pract Periodont Aesthet Dent 1999;11:95–106; quiz 108.

44. Esquivel-Upshaw JF, Young H, Jones J, Yang M, Anusavice KJ. Four-year clinical performance of a lithia disilicate-based core ceramic for posterior fixed partial dentures. Int J Prosthodont 2008;21:155–160.

45. Zeng K, Oden A, Rowcliffe D. Flexure tests on dental ceramics. Int J Prosthodont 1996;9:434–439.

46. Christel P, Meunier A, Heller M, Torre JP, Peille CN. Mechanical properties and short-term in-vivo evaluation of yttrium-oxide-partially-stabilized zirconia. J Biomed Mater Res 1989;23:45–61.

47. Chong KH, Chai J, Takahashi Y, Wozniak W. Flexural strength of In-Ceram alumina and In-Ceram zirconia core materials. Int J Prosthodont 2002;15:183–188.

48. McLaren EA, White SN. Survival of In-Ceram crowns in a private practice: a prospective clinical trial. J Prosthet Dent 2000;83:216–222.

49. Esquivel-Upshaw JF, Anusavice KJ, Young H, Jones J, Gibbs C. Clinical performance of a lithia disilicate-based core ceramic for three-unit posterior FPDs. Int J Prosthodont 2004;17:469–475.

50. Olsson KG, Furst B, Andersson B, Carlsson GE. A long-term retrospective and clinical follow-up study of In-Ceram Alumina FPDs. Int J Prosthodont 2003;16:150–156.

51. Vult von Steyern P, Jonsson O, Nilner K. Five-year evaluation of posterior all-ceramic three-unit (In-Ceram) FPDs. Int J Prosthodont 2001;14:379–384.

52. Fischer H, Weber M, Marx R. Lifetime prediction of all-ceramic bridges by computational methods. J Dent Res 2003;82:238–242.

53. Teixeira EC, Piascik JR, Stoner BR, Thompson JY. Dynamic fatigue and strength characterization of three ceramic materials. J Mater Sci Mater Med 2007;18:1219–1224.

54. Piconi C, Maccauro G. Zirconia as a ceramic biomaterial. Biomaterials 1999;20:1–25.

55. Luthardt RG, Holzhuter MS, Rudolph H, Herold V, Walter MH. CAD/CAM-machining effects on Y-TZP zirconia. Dent Mater 2004;20:655–662.

56. Filser F, Kocher P, Weibel F, Lüthy H, Schärer P, Gauckler LJ. Reliability and strength of all-ceramic dental restorations fabricated by direct ceramic machining (DCM). Int J Comput Dent 2001;4:89–106.

57. Tinschert J, Zwez D, Marx R, Anusavice KJ. Structural reliability of alumina-, feldspar-, leucite-, mica- and zirconia-based ceramics. J Dent 2000;28:529–535.

58. Lüthy H, Filser F, Loeffel O, Schumacher M, Gauckler LJ, Hämmerle CH. Strength and reliability of four-unit all-ceramic posterior bridges. Dent Mater 2005;21:930–937.

59. Guazzato M, Quach L, Albakry M, Swain MV. Influence of surface and heat treatments on the flexural strength of Y-TZP dental ceramic. J Dent 2005;33:9–18.

60. Papanagiotou HP, Morgano SM, Giordano RA, Pober R. In vitro evaluation of low-temperature aging effects and finishing procedures on the flexural strength and structural stability of Y-TZP dental ceramics. J Prosthet Dent 2006;96:154–164.

61. Lilley E. Review of low temperature degradation in Y-TZPs. In: Tressler RE, McNallan M (eds). Ceramic Transactions: Corrosion and Corrosive Degradation of Ceramics. Westerville, OH: American Ceramics Society, 1990:387–407.

62. Chevalier J. What future for zirconia as a biomaterial? Biomaterials 2006;27:535–543.

63. Guo X, He J. Hydrothermal degradation of cubic zirconia. Acta Mater 2003;51:5123–5130.

64. Ardlin BI. Transformation-toughened zirconia for dental inlays, crowns and bridges: chemical stability and effect of low-temperature aging on flexural strength and surface structure. Dent Mater 2002;18:590–595.

65. Raigrodski AJ. Contemporary materials and technologies for all-ceramic fixed dental protheses: a review of the literature. J Prosthet Dent 2004;92:557–562.

66. Nelsen RJ, Wolcott RB, Paffenbarger GC. Fluid exchange at the margins of dental restorations. J Am Dent Assoc 1952;44:288–295.

67. Barclay CW, Spence D, Laird WR. Intra-oral temperatures during function. J Oral Rehabil 2005;32:886–894.

68. Michailesco PM, Marciano J, Grieve AR, Abadie MJ. An in vivo recording of variations in oral temperature during meals: a pilot study. J Prosthet Dent 1995;73:214–218.

69. Palmer DS, Barco MT, Billy EJ. Temperature extremes produced orally by hot and cold liquids. J Prosthet Dent 1992;67:325–327.

70. Youngson CC, Barclay CW. A pilot study of intraoral temperature changes. Clin Oral Invest 2000;4:183–189.

71. Lee H, Carstens E, O'Mahony M. Drinking hot coffee: why doesn't it burn the mouth? J Sensory Stud 2003;18:19–32.

72. Creugers NH, Kayser AF, van 't Hof MA. A meta-analysis of durability data on conventional fixed bridges. Community Dent Oral Epidemiol 1994;22:448–452.

73. Scurria MS, Bader JD, Shugars DA. Meta-analysis of fixed partial denture survival: prostheses and abutments. J Prosthet Dent 1998;79:459–464.

74. Rekow ED, Harsono M, Janal M, Thompson VP, Zhang G. Factorial analysis of variables influencing stress in all-ceramic crowns. Dent Mater 2006;22:125–132.

75. Scherrer SS, de Rijk WG. The effect of crown length on the fracture resistance of posterior porcelain and glass-ceramic crowns. Int J Prosthodont 1992;5:550–557.

76. Anusavice KJ. Reducing the failure potential of ceramic-based restorations. Part 1: metal–ceramic crowns and bridges. Gen Dent 1996;44:492–494.

77. Anusavice KJ, Tsai YL. Stress distribution in ceramic crown forms as a function of thickness, elastic modulus and supporting substrate. In Bumgardner JD, Puckett AD (ed). Proceeding of the Sixteenth Southern Biomedical Engineering Conference. Biloxi, MS: IEEE, 1997:264–267.

78. Studart AR, Filser F, Kocher P, Gauckler LJ. Fatigue of zirconia under cyclic loading in water and its implications for the design of dental bridges. Dent Mater 2007;23:106–114.

79. Studart AR, Filser F, Kocher P, Lüthy H, Gauckler LJ. Mechanical and fracture behavior of veneer–framework composites for all-ceramic dental bridges. Dent Mater 2007;23:115–123.

80. Anusavice KJ (ed). Phillips' Science of Dental Materials, 10th edn. Philadelphia, PA: Saunders, 1996: 50–53.

81. Tinschert J, Natt G, Latzke P, Schulze K, Heussen N, Spiekermann H. Vollkeramische Bruecken aus DC-Zirkon: ein klinisches Konzept mit Erfolg? Deutsch Zahnaerztl Z 2005;60:435–445.

# Clinical Outcome of All-Ceramic Restorations

14

Matthias Kern

## Introduction

For many years, all-ceramic restorations made from feldspathic were mainly used for crowns cemented with conventional cements.[1,2] In the 1980s, glass-ceramic materials were introduced and this encouraged the use of all-ceramics. However, clinical failure rates were high when these were luted with conventional cements, particularly in posterior restorations.[3-5] Failure rates ranged from 15 to 35% for molar crowns after only 3–6 years of clinical service, which was unacceptably high when compared with the 'gold standard' of metal-ceramics, with failure rates of less than 5% within the first 5–10 years.[6]

In the 1990s, progress in adhesive luting technology[7] and the development of significantly stronger ceramic materials[8,9] broadly extended the indications for these materials. Computer-aided design and manufacture (CAD/CAM) provided the breakthrough needed for the production of high-strength all-ceramic restorations. Currently, high-strength all-ceramic materials exhibit fracture strengths and fracture toughness up to 10 times higher than those of traditional ceramic materials.[10,11] All-ceramic materials can now be used for a variety of fixed restorations, with the advantage of better esthetics and biocompatibility than metal-ceramic restorations. The purpose of this review is to summarize the published clinical success rates of all-ceramic restorations for a variety of clinical applications.

## Clinical Outcome

Clinical applications of all-ceramic materials include veneers, inlay, onlays, overlays, crowns, inlay- and crown-retained fixed dental prostheses (FDPs), resin-bonded FDPs, implant abutments, and implants. The restorations are made out of silicate ceramics (low to medium strength: 100–400 MPa) or oxide ceramics (high to very high strength: 400–1200 MPa).[12] When meta-analyses or systematic review articles on the clinical performance of a specific type of all-ceramic restorations are available, they are summarized below. Otherwise, clinical studies covering at least 3 years are included in this review.

### Inlays/Onlays

Ceramic inlays and onlays made by sintering, press-ceramic or CAD/CAM technologies are luted adhesively into the cavities, which provide enamel and dentin as bonding substrate (Fig 14-1). The IPS Empress pressed glass-ceramic system introduced at the beginning of the

195

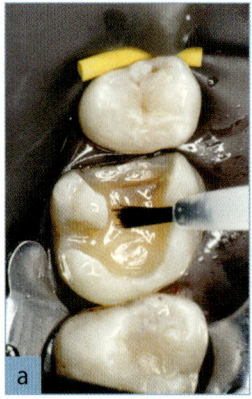
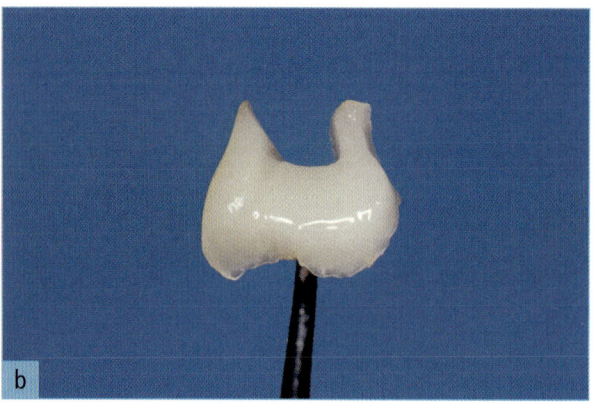
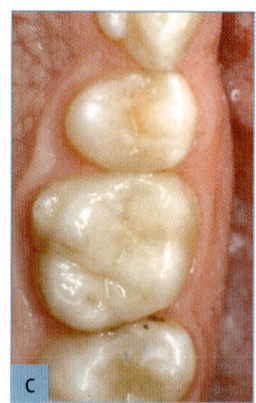

**Fig 14-1a–c** **(a)** Primer application to the cavity of an inlay preparation under rubber dam. **(b)** The silanated glass-ceramic inlay (IPS Empress). **(c)** The bonded inlay *in situ*.

1990s (Ivoclar-Vivadent) was the first glass-ceramic material providing high-end esthetics and perfectly fitting anatomical restorations in a simplified way.

A systematic review on the longevity of restorations in stress-bearing posterior cavities calculated annual failure rates.[13] These were 1.9% and 1.7%, respectively, for ceramic inlays and onlays when fabricated by CAD/CAM technology, which was only a little higher than that for cast gold inlays and onlays (1.4%). Direct fillings made from resin composite, amalgam, and glass-ionomer cement mostly had significantly higher annual failure rates, 2.2%, 3.0% and 7.2%, respectively.

Moreover, a recent systematic review on longevity and cost effectiveness of inlay restorations concluded that there were very similar failure-free survival rates for laboratory-fabricated ceramic, chairside CAD/CAM ceramic, and gold inlays, but the laboratory-fabricated ceramic inlays cost more to produce than the other two.[14] However, this comparison did not consider the esthetic outcome of the restorations.

Interestingly, recent studies on large patient groups in private practices have shown even better long-term success rates for CAD/CAM-produced ceramic restorations machined with the Cerec system (Sirona); success rates ranged from a 10-year survival rate of 90% (1010 restorations)[15] up to a 9-year survival rate of 95.5% (2328 restorations).[16]

It can be concluded that adhesively luted all-ceramic inlays and onlays provide an excellent clinical outcome and might replace gold inlays and onlays as the 'gold standard' in the treatment of posterior cavities, particularly when esthetics is also considered as an important function of posterior restorations.

## Veneers

Since the 1970s, all-ceramic veneers have been luted adhesively to the labial and/or lingual tooth surface, which is (mostly) enamel (Fig 14-2).[17] In contrast to inlays, the preparation design of veneers is usually without any mechanical retention.[18] Veneers are also made by sintering, press-ceramic or CAD/CAM technologies. In an early meta-analysis of veneers, all-ceramic veneers had a significantly higher survival rate than resin-based veneers after 3 years, at 92% and 74%, respectively.[19] In a more recent review on the longevity of all-ceramic veneers, the 10-year survival rate was 90%, which compares well with that for single crowns.[20] The preparation design (with or without incisal ceramic coverage) seems not to influence the clinical survival rate significantly.[21] However, an increased risk of failure was reported when veneers were bonded both to sound enamel and partially to dentin.[22,23] When at least 80% of each preparation is bonded to enamel, the survival of ceramic veneers was 96% at 5–6 years and still 91% at 12–13 years.[24]

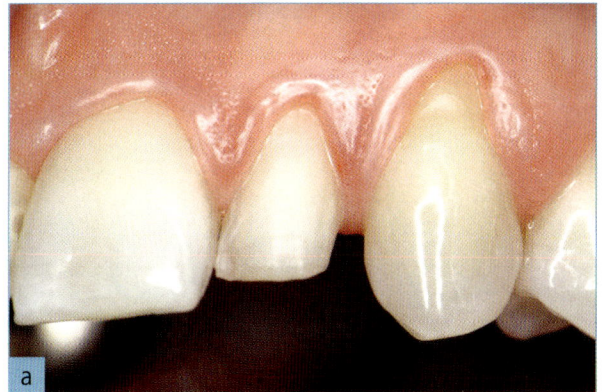

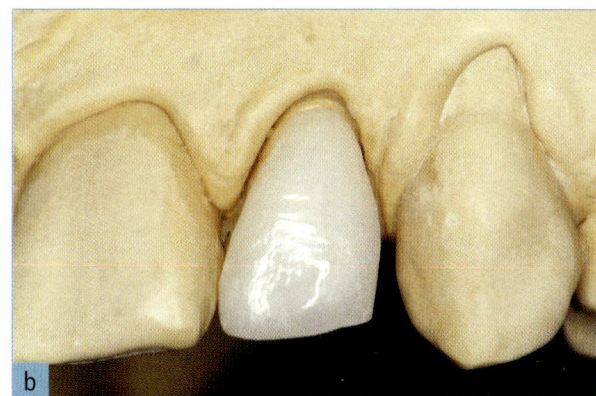

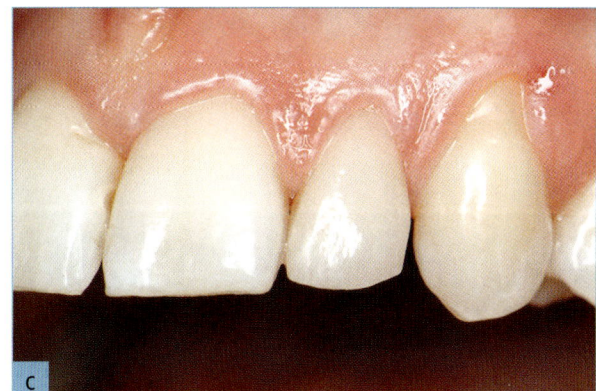

Fig 14-2a–c (a) Preparation of tooth 22 within the enamel for a ceramic veneer. (b) The glass-ceramic veneer (IPS Empress) on the master cast. (c) The bonded veneer *in situ*.

A clinical study on extended ceramic veneers made from IPS Empress and luted with Variolink II (both Ivoclar Vivadent) compared two preparation designs: an overlapping incisal edge preparation and a full-veneer preparation that extended on the palatal surface to the cingulum area.[25] After 5 years, the survival rate of the overlap veneers was 97.5% and that of full veneers was 100%.

In addition to the restoration of labial tooth surfaces, ceramic veneers can also be used to restore anterior guidance (Fig 14-3).[26,27] The survival rate of veneers restoring canine guidance was 76% after 6.5 years, which is very high considering the functional loading in this area.

In summary, it has been shown that ceramic veneers that are bonded mostly to enamel provide an excellent clinical outcome even when used with an extended palatal preparation design.

## Crowns

Early clinical trials with low-strength all-ceramic crowns showed dramatically improved clinical performance when crowns were luted adhesively.[28] Therefore, in most clinical situations, silicate ceramics of low to medium strength should be luted adhesively (Fig 14-4), while oxide ceramics of high to very high strength can often be luted with conventional cements.

In a recent meta-analysis, the overall 5-year survival of all-ceramic crowns was calculated at 93.3%, compared with 95.6% for metal-ceramic crowns.[29] A comparison based on the materials utilized showed that crowns made from densely sintered alumina (Procera, Noble Biocare), leucite-reinforced glass-ceramic (IPS Empress, Ivoclar-Vivadent), and glass-infiltrated alumina (In-Ceram, Vita) showed 5-year-survival rates of 96.4%, 95.4%, and 94.5%, respectively. A significantly lower survival rate of 87.5% was calculated for conventional glass-ceramic crowns after 5 years.

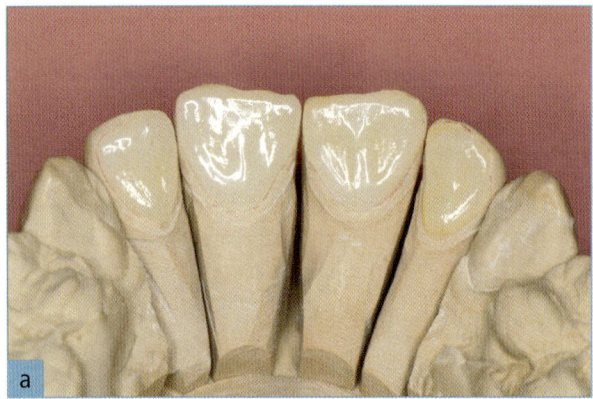

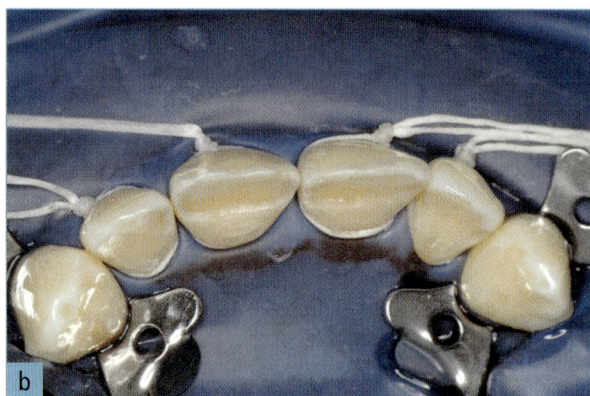

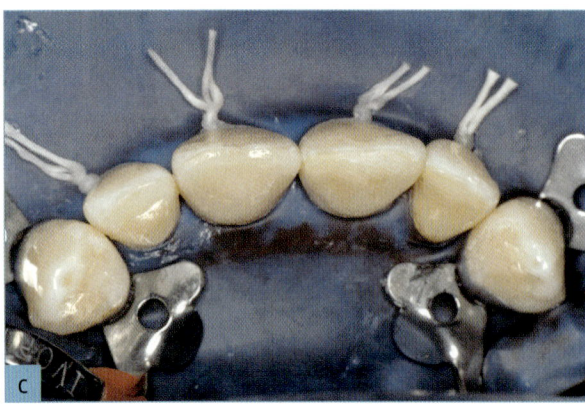

**Fig 14-3a–c** (a) Palatal veneers (IPS Empress) for the reconstruction of anterior guidance on the master cast, (b) The anterior teeth under rubber dam ready for bonding. (c) The bonded palatal veneers *in situ*.

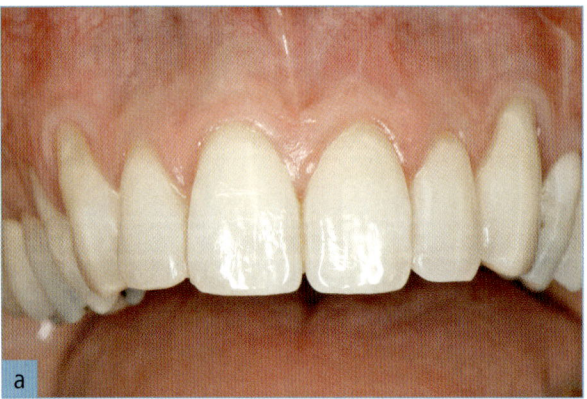

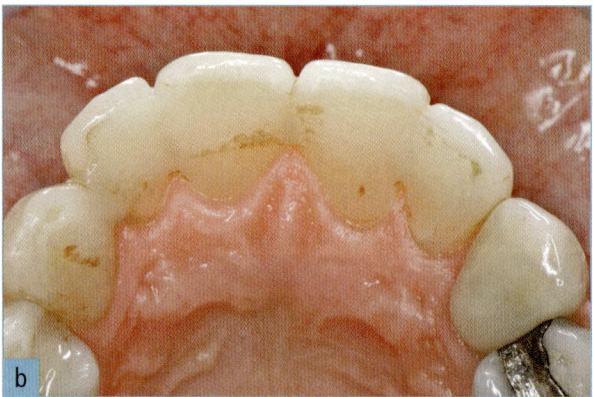

**Fig 14-4a–b** (a) Adhesively bonded glass-ceramic crown on the left canine (IPS Empress) after 9 years of clinical service. (b) The oral view shows discoloration of the resin fiber splint on the natural incisors. The ceramic shows no discoloration.

Using low-strength glass-ceramic crowns, failure rates were particularly high in the molar region but were mostly low in the anterior region (Table 14-1).[28,30–35] However, when using medium-strength glass-ceramics such as lithium disilicate (Empress 2, e.max press, Ivoclar-Vivadent), the survival rate became much better even in the molar region.[34,35] However, it must be emphasized that these positive outcomes can only be expected when the recommended preparation guidelines are followed. If the required thickness of the ceramic materials is not achieved, early failures can be expected (Fig 14-5).

Table 14-1 Failure rates of adhesively cemented crowns made from glass-ceramics related to their location.

| First author and year | N | Ceramic | Time (months) | Failure rate (%)[a] | | |
|---|---|---|---|---|---|---|
| | | | | Anterior teeth | Premolars | Molars |
| Hankinson 1994[56] | 95 | Optec | 30 | 0 | 2.3 | 24.0 |
| Lehner 1998[57] | 138 | Empress 1 | 73 | 15.6 | 5.4 | 10.8 |
| Malament 1999[28] | 1044 | Dicor | 168 | 5.8 | 10.8 | 29.0 |
| Sjogren 1999[58] | 110 | Empress 1 | 43 | 2.7 | 7.0 | 12.0 |
| Fradeani 2002[59] | 125 | Empress 1 | 132 | 1.1 | 15.6 | |
| Zimmer 2004[31] | 27 | Empress 2 | 38 | - | 0 | 0 |
| Edelhoff 2005[b 30] | 155 | Empress 2[b] | 37 | 0 | 0 | 0 |

[a]Failure rates excluded minor chippings of veneering ceramics that did not require repairs.
[b]In part luted with conventional cements.

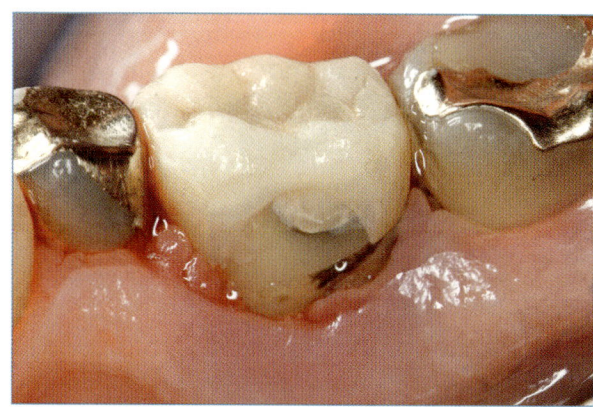

Fig 14-5 Fractured glass-ceramic crown on a maxillary molar with inadequate preparation (restored alio loco).

The survival rates of CAD/CAM crowns made with a glass-infiltrated alumina ceramic core (In-Ceram Spinell, Vita) or a mono-ceramic block (MK II, Vita) were 91.7% and 94.4%, respectively, after 45 months; however, this difference was not statistically significant.[36] High-strength oxide-containing ceramics can be luted with conventional cements without showing higher failure rates than metal-ceramics even in the molar region (Table 14-2).[37–48] However, chipping of the low-strength veneering ceramics was reported in several studies of high-strength oxide-ceramics. Nevertheless, for the posterior region, crowns made from oxide-ceramics can be recommended clinically even when used with conventional cements.

In conclusion, when using materials with adequate strength, all-ceramic crowns show survival rates comparable to those of metal-ceramic crowns. However, it must be noted that currently there are no clinical studies reporting the outcome of single crowns made from high-strength zirconia ceramic.

## Fixed Dental Prostheses (Crown Abutments)

Although all-ceramic FDPs using various all-ceramic systems were described as early as the 1980s,[49] it is only recently that clinical studies describing survival over 2–5 years have been reported.[50,51]

In a recent meta-analysis on the longevity of all-ceramic FDPs, the 5-year survival was 88.6%, which

Table 14-2 Failure rates of conventionally cemented crowns made from oxide ceramics related to their location.

| First author and year | N | Ceramic | Time (months) | Failure rate (%)[a] | | |
|---|---|---|---|---|---|---|
| | | | | Anterior teeth | Premolars | Molars |
| Pröbster 1996[60] | 95 | In-Ceram Al | 30 | 0 | 1.5 | |
| Rinke 1997[38] | 457 | In-Ceram Al | 72 | 5.0 | | |
| Odén 1998[61] | 100 | Procera Al | 60 | 0 | 3.6 | 7.3 |
| McLaren 2000[62] | 223 | In-Ceram Al | 36 | 2.1 | 6.5 | 6.2 |
| Haselton 2000[63] | 80 | In-Ceram Al | 48 | 7.7 | | |
| Odman 2001[64] | 87 | Procera Al | 120 | 6.5 | | |
| Segal 2001[65] | 546 | In-Ceram Al | 12-70 | 1.1 | 0.8 | |
| Fradeani 2002[66] | 40 | In-Ceram Sp | 50 | 2.5 | - | |
| Bindl 2002[67] | 43 | In-Ceram Al/Sp | 39 | - | 0 | 5.4 |
| Fradeani 2005[68] | 205 | Procera Al | 60 | 0 | 4.8 | |
| Galindo 2006[69] | 155 | Procera Al | 55 | 0 | 1.2 | |
| Walter 2006[70] | 107 | Procera Al | 72 | 3.3 | 3.3 | 8.7 |

[a]Failure rates excluded minor chippings of veneering ceramics that did not require repairs.

was significantly lower than that for metal-ceramic FDPs (94.4%).[50] Also the frequencies of material fractures, both framework and veneering material, were significantly higher for all-ceramic FDPs (6.5% and 13.6%, respectively) than for metal-ceramic FDPs (1.6% and 2.9%, respectively). In the review by Sailer and coworkers,[50] the most frequent reason for failure of FDPs made from glass-ceramics or ceramics was fracture of the framework or veneering ceramic. However, when zirconia ceramic was used as framework material, the reasons for failure were primarily biological and technical complications other than framework fracture.

If the location of the FDP was considered, medium-strength ceramics showed particularly high failure rates in the posterior region (Table 14-3).[34,35,52–59] For the lithi-um disilicate ceramic Empress 2, the clinical failure rate increased to an unacceptably high 45.9% when the FDP dimensions did not follow the recommendations of the manufacturer,[35] which included a mesiodistal width of the pontic < 9mm in the posterior region and < 11mm in the anterior region. The minimum connector size was 16mm$^2$ in the posterior region and 12 mm$^2$ in the anterior region.

When using the latest lithium disilicate ceramic (e.max press; Ivoclar Vivadent)[59,60] (Table 14-3) or zirconia-based high-strength ceramics[61–64] (Table 14-4) with the recommended dimensions,[10] the failure rates were comparable to those of metal-ceramic over a period of up to 7 years (Fig 14-6).[61–67] However, chipping of the veneering ceramic occurred in FDPs made from high-

Table 14-3 Failure rates of medium-strength all-ceramic fixed dental prostheses with crown abutments related to the pontic location.

| First author and year | N | Ceramic | Time (months) | Failure rate (%)[a] | | |
|---|---|---|---|---|---|---|
| | | | | Anterior teeth | Premolars | Molars |
| Hüls 1995[71] | 44 | In-Ceram Al | 36-72 | 0 | 19.0 | |
| Sorensen 1998[72] | 61 | In-Ceram Al | 36 | 0 | 11.0 | 24.0 |
| Pospiech 2000[73] | 51 | Empress 2 | 24 | 0 | 9.1 | 25.0 |
| Vult v. Steyern 2001[74] | 20 | In-Ceram Al | 60 | - | 0 | 22.2 |
| Tinschert 2002[54] | 18 | In-Ceram Al | 42 | 5.6 | - | - |
| Olsson 2003[75] | 42 | In-Ceram Al | 76 | 12.0 | | |
| Zimmer 2004[31] | 40 | Empress 2 | 38 | 27.6 | - | |
| Edelhoff 2005[30] | 43 | Empress 2 | 52 | 27.2 | | |
| Marquardt 2006[76] | 31 | Empress 2 | 50 | 30.0 | | - |
| Eschbach 2007[37] | 37 | e.max Press | 60-78 | 0 | 0 | 0 |

[a]Failure rates excluded minor chippings of veneering ceramics that did not require repairs.

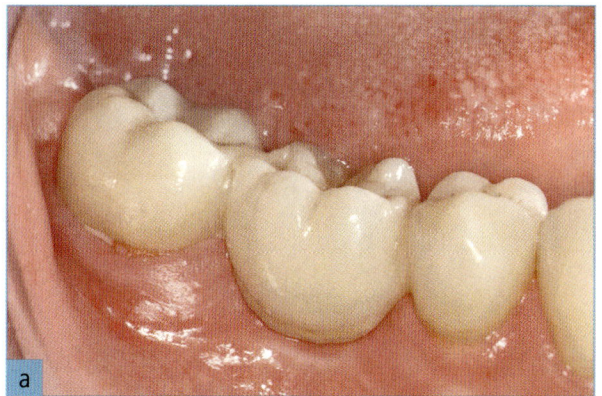
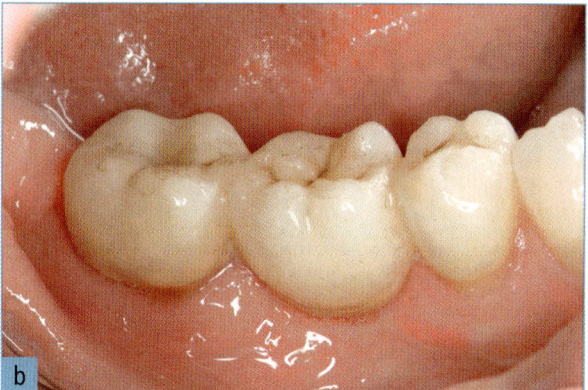

Fig 14-6a–b Posterior fixed dental prosthesis made from lithium disilicate (e.max press) after 4 years (a) and 8 years (b) in service.

strength ceramics to a similar or even higher extent as in metal-ceramics.[60–64,66] In one study, the overall failure rate with posterior zirconia-based ceramic FDPs after 5 years was 26.1%, as a result of loss of retention and biological complications such as caries and endodontic problems, although only one framework fracture occurred.[66]

In summary, medium-term results with FDPs made from the lithium disilicate ceramic e.max press and with zirconia-based ceramic are promising. However, in some studies, veneered zirconia-based ceramic FDPs showed a significant rate of chippings in the veneering ceramic.

| First author and year | N | Ceramic | Time (months) | Failure rate (%)[a] | | |
|---|---|---|---|---|---|---|
| | | | | Anterior teeth | Premolars | Molars |
| Pospiech 2004[38] | 35 | Lava | 36 | - | - | 0 |
| Suárez 2004[77] | 10 | In-Ceram Zr | 36 | 0 | 5.5 | |
| Kern 2006[39] | 60 | In-Ceram Zr | 36 | - | 0 | 2.2 |
| Sailer 2007[42] | 33 | DCM | 53 | - | 26.1 | |
| Molin 2008[40] | 19 | Denzir | 60 | 0 | 0 | 0 |
| Tinschert 2008[41] | 65 | DCS | 37 | 0 | 0 | |
| Wolfart 2008[78] | 24 | Cercon | 45 | - | 4.0 | |

**Table 14-4** Failure rates of high-strength all-ceramic fixed dental prostheses with crown abutments related to the pontic location.

[a]Failure rates excluded minor chippings of veneering ceramics that did not require repairs.

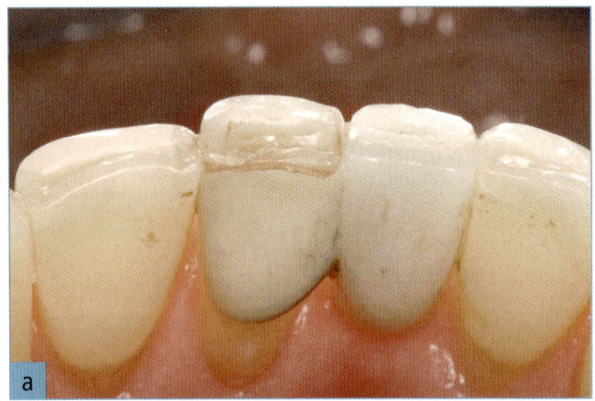
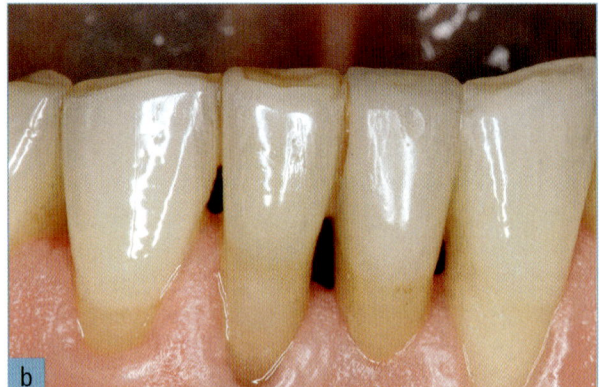

**Fig 14-7a–b** Resin-bonded all-ceramic fixed dental prosthesis with unilateral retainer wing (In-Ceram alumina, Vita, Bad Säckingen) after 10 years of clinical service.

## Minimally Invasive Resin-Bonded Fixed Dental Prostheses

All-ceramic resin-bonded FDPs were introduced in the early 1990s as a minimally invasive treatment option for missing incisors.[68] Resin-bonded FDPs with two retainers had a relatively high fracture rate within the first year of clinical service, but they mostly remained in function in cantilever restorations.[69] Therefore, in 1997, the cantilevered resin-bonded all-ceramic FDPs were

introduced as a new treatment modality (Fig 14-7).[70] Medium-term results with single-retainer resin-bonded FDPs made from glass-infiltrated alumina ceramic were quite promising (Table 14-5).[35,60,71,72] However, the clinical outcome might be improved further if high-strength zirconia-based ceramics such as e.max ZirCAD (Ivoclar-Vivadent) were used for resin-bonded FDPs (Fig 14-8).

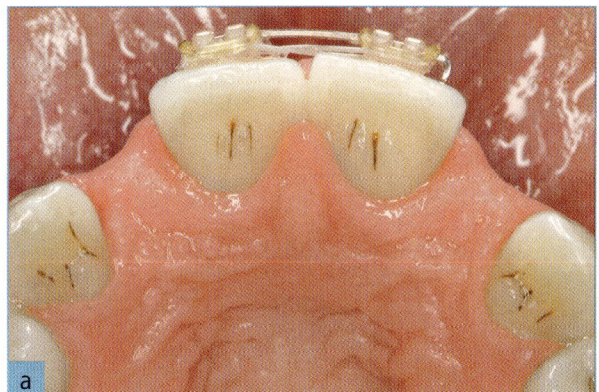
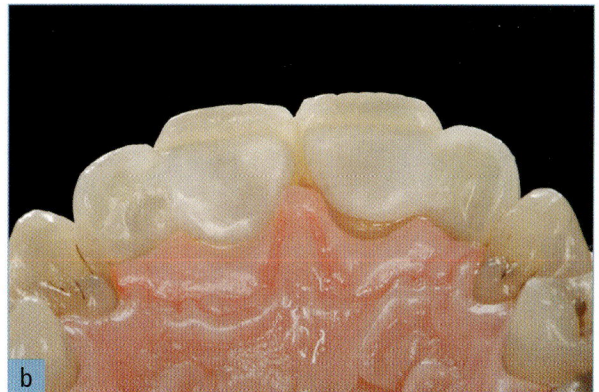
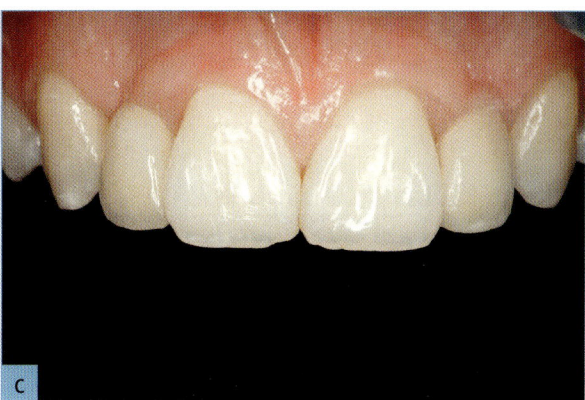

**Fig 14-8a–c** Congenitally missing lateral incisors.
**(a)** Preoperative view. **(b)** The resin-bonded all-ceramic fixed dental prosthesis with unilateral retainer wings (e.max. ZirCAD) replacing the missing teeth. **(c)** The frontal view of the restored anterior dentition.

**Table 14-5** Failure rates of all-ceramic fixed dental prostheses retained by resin-bonded retainer wings or inlays related to the pontic location.

| First author and year | N | Retainer | Ceramic | Time (months) | Failure rate (%)[a] Anterior teeth | Premolars | Molars |
|---|---|---|---|---|---|---|---|
| Dumfahrt 1995[19] | 19 | 2 wings | Optec HSP | 34 | 5.3 | – | – |
| Edelhoff 2002[30] | 15 | 2 wings/2 inlays | Empress 2 | 26 | 0 | 18.2 | – |
| Kern 2005[46] | 16 | 2 wings | In-Ceram Al | 60 | 26.1 | – | – |
| Kern 2005[46] | 21 | 1 wing | In-Ceram Al/Zr | 60 | 7.7 | – | – |
| Wolfart 2005[36] | 45 | 2 inlays | e.max press | 37 | – | 12.5 | 13.3 |

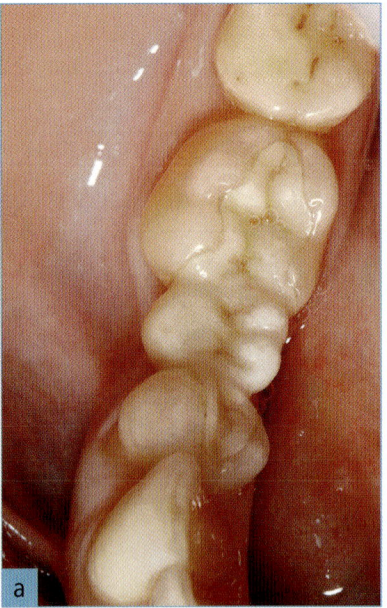
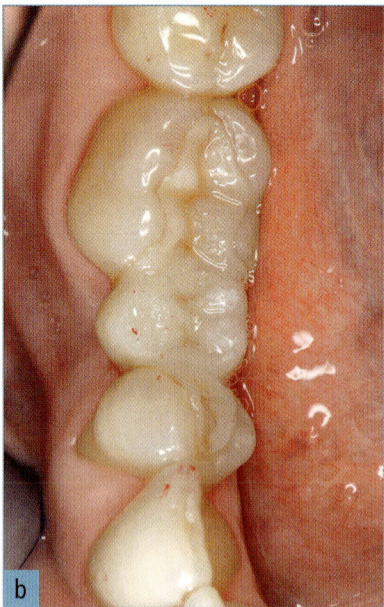
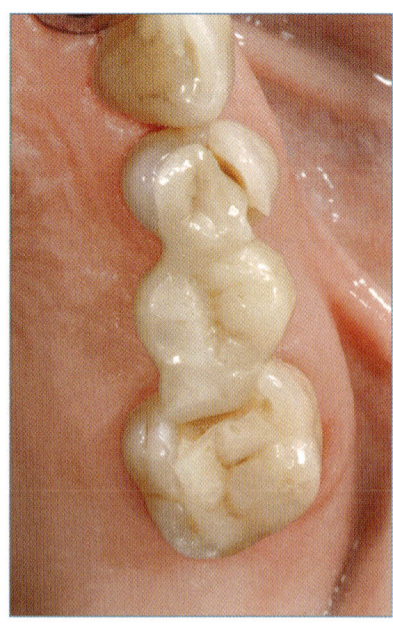

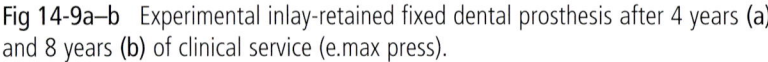

Fig 14-9a–b   Experimental inlay-retained fixed dental prosthesis after 4 years (a) and 8 years (b) of clinical service (e.max press).

Fig 14-10   An experimental inlay-retained fixed dental prosthesis that fractured after 3 years of clinical service (e.max press).

At the beginning of the twenty-first century, all-ceramic inlay-retained FDPs were evaluated experimentally as a minimally invasive treatment method for the replacement of missing posterior teeth;[60,73] however, they exhibited relatively high failure rates (12–18%) within the first 3 years (Table 14-5). Although some restorations served without problems for more than 8 years (Fig 14-9), after 5–8 years of clinical service the overall failure rate had increased to 46%, which seems unacceptably high (Fig 14-10; M Kern, unpublished data, June 2008).

Interestingly, inlay-retained FDPs made from the lithium disilicate ceramic e.max press failed not only because of ceramic fractures at the connector but also, and mostly, through loss of retention in the proximal inlay area, with fracture in the isthmus of the inlay.[60] So not only the fracture strength of the all-ceramic material but also sufficient adhesive retention of the restoration seem to be requisites for the clinical success of inlay-retained FDPs. Therefore, a new minimally inva-

sive retainer design has been described for posterior resin-bonded all-ceramic FDPs that combines increased strength and increased retention of the FDPs.[74] The strength of the restorations is improved by using zirconia-ceramic blocks (e.g. e.max ZirCAD, Ivoclar-Vivadent) in the Cerec InLab system, and the adhesive retention of the inlay retainer is increased by using additional retainer wings on the buccal and oral abutment surface (Fig 14-11). However, clinical studies have yet to show whether this design will result in an acceptable clinical outcome of inlay-retained all-ceramic FDPs.

In summary, while anterior all-ceramic resin-bonded FDPs with retainer wings show promising medium-term clinical results, posterior inlay-retained all-ceramic FDPs cannot be recommended as a viable treatment option as yet, independent of the ceramic material used.

## Implant Abutments

Implant abutments made from alumina ceramics were developed at the beginning of the 1990s, but only rela-

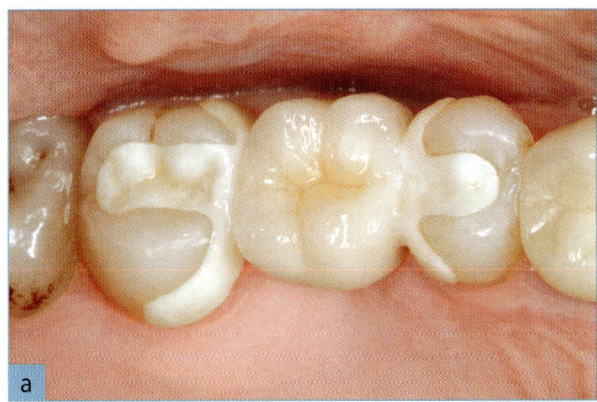
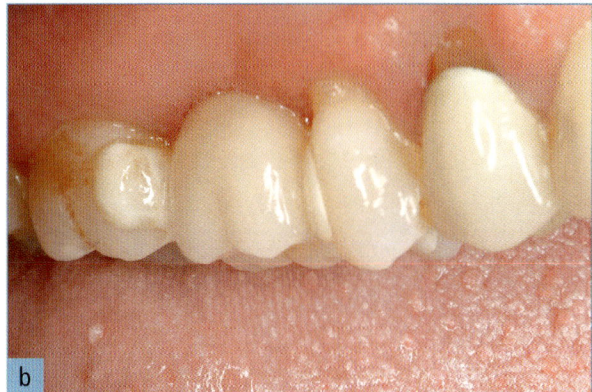

**Fig 14-11a–b** (a) Experimental inlay-retained fixed dental prosthesis made from zirconia ceramic with additional retainer wings for improved retention by increasing the bonding surface within the enamel. (b) The visibility of the retainer wings is an esthetical compromise.

tively short-term clinical data have been published. These show a fracture rate of 7% within the first year of clinical service for single-implant restorations.[75] No longer-term follow-up studies have been published and the alumina-ceramic implant abutments have been withdrawn from the market, suggesting that the clinical outcome has not been as expected (Fig 14-12).

Because densely sintered zirconia-ceramic has much better physical properties than alumina-ceramic,[76] zirconia-ceramic is now mainly used for implant abutments. An experimental zirconia-ceramic abutment has shown a promising clinical outcome over 4 years, without any abutment fractures.[77] However, in order to avoid technical complications when connecting ceramic abutments with screws to titanium implants, it might be advantageous to sinter or to bond a zirconia-ceramic abutment to a titanium base that is then screwed into or on to the implant (Fig 14-13).[78] However, no comparative clinical studies on the outcome of different all-ceramic abutment designs are available as yet. In view of the limited amount of available data, no general conclusions on all-ceramic abutments can yet be drawn.

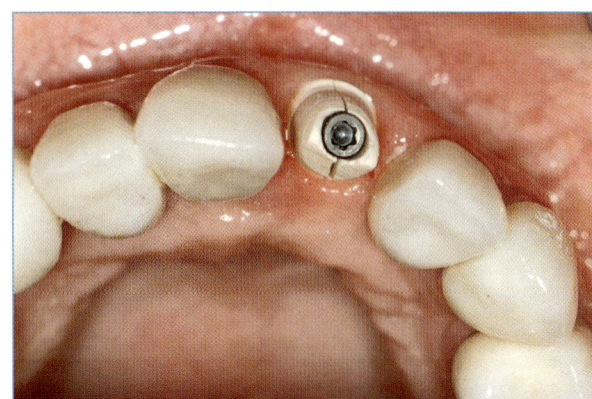

**Fig 14-12** Fractured alumina ceramic abutment.

## Implants

In the 1970s, all-ceramic implants made from densely sintered alumina-ceramic had been introduced to dentistry.[79] However, they showed a relatively high fracture rate (Fig 14-14) and were redrawn from the market.[80]

Because of the excellent physical properties of densely sintered zirconia-ceramic, several companies have recently introduced zirconia-ceramic implants (Fig 14-15). However, there is not as yet a systematic review providing longer-term data on the clinical outcome of zirconia-ceramic implants.[81] Consequently, the clinical application of all-ceramic implants must be considered experimental at present.

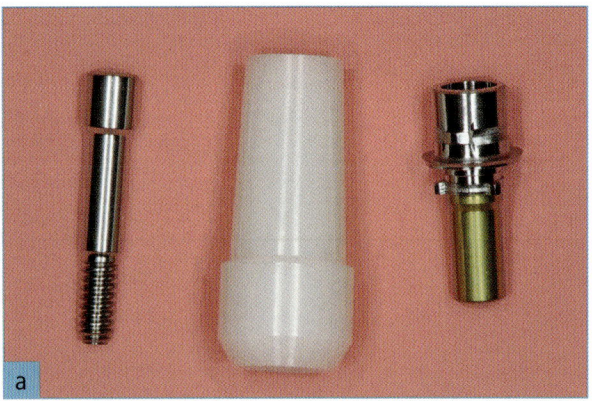

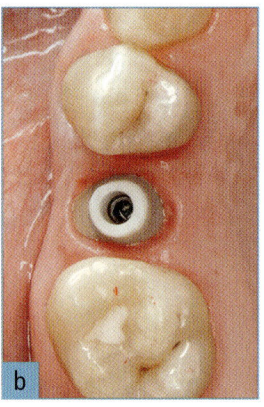

**Fig 14-13a–b** (a) The zirconia-ceramic abutment (Camlog Biotechnologies) is resin-bonded to a titanium base. (b) The zirconia ceramic abutment *in situ*.

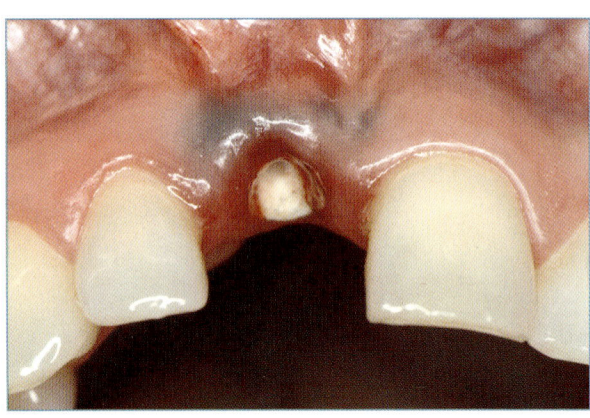

**Fig 14-14** Fractured alumina-ceramic implant after several attempted repairs.

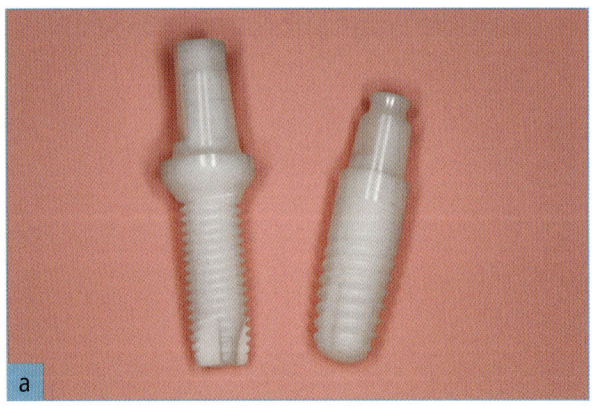

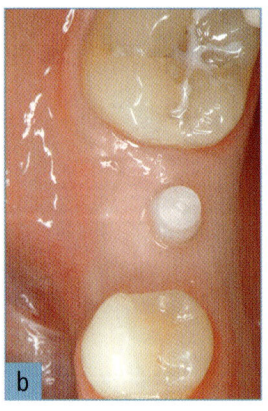

**Fig 14-15a–b** (a) Single part zirconia-ceramic implants. (b) The inserted zirconia-ceramic implant.

# Conclusions

Excellent long-term clinical data are available for all-ceramic restorations such as inlays, onlays, veneers, crowns, and anterior FDPs; these data support their use as an alternative to conventional metal-based restorations. However, for FDPs in the posterior area and for implants and implant abutments, insufficient long-term data have been published to recommend these restorations yet as a proven substitute for the established metal-based conventional counterpart.

# References

1. McLean JW, Schmidseder J. Hochfeste Keramiken. [High-density ceramics.] Phillip J Restaur Zahnmed1984;1:137–141.

2. Kelly JR, Nishimura I, Campbell SD. Ceramics in dentistry: Historical roots and current perspectives. J Prosthet Dent 1996;75:18–32.

3. Moffa JP. Porcelain materials. Adv Dent Res 1988;2:3–6.

4. Meier M, Richter E-J, Küpper H, Spiekermann H. Klinische Befunde bei Kronen aus Dicor-Glaskeramik. Dtsch Zahnärztl Z 1992;47:610–614.

5. Borchard R, Erpenstein H, Kerschbaum T. Langzeitergebnisse von galvanokeramischen und glaskeramischen (Dicor) Einzelkronen unter klinischen Bedingungen. Dtsch Zahnärztl Z 1998;53:616–619.

6. Walton TR. A 10-year longitudinal study of fixed prosthodontics: clinical characteristics and outcome of single-unit metal–ceramic crowns. Int J Prosthodont 1999;12:519–526.

7. Blatz MB, Sadan A, Kern M. Resin-ceramic bonding: a review of the literature. J Prosthet Dent 2003;89:268–274.

8. Kappert HF. Dental materials: new ceramic systems. Trans Acad Dent Mater 1996;9:180–199.

9. Kelly JR. Dental ceramics: current thinking and trends. Dent Clin North Am 2004;48:513–530.

10. Kunzelmann KH, Kern M, Pospiech P, Raigrodski AJ, Strassler HE, Mehl A, Frankenberger R, Reiss BWK. All-ceramics at a glance. 1. Auflage ed. Ettlingen: Arbeitsgemeinschaft für Keramik in der Zahnheilkunde, 2007.

11. Kelly JR, Denry I. Stabilized zirconia as a structural ceramic: an overview. Dent Mater 2008;24:289–298.

12. Kappert HF. Zur Festigkeit von Dentalkeramiken. Zahnärztl Mitt 2003;93:802–806.

13. Manhart J, Chen H, Hamm G, Hickel R. Buonocore Memorial Lecture. Review of the clinical survival of direct and indirect restorations in posterior teeth of the permanent dentition. Oper Dent 2004;29:481–508.

14. Gandjour A, Kerschbaum T, Reis A, Lauterbach KW. Technology assessment in dentistry. A comparison of the longevity and cost-effectiveness of inlays. Int J Technol Assess Health Care 2005;21:319–325.

15. Reiss B, Walther W. Clinical long-term results and 10-year Kaplan–Meier analysis of Cerec restorations. Int J Comput Dent 2000;3:9–23.

16. Posselt A, Kerschbaum T. Longevity of 2328 chairside Cerec inlays and onlays. Int J Comput Dent 2003;6:231–248.

17. Rochette AL. A ceramic bonded by etched enamel and resin for fractured incisors. J Prosthet Dent 1975;33:287–293.

18. Edelhoff D, Sorensen JA. Tooth structure removal associated with various preparation designs for anterior teeth. J Prosthet Dent 2002;87:503–509.

19. Kreulen CM, Creugers NH, Meijering AC. Meta-analysis of anterior veneer restorations in clinical studies. J Dent 1998;26:345–353.

20. Kerschbaum T. Langzeitüberlebensdauer von Zahnersatz. Eine Übersicht. Quintessenz 2004;55:1113–1126.

21. Smales RJ, Etemadi S. Long-term survival of porcelain laminate veneers using two preparation designs: a retrospective study. Int J Prosthodont 2004;17:323–326.

22. Dumfahrt H, Schäffer H. Porcelain laminate veneers. A retrospective evaluation after 1 to 10 years of service: Part II. Clinical results. Int J Prosthodont 2000;13:9–18.

23. Friedman MJ. Porcelain veneer restorations: a clinician's opinion about a disturbing trend. J Esthet Restor Dent 2001;13:318–327.

24. Layton D, Walton T. An up to 16-year prospective study of 304 porcelain veneers. Int J Prosthodont 2007;20:389–396.

25. Guess PC, Stappert CF. Midterm results of a 5-year prospective clinical investigation of extended ceramic veneers. Dent Mater 2008;24:804–813.

26. Schäffer H, Kulmer S. Functional reconstruction of abraded canines by resin-bonded all-ceramic guiding elements. Int J Prosthodont 1990;3:538–544.

27. Sieweke M, Salomon-Sieweke U, Zofel P, Stachniss V. Longevity of oroincisal ceramic veneers on canines. A retrospective study. J Adhes Dent 2000;2:229–234.

28. Malament KA, Socransky SS. Survival of Dicor glass-ceramic dental restorations over 14 years: Part I. Survival of Dicor complete coverage restorations and effect of internal surface acid etching, tooth position, gender, and age. J Prosthet Dent 1999;81:23–32.

29. Pjetursson BE, Sailer I, Zwahlen M, Hämmerle CHF. A systematic review of the survival and complication rates of all-ceramic and metal–ceramic reconstructions after an observation period of at least 3 years. Part I: single crowns. Clin Oral Implants Res 2007;18:73–85.

30. Hankinson JA, Cappetta EG. Five years' clinical experience with a leucite-reinforced porcelain crown system. Int J Periodontics Restorative Dent 1994;14:138–153.

31. Lehner CR, Studer S, Schärer P. Seven-year results of leucite-reinforced glass-ceramic crowns. J Dent Res 1998;77:802, Abstr 1368.

32. Sjogren G, Lantto R, Granberg A, Sundstrom BO, Tillberg A. Clinical examination of leucite-reinforced glass-ceramic crowns (Empress) in general practice: a retrospective study. Int J Prosthodont 1999;12:122–128.

33. Fradeani M, Redemagni M. An 11-year clinical evaluation of leucite-reinforced glass-ceramic crowns: a retrospective study. Quintessence Int 2002;33:503–510.

34. Zimmer D, Gerds T, Strub JR. Überlebensraten von IPS-Empress 2-Vollkeramikkronen und -brücken: Drei-Jahres-Ergebnisse. Schweiz Monatsschr Zahnmed 2004;114:115–119.

35. Edelhoff D, Spiekermann H, Brauner J, Yildirim M. IPS Empress 2: adhäsiv und konventionell befestigt. Vollkeramische Kronen und Brücken nach dreijähriger Tragedauer. Dent Labor 2005;63:1223–1235.

36. Bindl A, Mörmann WH. Survival rate of mono-ceramic and ceramic-core CAD/CAM-generated anterior crowns over 2–5 years. Eur J Oral Sci 2004;112:197–204.

37. Pröbster L. Four year clinical study of glass-infiltrated, sintered alumina crowns. J Oral Rehabil 1996;23:147–151.

38. Rinke S, Hüls A. Glass-infiltrated ceramic restorations. Clinical outcome after seven years. Lecture, 30th symposium of the German Society for Prosthodontics and Dental Materials (DGZPW), Gotha, Germany, May 1997.

39. Odén A, Andersson M, Krystek Ondracek I, Magnusson D. Five-year clinical evaluation of Procera AllCeram crowns. J Prosthet Dent 1998;80:450–456.

40. McLaren EA, White SN. Survival of In-Ceram crowns in a private practice: A prospective clinical trial. J Prosthet Dent 2000;83:216–222.

41. Haselton DR, Diaz-Arnold AM, Hillis SL. Clinical assessment of high-strength all-ceramic crowns. J Prosthet Dent 2000;83:396–401.

42. Odman P, Andersson B. Procera AllCeram crowns followed for 5 to 10.5 years: a prospective clinical study. Int J Prosthodont 2001;14:504–509.

43. Segal BS. Retrospective assessment of 546 all-ceramic anterior and posterior crowns in a general practice. J Prosthet Dent 2001;85:544–550.

44. Fradeani M, Aquilano A, Corrado M. Clinical experience with In-Ceram Spinell crowns: 5-year follow-up. Int J Periodontics Restorative Dent 2002;22:525–533.

45. Bindl A, Mörmann WH. An up to 5-year clinical evaluation of posterior In-ceram CAD/CAM core crowns. Int J Prosthodont 2002;15:451–456.

46. Fradeani M, D'Amelio M, Redemagni M, Corrado M. Five-year follow-up with Procera all-ceramic crowns. Quintessence Int 2005;36:105–113.

47. Galindo ML, Hagmann E, Marinello CP, Zitzmann NU. Klinische Langzeiterfahrungen mit Procera-AllCeram-Vollkeramikkronen. Schweiz Monatsschr Zahnmed 2006;116:804–809.

48. Walter MH, Wolf BH, Wolf AE, Boening KW. Six-year clinical performance of all-ceramic crowns with alumina cores. Int J Prosthodont 2006;19:162–163.

49. Graser GN, Myers ML, Grossman DG, Cammarato VT. Preliminary clinical evaluation of cast ceramic fixed partial dentures. J Dent Res 1985;64:362.

50. Sailer I, Pjetursson BE, Zwahlen M, Hämmerle CHF. A systematic review of the survival and complication rates of all-ceramic and metal–ceramic reconstructions after an observation period of at least 3 years. Part II: fixed dental prostheses. Clin Oral Implants Res 2007;18:86–96.

51. Denry I, Kelly JR. State of the art of zirconia for dental applications. Dent Mater 2008;24:299–307.

52. Hüls A. Vollkeramischer Zahnersatz aus In-Ceram. 6 Jahre klinische Praxis. Bad Säckingen: Vita, 1995.

53. Sorensen JA, Kang SK, Torres TJ, Knode H. In-Ceram fixed partial dentures: three-year clinical trial results. J Calif Dent Assoc 1998;26:207–214.

54. Tinschert J. Werkstoffkundliche und klinische Untersuchungen zu vollkeramischen Kronen und Brücken aus Hartkern-Systemen [Med. Habil.]. University of Aachen; 2002.

55. Pospiech P, Kistler S, Frasch C, Rammelsberg P. Clinical evaluation of Empress 2 bridges: first results after two years. J Dent Res 2000;79:334, Abstr 1527.

56. Vult von Steyern P, Jonsson O, Nilner K. Five-year evaluation of posterior all-ceramic three-unit (In-Ceram) FPDs. Int J Prosthodont 2001;14:379–384.

57. Olsson KG, Furst B, Andersson B, Carlsson GE. A long-term retrospective and clinical follow-up study of In-Ceram Alumina FPDs. Int J Prosthodont 2003;16:150–156.

58. Marquardt P, Strub JR. Survival rates of IPS empress 2 all-ceramic crowns and fixed partial dentures: results of a 5-year prospective clinical study. Quintessence Int 2006;37:253–259.

59. Eschbach S, Wolfart S, Kern M. Five years outcome of FPDs made from IPS e.max press. J Dent Res 2007;86(Special Issue A):Abstr 1968.

60. Wolfart S, Bohlsen F, Wegner SM, Kern M. A preliminary prospective evaluation of all-ceramic crown-retained and inlay-retained fixed partial dentures. Int J Prosthodont 2005;18:497–505.

61. Pospiech P, Nothdurft FP. Long-term behavior of zirconia-based bridges: three years results. J Dent Res 2004;83(Special Issue B):Abstr 0230.

62. Kern M, Bohlsen F, Eschbach S, Wolfart S. Outcome of posterior fixed partial dentures made from In-Ceram zirconia. J Dent Res 2006;85(Special Issue A):Abstr 0214.

63. Molin MK, Karlsson SL. Five-year clinical prospective evaluation of zirconia-based Denzir 3-unit FPDs. Int J Prosthodont 2008;21:223–227.

64. Tinschert J, Schulze KA, Natt G, Latzke P, Heussen N, Spiekermann H. Clinical behavior of zirconia-based fixed partial dentures made of DC-Zirkon: 3-year results. Int J Prosthodont 2008;21:217–222.

65. Suárez MJ, Lozano JF, Paz Salido M, Martinez F. Three-year clinical evaluation of In-Ceram Zirconia posterior FPDs. Int J Prosthodont 2004;17:35–38.

66. Sailer I, Feher A, Filser F, Gauckler LJ, Lüthy H, Hämmerle CH. Five-year clinical results of zirconia frameworks for posterior fixed partial dentures. Int J Prosthodont 2007;20:383–388.

67. Wolfart S, Harder S, Eschbach S, Kern M. Outcome of posterior FPDs of veneered zirconia ceramic (Cercon). J Dent Res 2008;86:Abstr 576.

68. Kern M, Knode H, Strub JR. The all-porcelain, resin-bonded bridge. Quintessence Int 1991;22:257–262.

69. Kern M, Strub JR. Bonding to alumina ceramic in restorative dentistry over up to five years. J Dent 1998;26:245–249.

70. Kern M, Gläser R. Cantilevered all-ceramic, resin-bonded fixed partial dentures. A new treatment modality. J Esthet Dent 1997;9:255–264.

71. Kern M. Clinical long-term survival of two-retainer and single-retainer all-ceramic resin-bonded fixed partial dentures. Quintessence Int 2005;36:141–147.

72. Dumfahrt H, Schäffer H. Vollkeramische Adhäsivbrücken aus Optec HSP im klinischen Versuch. Dtsch Zahnärztl Z 1995;50:375–378.

73. Edelhoff D, Spiekermann H, Yildirim M. Metal-free inlay-retained fixed partial dentures. Quintessence Int 2001;32:269–281.

74. Wolfart S, Kern M. A new design for all-ceramic inlay-retained FPDs. A report of two cases. Quintessence Int 2006;37:27–33.

75. Andersson B, Taylor A, Lang BR, Scheller H, Schärer P, Sorensen JA, Tarnow D. Alumina ceramic implant abutments used for single-tooth replacement: a prospective 1- to 3-year multicenter study. Int J Prosthodont 2001;14:432–438.

76. Yildirim M, Fischer H, Marx R, Edelhoff D. In vitro fracture resistance of implant-supported all-ceramic restorations. J Prosthet Dent 2003;90:325–331.

77. Glauser R, Sailer I, Wohlwend A, Studer S, Schibli M, Schärer P. Experimental zirconia abutments for implant-supported single-tooth restorations in esthetically demanding regions: 4-year results of a prospective study. Int J Prosthodont 2004;17:285–290.

78. Ebert A, Hedderich J, Kern M. Retention of zirconia ceramic copings bonded to titanium abutments. Int J Oral Maxillofac Implants 2007;22:921–917.

79. Schulte W, Heimke G. Das Tübinger Sofortimplantat. Quintessenz 1976;27:17–23.

80. Schlegel A, Leitenstorfer B, Jakobsen M, Toutenburg H. Zur klinischen Bruchfestigkeit von $Al_2O_3$-Implantaten. Z Zahnärztl Implantol 1994;10 68–70.

81. Wenz H-J, Bartsch J, Wolfart S, Kern M. Osseointegration and clinical success of zirconia dental implants. A systematic review Int J Prosthodont 2008;21:21–36.

# Are Composites at the End of Development? Requirements of Clinicians versus Technical Possibilities

**15**

Reinhard Hickel, David Watts, Franz-Xaver Reichl and Nicoleta Ilie

## Introduction

Since the late 1970s, many innovative improvements in direct restorative composite materials have been made, leading to the current situation where there is excellent acceptance of methacrylate-based direct restorative materials. The most significant changes in commercial composites by far have been made through improvements in the filler system. Filler not only directly determines the mechanical properties of composite materials but also allows reduction in the monomer content. This reduces polymerization shrinkage and optimizes wear, translucency, opalescence, radiopacity, and intrinsic surface roughness, and thus polishability. It also enhances esthetics and improves handling properties.

The size of filler particles incorporated in the resin matrix of commercial composites has continuously decreased over the years, from the traditional composites to the nano-hybrid materials. Modification of composites size and morphology has resulted in improved mechanical properties and esthetics compared with the early composite materials. The smaller the particles, the better the polishing and gloss; however, reducing filler size, and subsequently increasing the surface area to volume ratio, has limited the achievable filler loading, leading to less good handling and mechanical proper-

ties.[1] The larger surface area to volume ratio of the fillers present in the nano-filled materials also increases water uptake and resultant degradation of the filler/matrix interface, thus adversely affecting the mechanical properties when compared with a microhybrid composite (Filtek Z250).[2] Against this must be balanced the desire to have better polishing of a composite and thus improved esthetics, which is strongly determined by the size of the reinforced particles in the composite. On the other side, a better polishability of a composite and thus improved aesthetics are strongly determined by the size of the filler particles in the composite. Consequently, it is hard to achieve the goal of a really universal composite, combining the excellent mechanical properties necessary for a filling to survive in a load-bearing area with the esthetic requirements for anterior restorations.

## Classification Systems

Classification criteria have been developed to attempt to provide a clear clinical indication for commercial composites, which is most influenced by the filler system.[3–6] These criteria are primarily based on the fraction of inorganic filler as a percentage by volume or as a mean particle size. In addition, the Young's modulus

209

| Classification system | Composite type | Average particle size (µm) |
|---|---|---|
| Lutz and Phillips 1983[4] | Traditional | 1–15 |
| | Hybrid | 5 (glass) and 0.04 |
| | Microfill | 0.04–0.1 |
| Willems et al. 1992[5] | Densified | – |
| | Microfine | – |
| | Miscellaneous | – |
| | Traditional | – |
| | Fiber-reinforced | – |
| Bayne 1994[3] | Microfill | 0.01–0.10 |
| | Minifill | 0.10–1.0 |
| | Midfill | 1.00–10.0 |
| Hickel et al. 1998[6] | Pyrogenic $SiO_2$ | 0.0002–0.04 |
| | Ba-Sr-Silicat glass | Microfine |
| | Quarz | Fine ground |
| | $ZrO_2$ | 0.7–1.5 |
| | $YF_3/YbF_3$ | 0.7–1.5 |

**Table 15-1** Classification systems of composites.

and the intrinsic surface roughness are considered valuable classification parameters[5] in view of the crucial role the modulus of elasticity plays in the deformability of a material under masticatory stresses, particularly in posterior regions, and the role low intrinsic surface roughness plays in achieving esthetical demands.

The classical system introduced by Lutz and Phillips (1983)[4] offers a valuable overview of the development and diversity of composites. This classification is based on the specific filler size distribution and the amount of incorporated filler. It divides the composites into traditional, hybrids, containing a mixture of ground glass and microfill particles, and microfill composites (Table 15-1). The microfills are further subdivided, including the type of pre-polymerized resin fillers incorporated (i.e., splintered, agglomerated, or spherical), since the properties of a composite are influenced by filler shape

as well as by filler size and amount. Spherical fillers can be incorporated in a composite in a higher amount than irregular fillers of the same size, but spherical fillers allow higher wear.[7] The generally accepted view at present is that microfill composites have the ideal esthetic qualities, owing to their excellent polishability and for retaining surface smoothness over time. However, it is also accepted that, because of their poor mechanical properties, these materials are contraindicated for stress-bearing restorations such as Class 4 and moderate-to-large Classes 1 and 2 restorations in occlusal contact with opposing cusps.[1]

A more recent classification system[5] based on the filler volume fraction and the filler size distinguishes between densified composites, microfine composites, miscellaneous composites, traditional composites, and fiber-reinforced composites. Based on the Young's modulus of dentin, an equivalent filler percentage by volume of 60% was calculated as corresponding to this modulus for a filled composite. Since composites intended for posterior use should have a Young's modulus at least equal to that of dentin, the densified composites were subdivided into two classes: midway filled (< 60% by volume) and compact filled (> 60% by volume). A further subgrouping is based on the mean particle size of the composites, dividing this into ultrafine (< 3 mm) and fine (> 3 mm). A material with a low Young's modulus, particularly if placed in posterior regions, will have a higher deformability under masticatory stresses and this could lead to catastrophic failure in the restoration.

The single term 'hybrid' is no longer used in this classification since nearly all dental composites are now 'hybrids', with particles of two size ranges as some amorphous silica is added to improve handling by reducing stickiness.[1]

A much simpler classification system distinguishes three types of composite based on the size of their largest fillers; this has three groups: microfills (average particle size 0.01–0.1 μm), minifills (average particle size 0.1–1.0 μm), and midifills (average particle size 1.0–10.0 μm).[3] A system based only on the filler system has also been proposed by the FDI Commission Project 1998.[6]

# Properties

## Fatigue

Despite excellent improvement in composite materials, there still remain problems to be solved. Fatigue continues to be a major drawback of restorative materials when these are subjected to stress or strain over a long period of time. In dental restorations, fatigue became apparent as wear, fractured margins, or bulk fracture. The mechanisms responsible for fatigue-induced failure depend on material ductility. Whereas brittle materials are susceptible to catastrophic failure, the plasticity of ductile materials reduces stress concentrations at the crack tip.

Packable composites were developed in an attempt to limit wear, the fracture of the restoration within the body and at the margins, and marginal leakage owing to polymerization shrinkage. They also attempted to answer technical needs, including the ability to obtain adequate proximal contact in the final restoration and to create a substitute for amalgam. Studies have shown, however, that composites with very low or high filler content (< 60% or > 80% by weight) have significantly lowered tensile fatigue resistance when evaluated by the staircase method.[8] Trials to reduce the wear of the antagonist led to the development of porous glass fillers as a replacement for compact fillers (Solitaire). It was thought that a larger amount of a bigger filler could be incorporated into the organic matrix if a porous filler was used, creating a higher total inorganic filler amount. However, one problem with porous fillers was their susceptibility to staining. In addition, they also showed fatigue problems, which manifested as fractured margins.[9]

Using resin composite successfully in load-bearing surfaces of posterior teeth implies the use of a material with high mechanical properties, good wear resistance, high fracture toughness, small inherent flaw size and a high fatigue resistance. A review of published longitudinal studies for the reasons given for fractures showed a change in reasons for failures in composite fillings placed in load-bearing areas (Table 15-2). Because of the extension of the indication for composites to larger multisurface Class 2 cavities (contrary to earlier studies) instead of being restricted to secondary caries, the most frequent reason for failure in studies published since the mid-1990s is fracture of the restorations. The success or failure of different materials is indicated by calculated annual failure rates. Comparing the annual failure rates of all studies with at least 2 years of observation time with the ones having an observation time of at least 10 years, gold inlays/onlays always performed best and amalgam was in second place (Table 15-3). One problem with pooling data from different studies is that the conditions in the studies are not usually the same and it may be difficult to compare the results. Therefore, studies with direct comparison of different groups of materials were ana-

| Material | Median AFR (%) at | | Difference (median) |
|---|---|---|---|
| | 2 years | 10 years | |
| Amalgam | 1.2 | 1.5 | +0.3 |
| Composite | 1.9 | 1.9 | 0 |
| Composite inlay | 2.2 | 1.6 | −0.6 |
| Laboratory ceramic inlay | 1.6 | 1.3 | −0.3 |
| CAD/CAM-produced ceramic inlay | 1.5 | 1.1 | −0.4 |
| Gold inlay | 0.5 | 0.5 | 0 |
| AFR, annual failure rate; CAD/CAM, computer-aided design and manufacture. | | | |

**Table 15-2** Comparison of annual failure rates for restorations in studies with an observation period of at least 2 and 10 years

**Table 15-3** Main reasons for failure of restorations in studies with at least 2 years of observation time. (publications 1998–2007)

| Material | Functional reasons | | | Biological reasons | |
|---|---|---|---|---|---|
| | Filling fracture | Loss of fillings | Tooth fracture/crack | Secondary caries | Sensitivity/endodontic |
| Amalgam filling | 20.8 | 15.0 | 28.0 | 20.9 | 7.9 |
| Composite filling | 23.8 | 17.2 | 9.4 | 20.7 | 6.2 |
| Composite inlay/onlay | 30.2 | 1.0 | 15.2 | 16.4 | 15.6 |
| Ceramic inlay/onlay | 50.7 | 10.0 | 5.0 | 10.1 | 10.9 |
| Gold inlay/onlay | 0 | 25.4 | 7.9 | 23.5 | 6.9 |

lyzed. In the period 1998–2007, three studies were published with direct comparison of amalgam and composite and at least 10 years of observation.[10–12] Interestingly, all three show nearly identical results (Table 15-4).

## Polymerization Shrinkage

Polymerization shrinkage stress is still considered as the main drawback of methacrylate-based restorative dental materials. Several *in vitro* studies have found a significant correlation between marginal adaptation of dental composite, or microleakage, and reduced shrinkage stress.[13–16] Suggested manipulations to reduce shrinkage stress for a composite material at the interface of filling and tooth include slowing the composite polymerization rate,[13,17] replacing dual-cure resin cements with self-

cure cements,[15] placing thicker adhesive layers under the composite,[14] and using an incremental placement technique[18] or intermediate layers of low modulus.[19]

The main approaches adopted so far by manufacturers to reduce shrinkage are to change the monomer structure or chemistry or to change the filler amount, shape, or surface treatment. The literature offers comprehensive reviews of monomer development for reduced shrinkage.[1,20–23] Versatile methods to modify the monomer matrix have been developed, starting with typical dimethacrylate monomers being replaced by methacrylates with a reduced reactive group (e.g. hydroxyl-free bisphenol A glycidyl methacrylate [bis-GMA]) or altered structure (e.g. urethane dimethacrylate [UDMA]). Other proposed approaches include the

Table 15-4  Direct comparisons of amalgam and composite in three studies with an observation period of at least 10 years

| Study | Observation period (years) | Annual failure rate (%) | Reason for failure (%) | | |
|---|---|---|---|---|---|
| | | | Functional | Biological | Not specified |
| **Composite** | | | | | |
| Opdam et al. 2007[11] | 10 | 1.8 | 8.0 | 67.0 | 25.0 |
| van Nieuwenhuysen et al. 2003[12] | 16 | 1.9 | 75.7 | 24.3 | 0 |
| Mair 1998[10] | 10 | 0.7 | 100 | 0 | 0 |
| Composite median | 10 | 1.8 | 75.7 | 24.3 | 0 |
| **Amalgam** | | | | | |
| Opdam et al. 2007[11] | 10 | 2.1 | 10.0 | 66.0 | 24.0 |
| van Nieuwenhuysen et al. 2003[12] | 16 | 1.8 | 33.1 | 63.4 | 3.5 |
| Mair 1998[10] | 10 | 0.6 | 100 | 0 | 0 |
| Amalgam median | 10 | 1.8 | 33.1 | 63.4 | 3.5 |

development of liquid crystal monomers or ring-opening systems in order to achieve non-shrinking or minimally shrinking composites, for example addition of spiro-orthocarbonates to dimethacrylate or epoxy-based resins.[1,20–23] However, only a few of the new monomers have been launched in commercial composite materials, and the majority of conventional composite-type materials in use today continues to be based on the dimethacrylate resins introduced in the 1960s and 1970s.

In an attempt to overcome the problems created by polymerization shrinkage of conventional composites, new material classes have been developed. The ormocers (organically modified ceramics, first produced in 1998), having a very similar coefficient of thermal expansion to natural tooth structure, were formulated as a novel three-dimensionally cross-linked inorganic–organic polymer. They are synthesized from multifunctional UDMA and thioether(meth)acrylate alkoxysilanes as sol-gel precursors. The alkoxysilyl groups of the silane permit the formation of an inorganic Si–O–Si network by hydrolysis and polycondensation reactions. The

methacrylate groups are available for photochemical polymerization. These materials have a lower wear rate than the composites[24–26] and shrinkage equal to that of hybrid composites, despite having less filler content.[27] However, owing to problems with upscaling of prototypes and handling properties, conventional methacrylate has had to be added to the ormocer matrix and, therefore, no clear clinical improvement has been noted when using these restorative materials.

Although there were no data correlating contraction stress in dental composites and the clinical success of a composite restoration, new materials with reduced internal stress, as a result of low polymerization shrinkage, were predicted to dominate future markets even before the clinical consequences of shrinkage were fully understood.[28]

One of these new materials with low polymerization shrinkage is currently being introduced on the European market and is based on an innovative monomer system, silorane, obtained from the reaction of oxirane and siloxane.[29] The novel resin is claimed to have combined the two key advantages of the individual components: low polymerization shrinkage (achieved with the ring-opening oxirane monomer) and increased hydrophobicity (owing to the siloxane species). The mechanism of compensating polymerization shrinkage stress in this new system is achieved by opening of the oxirane ring during polymerization.[29] Rather than using the predominant radical-based polymerization initiation, as in conventional methacrylate-based composites, the silorane composite polymerizes by a cationic ring-opening process, which is insensitive to oxygen. This should overcome the disadvantage of the oxygen inhibition layer that is found in methacrylate-based composites as a result of deactivated polymerization-initializing radicals. Furthermore, the mutagenic potential of the various siloranes has been shown to be much lower than those of related oxiranes in diverse assessment systems.[30] Siloranes are also stable and insoluble in biological fluids, assessed using aqueous solutions containing epoxide hydrolase, porcine liver esterase, or dilute HCl.[31] The silorane-based composite had decreased water absorption, solubility and associated diffusion coefficient compared with conventional methacrylate-based composites.[32] Moreover, an *in vitro* study using extracted teeth for assessing restorations showed that cusp deflection caused by polymerization shrinkage was significantly lower for an experimental silorane material than for a methacrylate-based composite (Filtek Z250, 3M ESPE).[33] A comparison of the micromechanical properties of the siloranes with a well-known nano-hybrid composite (Tetric EvoCeram, Ivoclar-Vivadent) could demonstrate no differences between the two types of material in terms of hardness, but the modulus of elasticity of the silorane-based material was slightly lower and the creep resistance higher than the methacrylate-based composite. Therefore, the siloranes have good mechanical properties that are comparable to those of clinically successful methacrylate-based composite materials.[34] However, some disadvantages, such as the poor radiopacity, the lack of a flowable silorane and concerns regarding the compatibility with methacrylate-based composites in terms of repairs, have to be considered.

## Adhesion to Enamel and Dentin

At present, glass-ionomer cements are the only restorative materials capable of forming stable physicochemical bonds to both enamel and dentin. As a caries-restraining material, they are also capable of sustained long-term fluoride release. Other clinical advantages include good biocompatibility, resistance to microleakage and a low coefficient of thermal expansion. Nonetheless, conventional glass-ionomer cements are not without flaws and failures, having poor mechanical properties, which limit their clinical use as a permanent filling material in the posterior region. Since regular methacrylate materials are not able to bond by themselves on the tooth structure, interest in self-adhesive bioactive dental materials is high. Some functionalized methacrylates containing strong acidic monomers, such as 10-methacryloyloxidecyldihydrogen phosphate (MDP) or glycerol dimethacrylate dihydrogen phosphate (GDMX), are considered to be promising constituents in the development of self-adhesive luting cements.[35] The idea of self-adhesive composites was introduced in the late 1990s,[36] but implementation in a commercial composite has failed so far owing to problems caused by the poorer wetting ability of the more viscous materials on the tooth surface, which impedes the development of a intact adhesive interface.

## 'Smart' Composites

'Smart' composites, like the ion-releasing resin-based composite material (first product was Ariston pHc in 1998), were developed in order to reduce secondary caries formation at the margin of a restoration by inhibiting bacterial growth through the release of fluoride, hydroxyl, and calcium ions as the pH falls in the area immediately adjacent to the restorative material. Smart composites work by using an alkaline glass filler, which will reduce demineralization and will buffer the acid produced by caries-forming microorganisms.[37] The use of a dental adhesive was not recommended. The high water absorption of these materials, however, causes problems, which manifest in an increased fracture rate of the teeth.

Compomers (polyacid-modified resins) were developed as a mixture between composites and glass-ionomers. The compomer monomers contain acidic functional groups that can participate in an acid–base glass-ionomer reaction following polymerization of the resin molecule, and the materials can then release fluoride. Ion release (fluoride, calcium) could act to reduce demineralization, but the exchange of ions needs water uptake and so this may reduce the long-term stability of the materials. Another problem is with the surface treatment of the ion-releasing fillers, since an efficient release is only possible if the fillers are not, or are only partly, silanized. This leads to decreased mechanical properties.

Antimicrobial substances such as chlorhexidine or triclosane have also been added to restorative materials in order to impede secondary caries formation. The problem with physically bonded antimicrobial agents is that the drugs are released only in an initial phase in high amounts and not constantly during the whole function time of the filling. Other attempts have focused on the synthesis of antibacterial monomers that could be incorporated into a composite by copolymerization.[38] The disadvantage of this is that such a composite would only show an antimicrobial effect if in direct surface contact with the bacteria.

## Toxicology and Biocompatibility

Questions regarding the toxicology and biocompatibility of restorative materials have also attracted increasing interest. Direct evidence of (co)monomer release from resin composites and fissure sealants into the biophase was provided by Tanaka and coworkers,[39], Spahl and coworkers,[40] and Nalcaci and coworkers.[41] Released dental components can enter the body by two routes after resin placement: via the saliva and gastrointestinal tract and into the bloodstream via the dentin and pulp (if the material is placed on to dentin).[42]

Adverse effects, whether allergic or toxic, can arise only if the relevant compound can enter the organism and/or is able to cross physiological barriers such as the mucosal epithelium in the mouth or gastrointestinal tract if swallowed. Dental (co)monomers may cause a wide range of adverse health effects, for example irritation to skin, eyes or mucous membranes; and gastrointestinal complaints in dental workers and, to a much lesser extent, in patients.[36,43–46]

Dental personnel may be exposed to (co)monomers when handling non-reacted (co)monomers. Leachable components from dental polymeric materials have been implicated in allergic reactions in dental workers and, very rarely, in patients.[45,47–50] Gloves do not confer protection against skin contact; face masks do not prevent inhalation of monomers, and ordinary glasses do not protect the eyes against vapor from monomers.[44]

Studies have examined the uptake, distribution, excretion, and metabolism of the (co)monomers 2-hydroxyethylmethacrylate (HEMA), triethyleneglycoldimethacrylate (TEGDMA), and bis-GMA applied via gastric and intravenous administration in guinea pigs.[51–53] All were taken up rapidly from the stomach and intestine after gastric administration and were widely distributed in the body following administration by either route. The liver was the target organ for TEGDMA and HEMA and the lung for bis-GMA. Similar metabolisms of these (co)monomers were found *in vivo*. Over 24 hours, more than 70% of each administered (co)monomer was excreted through the lungs as carbon dioxide, while some 10% appeared in the urine.[51–53] The intermediate 2,3-epoxymethacrylic acid was clearly demonstrated during the metabolism of these (co)monomers.[54] Generally, most epoxides are regarded as toxic (mutagenic, carcinogenic) agents. In previous *in vitro* studies, teratogenic effects could be demonstrated for 2,3-epoxymethacrylic acid in mouse stem cells.[55] However, the peak (co)monomer equivalent level in the guinea pig tissues examined was at least 1000-fold less than known toxic levels.[51–53] Future research should focus on the development of composites with reduced elution of their components, which may lead to reduced (co)monomer burden in the body and, therefore, minimize health risks.

A further promising innovative approach in the development of bioactive dental materials is represented by the amorphous calcium phosphate (ACP) composites, which have the ability to supply the calcium and phosphate ions needed to reform damaged mineral structures. A problem with ACP-based composites, however, is their inability to resist cracking under masticatory stress because of their low strength and toughness. The uncontrolled aggregation of ACP particles was identified as one of the main reasons for a poor interfacial interaction with dental resin matrices, leading to lower mechanical properties when compared with glass-reinforced composites.[56]

## Conclusions and Future Needs

Despite many and remarkable improvements in recent years, much developmental change is still possible for the composites. Even if the application of tissue engineering approaches in dentistry could solve major dental problems by remineralizing carious lesions, or vaccination against caries and oral diseases could be developed, composites with improved characteristics will still have a valuable role in the time before, and during, the successful introduction of such innovative approaches.

From the perspective of clinicians, several future needs and wishes can be identified.

1. Functional properties to enhance the longevity of the restorations by achieving excellent mechanical properties
  ♦ high strength and fracture toughness
  ♦ surface hardness and low wear
  ♦ optimized modulus of elasticity
  ♦ low water sorption and solubility
  ♦ low polymerization shrinkage
  ♦ low fatigue and degradation
  ♦ high radiopacity.
2. Biological properties:
  ♦ good biocompatibility (systemic and local)
  ♦ no post-operative pain or hypersensitivity

  ♦ preservation of tooth integrity (no fractures, cracks etc.)
  ♦ caries-restraining properties.
3. Esthetical properties:
  ♦ good color matching and color stability (translucency, shades)
  ♦ optimized polishability
  ♦ long-term surface gloss
  ♦ no marginal or surface staining
  ♦ good long- term anatomical form
4. Handling properties:
  ♦ improved by optimized rheological behavior
  ♦ less stickiness to instruments
  ♦ less technique sensitivity
  ♦ ability to be placed in bulk or larger increments
  ♦ short curing time
  ♦ better detection during removal.

As all these wishes will be difficult to integrate into one material, different optimized composites for anterior and posterior restoration (high esthetics versus high strength) should be developed.

## References

1. Ferracane JL. Current trends in dental composites. Crit Rev Oral Biol Med 1995;6:302–318.
2. Curtis AR, Shortall AC, Marquis PM, Palin WM. Water uptake and strength characteristics of a nanofilled resin-based composite. J Dent 2008;36:186–193.
3. Bayne SC, Heymann HO, Swift El. Update on dental composite restorations. J Am Dent Assoc 1994;125:687–701.
4. Lutz F, Phillips RW. A classification and evaluation of composite resin systems. J Prosthet Dent 1983;50:480–488.
5. Willems G, Lambrechts P, Braem M, Celis JP, Vanherle G. A classification of dental composites according to their morphological and mechanical characteristics. Dent Mater 1992;8:310–319.
6. Hickel R, Dasch W, Janda R, Tyas M, Anusavice K. New direct restorative materials. FDI Commission Project. Int Dent J 1998;48:3–16.
7. Venhoven BA, de Gee AJ, Werner A, Davidson CL. Influence of filler parameters on the mechanical coherence of dental restorative resin composites. Biomaterials 1996;17:735–740.
8. Htang A, Ohsawa M, Matsumoto H. Fatigue resistance of composite restorations: effect of filler content. Dent Mater 1995;11:7–13.
9. Lohbauer U, Frankenberger R, Krämer N, Petschelt A. Time-dependent strength and fatigue resistance of dental direct restorative materials. J Mater Sci Mater Med 2003;14:1047–1053.

10. Mair LH. Ten-year clinical assessment of three posterior resin composites and two amalgams. Quintessence Int 1998;29:483–490.

11. Opdam NJ, Bronkhorst EM, Roeters JM, Loomans BA. A retrospective clinical study on longevity of posterior composite and amalgam restorations. Dent Mater 2007;23:2–8.

12. van Nieuwenhuysen JP, D'Hoore W, Carvalho J, Qvist V. Long-term evaluation of extensive restorations in permanent teeth. J Dent 2003;31:395–405.

13. Uno S, Asmussen E. Effect on bonding of curing through dentin. Acta Odontol Scand 1991;49:317–320.

14. Choi KK, Condon JR, Ferracane JL. The effects of adhesive thickness on polymerization contraction stress of composite. J Dent Res 2000;79:812–817.

15. Braga RR, Ferracane JL, Condon JR. Polymerization contraction stress in dual-cure cements and its effect on interfacial integrity of bonded inlays. J Dent 2002;30:333–340.

16. Irie M, Suzuki K, Watts DC. Marginal gap formation of light-activated restorative materials: effects of immediate setting shrinkage and bond strength. Dent Mater 2002;18:203–210.

17. Mehl A, Hickel R, Kunzelmann KH. Physical properties and gap formation of light-cured composites with and without 'softstart-polymerization'. J Dent 1997;25:321–330.

18. Lutz E, Krejci I, Oldenburg TR. Elimination of polymerization stresses at the margins of posterior composite resin restorations: a new restorative technique. Quintessence Int 1986;17:777–784.

19. Unterbrink GL, Liebenberg WH. Flowable resin composites as 'filled adhesives': literature review and clinical recommendations. Quintessence Int 1999;30:249–257.

20. Braga RR, Ferracane JL. Alternatives in polymerization contraction stress management. Crit Rev Oral Biol Med 2004;15:176–184.

21. Eick JD, Robinson SJ, Byerley TJ, Chappelow CC. Adhesives and non-shrinking dental resins of the future. Quintessence Int 1993;24:632–640.

22. Peutzfeldt A. Resin composites in dentistry: the monomer systems. Eur J Oral Sci 1997;105:97–116.

23. Rueggeberg FA. From vulcanite to vinyl, a history of resins in restorative dentistry. J Prosthet Dent 2002;87:364–379.

24. Tagtekin DA, Yanikoglu FC, Bozkurt FO, Kologlu B, Sur H. Selected characteristics of an Ormocer and a conventional hybrid resin composite. Dent Mater 2004;20:487–497.

25. Watts DC, Marouf AS. Optimal specimen geometry in bonded-disk shrinkage-strain measurements on light-cured biomaterials. Dent Mater 2000;16:447–451.

26. Yap AU, Tan CH, Chung SM. Wear behavior of new composite restoratives. Oper Dent 2004;29:269–274.

27. Cattani-Lorente M, Bouillaguet S, Godin C.H, Meyer J.M. Polymerization shrinkage of Ormocer based dental restorative composites. Eur Cell Mater 2001;1:25–26.

28. Ferracane JL. Developing a more complete understanding of stresses produced in dental composites during polymerization. Dent Mater 2005;21:36–42.

29. Weinmann W, Thalacker C, Guggenberger R. Siloranes in dental composites. Dent Mater 2005;21:68–74.

30. Schweikl H, Schmalz G, Weinmann W. The induction of gene mutations and micronuclei by oxiranes and siloranes in mammalian cells in vitro. J Dent Res 2004;83:17–21.

31. Eick JD, Smith RE, Pinzino CS, Kostoryz EL. Stability of silorane dental monomers in aqueous systems. J Dent 2006;34:405–410.

32. Palin WM, Fleming GJ, Burke FJ, Marquis PM, Randall RC. The influence of short and medium-term water immersion on the hydrolytic stability of novel low-shrink dental composites. Dent Mater 2005;21:852–863.

33. Palin WM, Fleming GJ, Nathwani H, Burke FJ, Randall RC. In vitro cuspal deflection and microleakage of maxillary premolars restored with novel low-shrink dental composites. Dent Mater 2005;21:324–335.

34. Ilie N, Hickel R. Silorane-based dental composite: behavior and abilities. Dent Mater J 2006;25:445–454.

35. Moszner N, Salz U, Zimmermann J. Chemical aspects of self-etching enamel-dentin adhesives: a systematic review. Dent Mater 2005;21:895–910.

36. Hickel R. Moderne Füllungswerkstoffe. Dtsch Zahnärztl Z 1997;52:572–585.

37. Kielbassa AM, Müller U, Garcia-Godoy F. In situ study on the caries-preventive effects of fluoride-releasing materials. Am J Dent 1999;12(Special Issue):S13–S14.

38. Imazato S, Ebi N, Tarumi H, Russell RR, Kaneko T, Ebisu S. Bactericidal activity and cytotoxicity of antibacterial monomer MDPB. Biomaterials 1999;20:899–903.

39. Tanaka K, Taira M, Shintani H, Wakasa K, Yamaki M. Residual monomers (TEGDMA and bis-GMA) of a set visible-light-cured dental composite resin when immersed in water. J Oral Rehabil 1991;18:353–362.

40. Spahl W, Budzikiewicz H, Geurtsen W. Determination of leachable components from four commercial dental composites by gas and liquid chromatography/mass spectrometry. J Dent 1998;26:137–145.

41. Nalcaci A, Ulusoy N, Atakol O. Time-based elution of TEGDMA and BisGMA from resin composite cured with LED, QTH and high-intensity QTH lights. Oper Dent 2006;31:197–203.

42. Hume WR, Gerzina TM. Bioavailability of components of resin-based materials which are applied to teeth. Crit Rev Oral Biol Med 1996;7:172–179.

43. Mathias CG, Caldwell TM, Maibach HI. Contact dermatitis and gastrointestinal symptoms from hydroxyethylmethacrylate. Br J Dermatol 1979;100:447–449.

44. Lonnroth EC, Shahnavaz H. Use of polymer materials in dental clinics, case study. Swed Dent J 1997;21:149–159.

45. Kanerva L. Cross-reactions of multifunctional methacrylates and acrylates. Acta Odontol Scand 2001;59:320–329.

46. Hamann CP, Rodgers PA, Sullivan KM. Occupational allergens in dentistry. Curr Opin Allergy Clin Immunol 2004;4:403–409.

47. Kanerva L, Estlander T, Jolanki R. Allergic contact dermatitis from dental composite resins due to aromatic epoxy acrylates and aliphatic acrylates. Contact Dermatitis 1989;20:201–211.

48. Jolanki R, Kanerva L, Estlander T. Occupational allergic contact dermatitis caused by epoxy diacrylate in ultraviolet-light-cured paint, and bisphenol A in dental composite resin. Contact Dermatitis 1995;33:94–99.

49. Lindstrom M, Alanko K, Keskinen H, Kanerva L. Dentist's occupational asthma, rhinoconjunctivitis, and allergic contact dermatitis from methacrylates. Allergy 2002;57:543–545.

50. Piirila P, Hodgson U, Estlander T, Keskinen H, Saalo A, Voutilainen R, et al. Occupational respiratory hypersensitivity in dental personnel. Int Arch Occup Environ Health 2002;75:209–216.

51. Reichl FX, Durner J, Kunzelmann KH, Hickel R, Spahl W, Hume WR, et al. Biological clearance of TEGDMA in guinea pigs. Arch Toxicol 2001;75:22–27.

52. Reichl FX, Durner J, Kehe K, Manhart J, Folwaczny M, Kleinsasser N, et al. Toxicokinetic of HEMA in guinea pigs. J Dent 2002;30:353–358.

53. Reichl FX, Seiss M, Kleinsasser N, Kehe K, Kunzelmann KH, Thomas P, et al. Distribution and excretion of BisGMA in guinea pigs. J Dent Res 2008;87:378–380.

54. Seiss M, Nitz S, Kleinsasser N, Buters JT, Behrendt H, Hickel R, et al. Identification of 2,3-epoxymethacrylic acid as an intermediate in the metabolism of dental materials in human liver microsomes. Dent Mater 2007;23:9–16.

55. Schwengberg S, Bohlen H, Kleinsasser N, Kehe K, Seiss M, Walther UI, et al. In vitro embryotoxicity assessment with dental restorative materials. J Dent 2005;33:49–55.

56. Skrtic D, Antonucci JM, Eanes ED, Eidelman N. Dental composites based on hybrid and surface-modified amorphous calcium phosphates. Biomaterials 2004;25:1141–1150.

# Dental Technology – Visions for Materials and Processes of the Future

**16**

Horst Fischer

## Introduction

In recent years, it has been apparent that there has been a considerable increase in dental prosthetic applications with ceramic components.[1] This is particularly seen with dental crowns and other fixed dental prostheses. Several reasons account for this. Of these, a major advantage is that ceramic and particularly glass-ceramic materials are highly biocompatible and exhibit wear characteristics that are close to those of natural enamel.[2] Moreover, recent dental glass-ceramic materials are excellent in terms of mimicking the esthetic appearance of a natural tooth.[3] However, ceramic materials have several shortcomings for use in dental restorative and prosthetic applications. In particular, the glass-ceramic materials that are favored for their esthetic advantages also exhibit relatively low strength and very low fracture toughness. Even the slightly tougher lithium disilicate glass-ceramics are mechanically inferior to dental alloys.[4] The brittleness of non-metallic inorganic materials results in increased sensitivity to tensile stress peaks. This behavior becomes even more critical because of the high Young's moduli of this class of materials and the mathematical relationship between stiffness and stress (Hook's law).

The mechanical, chemical, and biological properties of a material are critically important but are not the only criteria for a suitable and successful application of a material in dentistry. Another important issue is the nature of the manufacturing process, more precisely the process chain from raw material to final restoration. Key issues in this context are long-term availability, costs and quality assurance of raw materials, investments in machines and tools, complexity and sensitivity of the manufacturing process, time required for training in handling the material, the option of individual and rapid production, manufacturing time and costs, and, finally, the psychological acceptability of new materials and processes by clinicians and patients.

Therefore, comprehensive strategies must be utilized in the development of a successful new dental material. A major issue is the development of innovative dental materials that exhibit increased toughness and strength. These high-strength materials should also mimic the natural tooth in esthetic appearance. It should be possible to manufacture individually shaped dental components from these materials without costly and time-consuming processes. Furthermore, it has to be possible to adapt the material after insertion easily by grinding for an optimal occlusion. This final mechanical treatment, however, must not weaken the material by the introduction of microscopic cracks.

It is obvious that one single material and one specific manufacturing process cannot meet all these requirements and objectives and, as a result, the composite materials will play an increasingly dominant role. The inorganic non-metallic materials (i.e. ceramics) will nevertheless be of decisive importance in the near future. The first section below, Potential of Ceramic Materials, will describe in detail the possibilities for innovative ceramic materials in restorative and prosthetic dentistry. It will analyze the properties that can be achieved by high-performance ceramics, drawing on recent developments in orthopedic and traumatic surgery.

This is followed by a discussion of the conditions needed for implants as opposed to prosthetic applications (Functionalization of Surfaces). Specific interdisciplinary questions must be answered for the development of optimum dental implant material and promising trends and visions for this will be discussed.

The section on manufacturing techniques addresses the question of a cost-effective, rapid and individual production of dental replacements in the future. The key issue will be rapid prototyping and already there are many different generative manufacturing techniques in development. The section will highlight the techniques that have the highest potential, and the suitability of these for dental applications will be discussed.

As commented on above, the optimum dental material of the future will be a composite material that combines the required mechanical, biological and chemical properties that at present can only be achieved by different classes of material. Moreover, an intelligent material for tooth replacement should consist of both organic and inorganic phases. The best support for this statement is the natural tooth itself. The human tooth exhibits intricate architecture comprising organic and inorganic phases with a complex interaction between the phases. The final section, Mimicking Nature, describes potential options to mimic a complex structure such as natural tooth by synthetic means and processes.

# Potential of Ceramic Materials

The natural tooth, in particular enamel, has a high content of non-metallic inorganic phases. It is for this reason that ceramics and glasses can have such outstanding roles in the search for an optimum restoration material. Two subgroups of non-metallic inorganic materials are very important in this context: the high-strength polycrystalline oxide ceramics and the glass-ceramics. The latter are important because of their excellent esthetic appearance. No other class of material at present can mimic the appearance of a natural tooth crown as well. However, the brittleness of the glass-ceramics is a critical factor and will be an important issue for future research and development.

The lithium disilicate glass-ceramics have been developed to reduce the problem of brittleness while conserving the esthetic advantages of the glass-ceramics.[5] The crystals of lithium disilicate glass-ceramics form an interlaced microstructure that gives improved fracture toughness and strength.[6] Although these materials do not reach the strength of the polycrystalline materials, such as alumina and zirconia, they exhibit significantly higher strength than feldspathic porcelains. Although the development of this class of glass-ceramic materials has been a breakthrough in the dental field, the applications for which lithium disilicates can be used without a mechanical risk are still limited. Posterior crowns and wide-span fixed dental prostheses still require materials of higher strengths.

Consequently, methods to increase the strength of highly esthetic glass-ceramics are still being sought. One option for such an improvement is ion-exchange treatment. The exchange of ions with a large diameter for ones with smaller diameters in a glass-ceramic component can induce high compressive residual stresses in the surface layer and thereby help to improve the short- and long-term mechanical behavior. It has been shown that both short- and long-term strength is significantly increased by this tailored ion-exchange process performed in the molten salt. Moreover, the large strength scatter, which is another critical property of glass-ceramics, can be drastically decreased by ion-exchange treatments.[7–9]

A significant increase in the strength of non-metallic inorganic dental materials is only possible if the strength-decreasing glass phases can be completely avoided. The esthetics, however, will deteriorate in a switch to glass-free materials, for example alumina and zirconia. This is because of the reduced translucency of polycrystalline ceramic materials. The less-optimal esthetics of polycrystalline oxide ceramics can be acceptable if it allows, for example, the effective production of highly loaded dental ceramic components in wide-span posterior fixed dental prostheses or filigree inlay-retained FDPs.[10] Those developing dental materials have focused on zirconia in these contexts because of its very high toughness and strength. Much can be learnt, however, from the experiences of production of ceramic joint prosthetics. Zirconia was introduced to the joint prosthetic market in 1985. Subsequently, in the 1990s, an increasing number of these zirconia implants failed in patients. It was well known that special oxides (e.g. of yttria) are used to stabilize the (high-strength) high-temperature tetragonal phase. Where these prostheses had failed, the cause was the humidity inside the human body, which precipitated the stabilizer ($Y_2O_3$) at the grain boundaries. Massive phase transformations occurred (tetragonal to monoclinic), with pronounced crack formations and finally fractures of the bioceramic implant.

The high failure rates were the reason to initiate a search for tailored $Al_2O_3$–$ZrO_2$ dispersion ceramics for orthopedic joint surgery. The dental field will benefit from this initiative. The dispersion ceramics alumina-toughened zirconia (ATZ) and zirconia-toughened alumina (ZTA) exhibit properties that are also of interest for dental uses,[11,12] particularly the improved mechanical long-term reliability, and hence lifetime, of the dispersion ceramics compared with monolithic zirconia.[13]

Another challenging aspect of the development of effective dental ceramics is the need to create a transparent polycrystalline ceramic. As explained above, a high glass phase content can help to mimic the esthetic appearance of the natural tooth but strength decreases with increased glass amount. The polycrystalline ceramics exhibit suitable strengths but not adequate esthetics as they have insufficient translucency. A transparent polycrystalline ceramic material could merge the requirements for 'high strength' with those for 'dental-like esthetics'. Recent developments suggest that it is possible, in principle, to synthesize not only translucent but even transparent tetragonal zirconia polycrystal (TZP) ceramics.[14] Residual submicrometer pores in the zirconia material can be created in a tailored manufacturing process and are responsible for light transmission in the visible region. As a useful 'side-effect', the extremely fine-grained transparent zirconia ceramics also exhibit even higher strengths than traditional dental zirconia materials. A further major issue with respect to translucent high-strength ceramics is the manufacturing process. An optimum translucency can only be achieved using hot-isostatic pressing. In addition, the tailored ceramic process is very sensitive. This implies that further developments are needed to be able to manufacture high-strength transparent dental ceramics with reproducibility and cost effectiveness.

# Functionalization of Surfaces

Because of the good acceptance of the high-performance ceramics based on alumina and zirconia, further possible applications for these materials have been considered, particularly in dental implantology. The major argument for use of these white-colored oxide ceramics for dental implants is their esthetic appearance. The dark grey tone of a titanium implant can sometimes influence the esthetics, particularly in the subgingival area. It is difficult, however, to find good scientific arguments for replacing titanium and titanium alloys as materials for dental implants.[15] Recent studies have indicated that titanium has clear advantages over zirconia in terms of the molecular mechanisms that control bone formation,[16] and clinical studies show excellent long-term survival rates for dental implants made of titanium.[17,18] In contrast, long-term studies for ceramic dental implants are not yet available.

Alumina and zirconia are bioinert ceramic materials. This property is suitable for applications in joint prosthetics, for example for femoral head balls, and in some dental prosthetics, for example for dental crowns and other fixed dental prostheses. In situations where there is close contact between the biomaterial and bone tissue, the material needs to have a bioactive behavior that can stimulate osseoconductivity. Pronounced osseoconductivity is desirable not just to achieve initial stability but also, and most notably, to achieve a long-term tight interconnection between implant and bone. For this reason, developing high-performance ceramics with tailored functionalized surfaces for implantology applications is an important issue for the 'roadmap' for producing the dental materials of the future. The functionalized surfaces must be designed to bioactivate the adjacent hard tissue.

One possibility for bioactivation of inert ceramic implant surfaces is to coat them with bioactive calcium phosphate ceramics. These ceramics are said to activate cell attachment and osseointegration, leading to a tight interconnection between bone tissue and implant surface.[19,20] This strategy could achieve a combination of bioactivity at the surface plus good mechanical properties of the bulk material. Nevertheless, uncontrollable resorption dynamics of the coating are problematic. Furthermore, differing thermal expansion coefficients (coating versus bulk material) promote mechanical stresses in the interface and can eventually lead to spalling of the coated material.

Another approach to bioactivate inert high-strength oxide ceramics is to synthesize a zirconia–alumina nanocomposite with the addition of bioactive hydroxyapatite. Such a composite has been shown to be bioactive using *in vitro* cell culture tests with MG63 cell lines, where an increase in alkaline phosphatase production occurred. However, the strength of specimens of alumina–zirconia–hydroxyapatite composite materials drastically decreases with increased amount of the (bioactivating) hydroxyapatite phase.[21] In addition, the hydroxyapatite phase will probably have a deleterious effect on the subcritical crack growth behavior and thereby on the long-term strength of the component.

Other more promising approaches are to pursue the strategy of modifying the inert ceramic material at the surface by made-to-measure surface treatments. Recent developments in this area have successfully hydroxylated alumina by a thermal treatment in sodium hydroxide. Cell culture tests confirmed that a bioactive behavior of the oxide-ceramic surface can be achieved by this treatment.[22] Phosphates show even stronger bioactivity than hydroxy groups. Therefore, high-performance ceramics treated with phosphate could have even stronger osseoconductive properties.[23] Phosphatization of the surface of high-strength oxide ceramics was achieved by a tailored thermal treatment in monoaluminum phosphate. *In vitro* tests of such functionalized ceramics in simulated body fluid indicated bioactivity in that apatite-forming ability was confirmed.[24] It is an important task for developmental progress in dental implant ceramic materials to extend such made-to-measure surface treatments in order to create a functional implant surface that not only shows an initial burst of bioactivity but also exhibits a controlled long-term stimulating effect *in vivo*.

# Generative Manufacturing Techniques

Alongside the ongoing developments in dental materials described above, there will also need to be innovations in manufacturing techniques in order to produce restorations out of these novel materials. Two aspects will play an important role in this context. First, it is important to be able to manufacture dental restorations at low costs by developing innovative, rapid, and cost-effective manufacturing techniques. Second, there will be a demand for manufacturing techniques that enable production from completely novel composite materials with complex microstructures that cannot be manufactured by conventional production methods. These requirements lead to utilization of 'generative manufacturing processes' or 'rapid prototyping processes'. The term generative manufacturing processes covers additive manufacturing processes including rapid prototyping (rapid tooling and rapid manufacturing). The main advantage of generative processes is the possibility of realizing nearly unlimited geometries in a mass production methodology.

The application of such manufacturing techniques in production of dental restorations was initially performed by the use of the half-automatic hot-pressing technique for the material Empress in the early 1990s.[25] The technique and the glass-ceramic materials for use in this system have been improved continually over the last 20 years so that now short-time production of restorations with complex shapes is possible.[26]

When the high-performance oxide ceramics, in particular TZP (zirconia) were introduced in dentistry, it was necessary to develop other advanced processes. This led to development of computer-aided design and manufacturing (CAD/CAM) systems, which are now available on the market in a multitude of variations.[27–29] The drawbacks of the CAD/CAM milling systems, however, are widely known. The major issues with the systems that mill a white monoblock ('soft machining') with subsequent sintering are quality assurance of the green bodies, accuracy of fit of the sintered part, and reproducibility of the process. The main problems of the systems that mill a restoration out of a sintered monoblock ('hard machining') are long machining times, significant tool wear, and the risk of introducing microscopic cracks during the hard-machining process. Furthermore, both milling methods have a high amount of raw material waste, which is unwelcome in today's drive for careful use of resources, and the costs of investment in equip-

ment can be critical with respect to market success.

In contrast to the CAD/CAM milling systems, the generative manufacturing processes only use the amount of raw material that matches the geometry of the specific component. It was for this reason that the generative manufacturing technique of laser melting was developed for titanium-based dental materials some years ago. Crowns produced with laser melting technology exhibit a marginal fit and internal accuracy that are comparable to restorations that are manufactured by conventional production procedures.[30] It is clear that ceramics will play an even more dominant role in the future as dental materials and so it will be important to develop generative manufacturing techniques for ceramic materials. Two major fields can be identified in this context. The first is generative manufacturing techniques suited to building up locally graded three-dimensional structures. This is of particular interest for bone substitutes. The second is rapid prototyping techniques that allow individual complex shapes to be produced. This will be of particular use for the manufacturing of dental crowns and other fixed dental prostheses.

There are already developments ongoing with respect to rapid prototyping of bone substitutes. The three-dimensional printing (3D-P) technique – printing of a binder into a ceramic powder bed – has recently been developed for bioactive calcium phosphates.[31] Different scientific groups have succeeded in building up bone-like structures using this 3D-P technique and clinical computerized tomography data. The printed scaffolds could be of use particularly for maxillofacial surgery. Comparable bone substitutes have been manufactured using the rapid prototyping technique laser melting. In this case, tailored calcium phosphate–bioglass composite materials were synthesized and used for the process.[32]

Only porous ceramic components can be produced by 3D-P and laser melting and therefore these techniques are suitable and favored for bone substitutes. Dental prosthetic restorations, however, require dense microstructures to achieve high strengths and wear resistance. This can be achieved using the technique of 'direct inkjet printing'. Direct inkjet printing has so far only been used for the fabrication of patterns for the lost-wax casting technique from materials such as wax or resin.[33] As an innovation, the direct inkjet printing process is currently in development for high-strength ceramics, in particular for zirconia.[34] A ceramic suspension with a high solids content is directly printed on to a suitable substrate. With the help of a specific drying technique, it is then possible to build up a ceramic green body layer by layer. The three-dimensional component is subsequently sintered in a conventional ceramic furnace. Components exhibiting complex designs and high strengths can be manufactured by this method. It would be possible, in principle, to manufacture dental restorations made of monolithic zirconia by direct inkjet printing and then print additionally different color pigments and glass phases during the three-dimensional build up. In this way, the esthetic appearance of a natural tooth could be mimicked without an additional glaze layer.

# Mimicking Nature

It is a simple truth that the 'natural prototype' is always the optimum replacement for a defective part of the body. The strategy of mimicking natural structures in terms of biomimetics can be used not just in technical applications but also, of course, for medical implantology and prosthetics. Therefore, it will be helpful to analyze the microstructure of the natural tooth first if innovative synthetic dental materials are to be developed.

Using such an approach, the following facts should be considered.

1. The human body needs a period of several years to build up the intricate architecture of biological structures.

2. A naturally grown part of the body, such as the tooth, exhibits specific and versatile biological, chemical, and mechanical properties as a result of its complex microstructure.

3. The major advantage of biological structures compared with synthetic substitutes is that the natural prototype is able to regenerate itself (i.e. it has the capability to repair defects by itself).

4. Both soft and hard tissues exhibit the potential to regenerate. Differences between the regeneration processes for hard and soft tissue relate to the dynamics of the specific regeneration process, which is slower for hard tissues. The process is extremely slow for enamel, the hardest substance in the human body. While enamel as well is able to repair itself in terms of the remineralization process, amelogenesis is a process that occurs over a very long period.

5. All structures of the human body, such as enamel, consist of a complex of organic and inorganic phases. Protein–protein and protein–mineral interaction play crucial roles in the process of enamel formation.

From the analysis above, it can be seen that monolithic high-performance materials, such as titanium alloys, high-strength oxide ceramics, and selected high-performance polymers, can restore specific functions of the natural tooth. The materials available currently for dental restorations are not, however, the optimum substitutes for the natural dental hard tissue. It is likely, therefore, that the dental materials of the future will be assembled entirely differently to those in current use. In addition, the process technology to manufacture these innovative materials will also be entirely different.

Human enamel consists to (95%) of hydroxyapatite $(Ca_{10}(PO_4)_6(OH)_2)$. This does not mean, however, that it is possible to create a coequal substitute for the natural prototype by the conventional ceramic process technology using synthetic hydroxyapatite powders and granulates. Enamel exhibits its extraordinary properties (extreme hardness, abrasion resistance, strength, and toughness) not only because of its chemical composition but also, and primarily, because of its intricate microstructure. The human body generates such a microstructure by biomineralization.

Biomineralization is characterized by a complex interaction between organic and inorganic substances.

The proteins amelogenin, enamelin, ameloblastin, and enamelysin are known to play a vital role in proper enamel mineral formation.[35] This finding may be of use in mimicking biomineralization. Different scientific teams have been successful in synthesizing a variety of unusual calcium phosphate structures by adsorbing specific proteins to crystal faces.[36–38] Furthermore, made-to-measure hydroxyapatite nanorods have been created by using amelogenin-like proteins. These nanorods self-assembled into enamel-like prisms.[39]

The major issue regarding these challenging developments is that only very small amounts of biomineralized materials can be synthesized at present. Biomineralization is an evolutionary, long-term process. This means that it will not be possible within the next few years to manufacture components on the cubic centimeter scale as dental crowns or inlays with the help of techniques of biomineralization. However, biomineralization has already been used to induce bioactive processes at the interface between the restorative material and dental hard tissue. A tailored calcium aluminate-based filling materials has been shown to form a tight bond between material and tooth and to generate apatite *in situ* during hardening through precipitation.[40] Another promising approach is the development of a hydroxyapatite–protein paste that can repair tiny early caries lesions by biomineralization.[41] Comparable successful results have also been obtained by the infiltration of tiny caries lesions with special peptides that can induce hydroxyapatite nucleation *in situ*.[42]

# Conclusions

Dispersion ceramics as alumina-toughened zirconia and zirconia-toughened alumina that were initially developed for components of joint replacement will probably play an important role for dental prosthetic restorations in the future. A further advance will be production of high-strength polycrystalline ceramics that exhibit the additional feature of translucency, achievable at present

only with glass-ceramic materials. Functionalization methods to bioactivate high-strength ceramic surfaces are in development to improve the osseoconductivity of ceramic dental implant materials. It can be foreseen that generative manufacturing techniques will 'squeeze' the 'subtractive methods' –CAD/CAM milling techniques – out of the market as soon as they are sufficiently developed. The long-term future for dental materials, however, will be organic–inorganic functionalized composite materials that can stimulate the dental tissue to restore a defect by itself through an externally controlled biomineralization process.

# References

1. The Freedonia Group. Dental Products and Materials: Market Research, Market Share, Market Size, Sales, Demand Forecast, Market Leaders, Company Profiles, Industry Trends. Study 2044. Cleveland, OH: The Freedonia Group, 2006.
2. Krejci I, Lutz F, Reimer M, Heinzmann JL. Wear of ceramic inlays, their enamel antagonists, and luting cements. J Prosthet Dent 1993;69:425–430.
3. Edelhoff D, Spiekermann H, Yildirim M. A review of esthetic pontic design options. Quintessence Int 2002;33:736–746.
4. Fischer H, Marx R. Mechanische Eigenschaften von Empress 2. Acta Med Dent Helv 1999;4:141–145.
5. Schweiger M, Höland W, Frank M, Drescher H, Rheinberger V. IPS Empress 2:A new pressable high strength glass-ceramic for esthetic all ceramic restorations. Quint Dent Tech 1999;22:143–152.
6. Höland W, Schweiger M, Frank M, Rheinberger V. A comparison of the microstructure and properties of the IPS Empress 2 and the IPS Empress glass-ceramics. J Biomed Mater Res (Appl Biomater) 2000;53:297–303.
7. Fischer H, Marx R. Improvement of strength parameters of a leucite reinforced glass ceramic by dual ion-exchange. J Dent Res 2001;80:336–339.
8. Fischer H, Marx R. Suppression of subcritical crack growth in a leucite reinforced dental glass by ion-exchange. J Biomed Mater Res 2003;66A:885–889.
9. Fischer H, de Souza RA, Wätjen AM, Richter S, Edehoff D, Mayer J, et al. Chemical strengthening of a dental lithium disilicate glass-ceramic material. J Biomed Mater Res A 2008;epub 10.1002/jbm.a.31798. PMID 18186047.
10. Edelhoff D, Spiekermann H, Yildirim M. Metal-free inlay-retained fixed partial dentures. Quintessence Int 2001;32:269–281.
11. Morita Y, Nakata K, Kim YH, Sekino T, Niihara K, Ikeuchi K. Wear properties of alumina/zirconia composite ceramics for joint prostheses measured with an end-face apparatus. Biomed Mater Eng 2004;14:263–270.
12. Begand S, Oberbach T, Glien W. Characteristic properties of a new dispersion ceramic. Key Eng Mater 2007;330–332:1207–1210.

13. De Aza AH, Chevalier J, Fantozzi G, Schehl M, Torrecillas R. Crack growth resistance of alumina, zirconia and zirconia toughened alumina ceramics for joint prostheses. Biomaterials 2002;23:937–945.

14. Tsukuma K, Yamashita I, Kusunose T. Transparent 8 mol% $Y_2O_3–ZrO_2$ (8Y) ceramics. J Am Ceram Soc 2008;91:813–818.

15. Le Guehennec L, Lopez-Heredia MA, Enkel B, Weiss P, Amouriq Y, Layrolle P. Osteoblastic cell behaviour on different titanium implant surfaces. Acta Biomater 2008;4:535–543.

16. Palmieri A, Pezzetti F, Brunelli G, Muzio LL, Scarano A, Scapoli L, et al. Short-period effects of zirconia and titanium on osteoblast microRNAs. Clin Implant Dent Relat Res, 2008;epub. PMID 18241218.

17. Levine RA, Clem D, Beagle J, Ganeles J, Johnson P, Solnit G, et al. Multicenter retrospective analysis of the solid screw ITI implant for posterior single-tooth replacements. Int J Oral Maxillofac Implants 2002;17:550–556.

18. Melo MD, Shafie H, Obeid G. Implant survival rates for oral and maxillofacial surgery residents: A retrospective clinical review with analysis of resident level of training on implant survival. J Oral Maxillofac Surg 2006;64:1185–1189.

19. Takaoka T, Okumura M, Ohgushi H, Inoue K, Takaura Y, Tamai S. Historical and biomechanical evaluation of osteogenetic response in porous hydroxyapatite coated alumina ceramics. Biomaterials 1996;17:1499–1505.

20. Suzukia T, Fujibayashia S, Nakagawaa Y, Nodab I, Nakamuraa T. Ability of zirconia double coated with titanium and hydroxyapatite to bond to bone under load-bearing conditions. Biomaterials 2006;27:996–1002.

21. Kong YM, Bae CJ, Lee SH, Kim HW, Kim HE. Improvement in bio-compatibility of ZrO2–Al2O3 nano-composite by addition of HA. Biomaterials 2005;26:509–517.

22. Fischer H, Niedhart C, Kaltenborn N, Prange A, Marx R, Niethard FU, et al. Bioactivation of inert alumina ceramics by hydroxylation. Biomaterials 2005;26:6151–6157.

23. Tanahashi M, Matsuda T. Surface functional group dependence on apatite formation on self-assembled monolayers in a simulated body fluid. J Biomed Mater Res 1997;34:305–315.

24. Kaltenborn N, Sax M, Müller FA, Müller L, DiekerH, Kaiser A, Teller R, Fischer H. Coupling of phosphates on alumina surfaces for bioactivation. J Am Ceram Soc 2007;90:1644–1646.

25. Beham G. IPS-Empress: Eine neue Keramiktechnologie. ZWR 1991;100:404–408.

26. Höland W, Rheinberger V, Apel E, van 't Hoen C, Höland M, Dommann A, et al. Clinical applications of glass-ceramics in dentistry. J Mater Sci Mater Med 2006;17:1037–1042.

27. Tinschert J, Natt G, Hassenpflug S, Spiekermann H. Status of current CAD/CAM technology in dental medicine. Int J Comput Dent 2004;7:25–45.

28. McLaren EA, Terry DA. CAD/CAM systems, materials, and clinical guidelines for all-ceramic crowns and fixed partial dentures. Compend Contin Educ Dent 2006;23:637–641.

29. Beuer F, Schweiger J, Edelhoff D. Digital dentistry: an overview of recent developments for CAD/CAM generated restorations. Br Dent J 2008;204:505–511.

30. Quante K, Ludwig K, Kern M. Marginal and internal fit of metal-ceramic crowns fabricated with a new laser melting technology. Dent Mater 2008;epub 31.03.2008. PMID 18685891.

31. Khalyfa A, Vogt S, Weisser J, Grimm G, Rechtenbach A, et al. Development of a new calcium phosphate powder-binder system for the 3D printing of patient specific implants. J Mater Sci Mater Med 2007;18:906–916.

32. Fischer H, Wilkes J, Bergmann C, Kuhl I, Meiners W, Wissenbach K, et al. Bone substitute implants made of TCP/glass composites using selective laser melting technique. cfi/Ber DKG 2006;83:57–60.

33. Witkowski S, Lange R. Stereolithography as an additive technique in dentistry. Schweiz Monatsschr Zahnmed 2003;113:868–884.

34. Uibel K, Telle R, Fischer H. Verfahren und Vorrichtung zur Herstellung dreidimensionaler keramischer Formkörper. Patent DE 102006015014 (2006).

35. Margolis HC, Beniash E, Fowler CE. Role of macromolecular assembly of enamel matrix proteins in enamel formation. J Dent Res 2006;85:775–793.

36. Bertoni E, Bigi A, Falini G, Panzavolta S, Roveri N. Hydroxyapatite/polyacrylic acid nanocrystals. J Mater Chem 1999;9:779–782.

37. Burke EM, Guo Y, Colon L, Rahmia M, Veis A, Nancollas GH. Influence of polyaspartic acid and phosphophoryn on octacalcium phosphate growth kinetics. Colloids Surf B Biointerfaces 2000;17:49–57.

38. Peytcheva A, Cölfen H, Schnablegger H, Antonietti M. Calcium phosphate colloids with hierarchical structure controlled by polyaspartates. Colloid Polym Sci 2002;280:218–227.

39. Chen H, Clarkson BH, Sun K, Mansfield JF. Self-assembly of synthetic hydroxyapatite nanorods into an enamel prism-like structure. J Colloid Interface Sci 2005;288:97–103.

40. Engquist H, Schultz-Walz JE, Loof J, Botton GA, Mayer D, Phaneuf MW, et al. Chemical and biological integration of a mouldable bioactive ceramic material capable of forming apatite in vivo in teeth. Biomaterials 2004;25:2781–2787.

41. Yamagishi K, Onuma K, Suzuki T, Okada F, Tagami J, Otsuki M, et al. A synthetic enamel for rapid tooth repair. Nature 2005;433:819.

42. Kirkham J, Firth A, Vernals D, Boden N, Robinson C, Shore RC, et al. Self-assembling peptide scaffolds promote enamel remineralization. J Dent Res 2007;86:426–430.

# The Future of Dental Medicine

17

Heinrich F. Kappert and Jean-François Roulet

*He Who Does Not Think About the Future Does Not Have Any!*

## Introduction

There is a widespread agreement that our society is subject to profound processes of change. Furthermore, the speed of change has dramatically accelerated, supported by the possibility of worldwide scientific information exchange and the access to data through the internet. This presents a new challenge to scientists and engineers to use their creativity to develop beneficial conditions for the environment and future life of human beings.

To prepare ourselves for the demands of the future, there is firstly a need to gain deep insight into today's scientific knowledge. Science means to know and preserve valid principles and to develop a new theoretical framework for future demands, problems and questions. On one hand, strong visions for the future can be developed by extrapolating today's technologies into the upcoming potential technological environment. However, to predict what lies ahead, one must often rely on guesswork. On the other hand – and this might be even more effective – one must imagine what the way of life will be in the future. Nothing is more powerful than the right idea at the right time. Today's imag-

ination and visions coupled with passion are the right tools to maintain the motivation needed to pursue innovative ideas. When James Watt built the first steam engines 200 years ago, he had intuition but not the laws of thermodynamics to guide him. However, visions must be transformed into concepts, and finally – in terms of industrial development – they must be realized as a product. It takes courage to transform a clever invention into a business success. However, when the time is ready, far-fetched ideas may be realized.

In the past, future developments were more-or-less restricted to localized populations. The more generally important innovations were and the better the worldwide information flow functioned, the faster innovations spread around the world. Today we are living in a global world, with companies functioning on a global scale. Nevertheless, not all nations/markets are on the same technological and social level. Therefore there will be always a marketing force driving innovations at a local level, with the consequence that innovations will be introduced at different times in different regions. In the long term, every innovative technology will be available globally, but at different times. In other words, at a given time, different innovations will be important for different regions. This is important to realize when planning innovations for global companies.

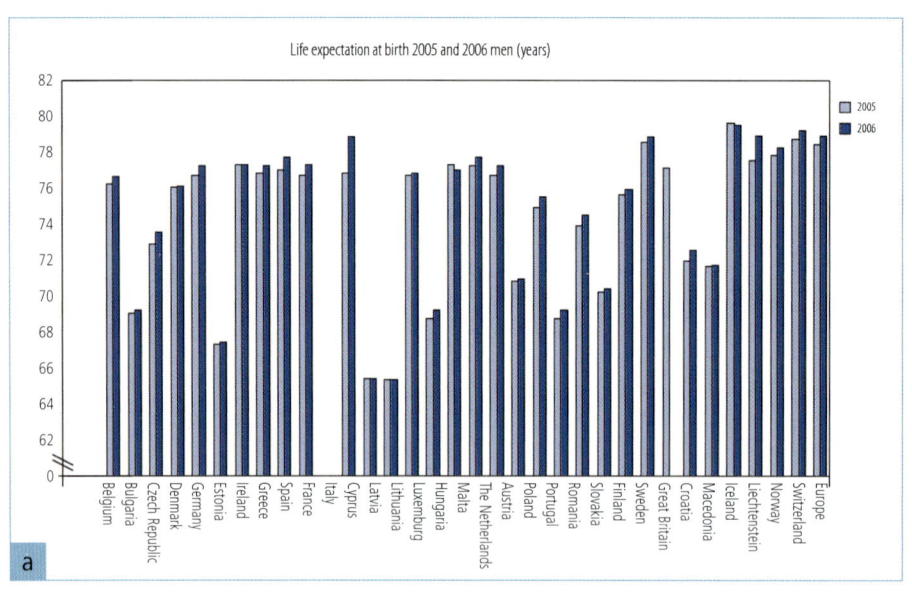

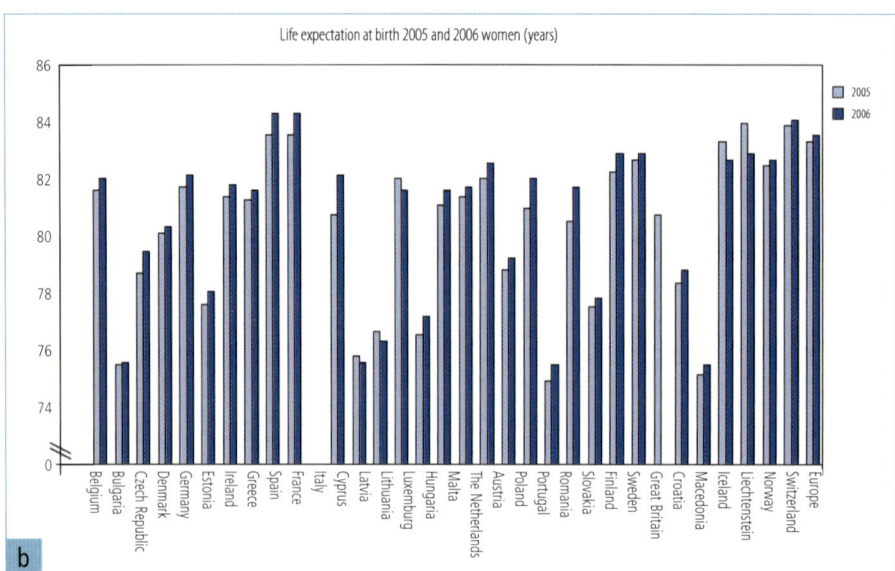

**Fig 17-1a-b** Life expectancy in Europe: **(a)** males; **(b)** females.

# Global Changes that Influence the Future of Dental Medicine

## Demographic Changes

Two major changes have occurred in the last 100 years. First, the global population has increased dramatically (at July 2008, approximately $6.7 \times 10^9$),[1] and second, the life expectancy for people living in industrialized nations, with good access to healthcare, has almost doubled in the last 100 years. Today's life expectancy for the average US citizen is 75.2 years for a male and 81.0 years for a female.[2] On average, in 2006 life expectancy across Europe was similar: 79.0 years for males and 83.5 years for females. However, among the different European nations there are differences in life expectancy (Fig 17-1).[3] Similar data are available for all populations in industrialized nations, whereas in China the average life expectancy is only 68.0 years for males and 73.0 years for females. In the last 50 years, the average

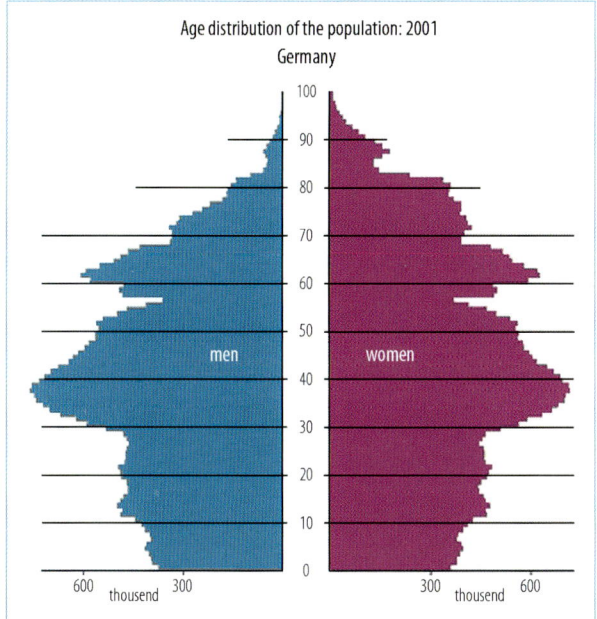

Fig 17-2   Age pyramid for Germany in 2001.

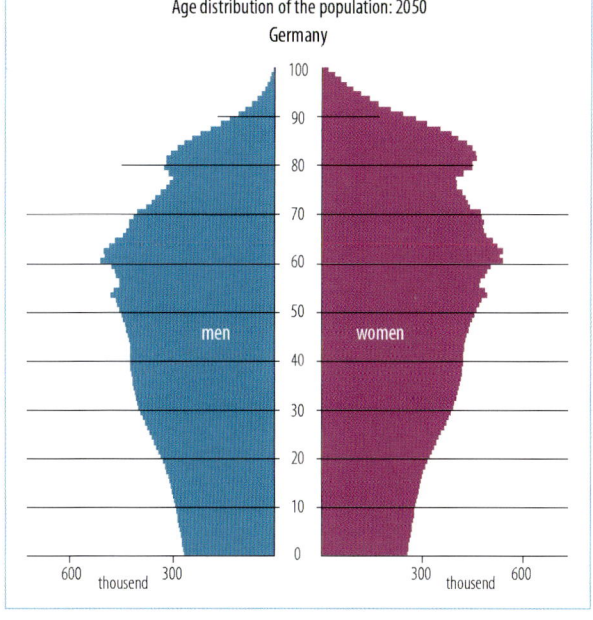

Fig 17-3   Estimated age pyramid for Germany in 2050.

Fig 17-4   Age pyramids of developed world countries and developing world countries. Note that the majority of the world population is living in developing nations. The top figure shows the population-age pyramid for the developed world and the bottom figure is for the developing world. The figure illustrates the pyramids for the year 1975 (pink) and 2000 (blue).

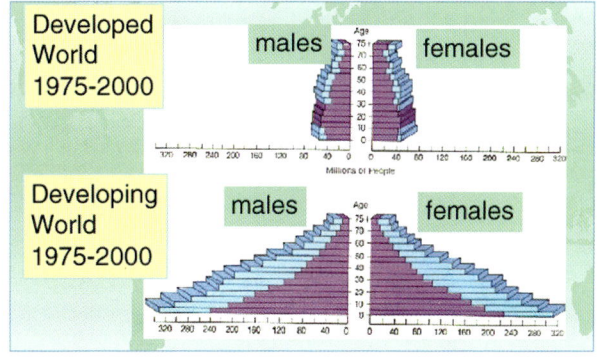

family size has decreased and the age of parents when they have their children has increased. Consequently, the age distribution of populations changed from a pyramid to a mushroom shape, as seen in Germany (Figs 17-2 and 17-3).[4] This is valid at least for industrialized countries, the so-called developed world, in contrast to the developing world (Fig 17-4).[5] Therefore, the populations treated by dentists in the developed world will dramatically change in the near future. Owing to the increased longevity of their patients, US clinicians estimate that there is a need for one more reconstruction of the dentition per patient compared with the

past.[6] Combined with the effects of prevention, in the future, elderly patients with their own teeth and perhaps with more implant-supported reconstructions will be the rule. While 50 years ago edentulism was an accepted sequela of aging, this has completely changed in recent decades. There has been a dramatic reduction in the prevalence of edentulism and incidence of tooth loss in industrialized countries.[7-9] As an example, in Switzerland today only 13.8% of the 65- to 74-year-olds are edentulous.[10] Mojon et al.[9] have published a prediction of the prevalence of edentulism based on data of four nations (USA, Finland, UK, and Sweden).

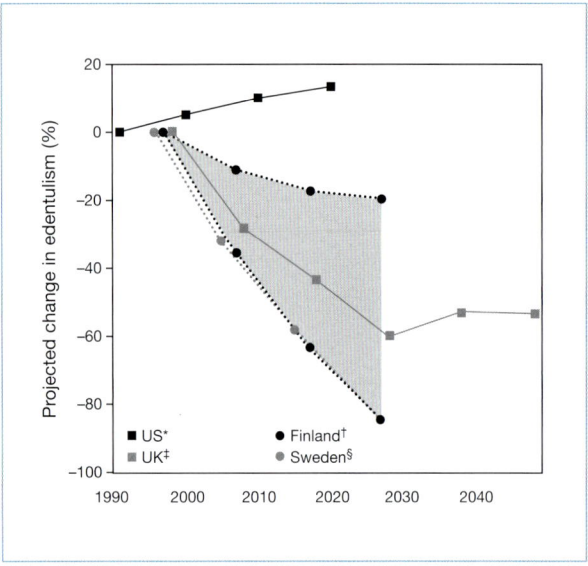

Fig 17-5 Prediction of the prevalence of edentulism in four countries. *(reproduced from Mojon et al.[11])*

It shows a dramatic decrease until the year 2030 (Fig 17-5). This will lead to new needs for dentistry: as citizens age, the more their dexterity diminishes. Therefore the level of self-administrated oral hygiene will decrease. Combined with a physiologic decrease in saliva secretion, it can be assumed that the growing elderly population will have increased caries rates, especially root caries. There will also be an increase in periodontal diseases, including periimplantitis, in the mid-term future. Manufacturers of dental materials, suppliers of dental care, and the society (healthcare politics) must adapt to these changes.

In the long term, developing countries will follow the same route. However, at present most developing countries are still growing at an accelerated rate, with the consequence that their populations are dominated by children, adolescents and young adults. The average age of the world population according to WHO was 27.6 in 2004 (whereas the average age in the US was 35.3 years in 2000)[2]. The 'dental route' of the populations in developing countries will be strongly dependent on the ability of their societies to install preventive programs and thus generate populations with good oral health within a few years. The alternative is that we will observe a repeat of the changes in industrialized nations over the last 100 years: a tremendous increase in the demand for restorative treatment, followed by the urgent need for prevention in order to avoid costly restorative treatment. Depending on the developments that take place in the different nations/cultures, dental manufacturers must be ready to react to different possible scenarios: either to offer good and efficient systems for restorative care or to be ready to support the societies to set up effective prevention programs for healthy teeth and periodontal tissues.

## Social Changes

Technological advancement in the last century gave us the industrial revolution, and, with it, an abundance of food. Knowledge in medicine (eg, antibiotics, surgical techniques, enhanced diagnostics, especially at the biochemical level) has prolonged the average life expectancy substantially. However, with this development came a severe cost: in industrialized nations worldwide the healthcare expenses have steadily increased. In some industrialized nations the healthcare expenditures have reached more than 10% of the gross domestic product (GDP) (Fig 17-6).[12] Dentistry, as part of the medical care community, is also concerned with this development, on one hand by contributing to these increased costs, and on the other by being a victim of prioritization. Bad teeth (caries and periodontal disease) are not

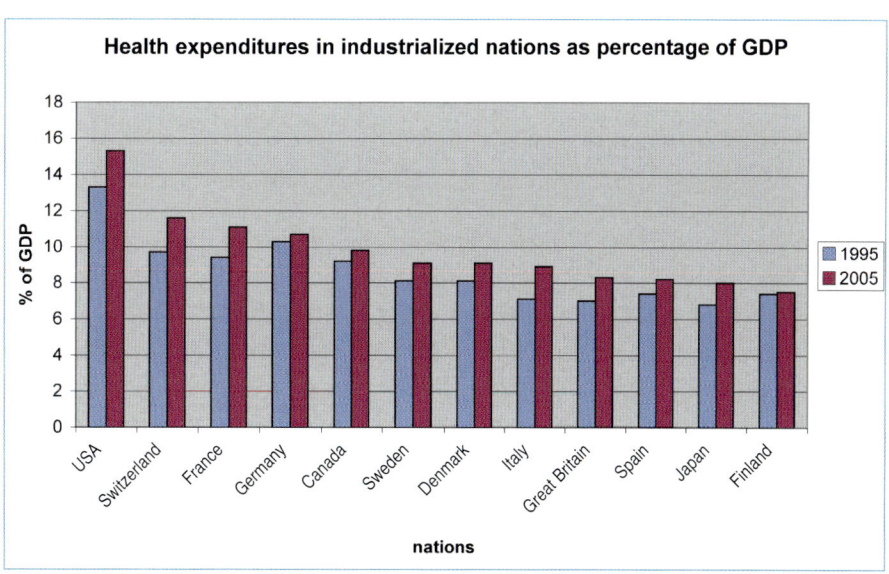

**Fig 17-6** Health expenditure in industrialized nations as percentage of GDP.

a life-threatening disease, so in the fight for the health-care resources, dentistry has a weak position. You can live without teeth, but not without a heart, a liver, or functioning kidneys. This controversy will be more accentuated in the future, because the lifestyle in industrialized countries leads to obesity, which will dramatically increase the need for healthcare. Some scientists predict that life expectancy in the US will decrease by 2 to 5 years until 2050 because of the increase in obesity. In the US, obesity is already the second most common cause of death.[13,14]

Obesity leads to a higher risk for coronary heart disease, diabetes and problems with movement (eg, wear of the joints). Furthermore, today's trend in dentistry is that many clinicians opt to treat only the top 5% of the population, who can afford extremely expensive, highly 'esthetic' treatment, such as implants with bone grafts and soft tissue transplants, followed by full-ceramic reconstructions. Palla[15] stated: 'Dentists must serve the complete population and not only the most upper small segment that can afford extremely expensive treatments. If dentistry as a profession misses fulfilling this request, it will exclude itself from the medical professional community!' The clinicians who have tried to link dental disease, such as periodontitis, with other general diseases such as coronary heart disease, premature birth or

apoplexia, are doing dental medicine a great favor, because they help to anchor it in the general healthcare system. Dentists, as part of the medical community, must serve the whole population.

These thoughts seem logical; however, there are some problems. Traditionally, healthcare is seen as the responsibility of the nation. It is a public duty to ensure the health of the population. Depending on the philosophy, this is more or less true in most countries. But the common trend, independent from the political system, is that healthcare expenditures are rising. Therefore, the state and private insurance companies are trying to reduce expenditure. Since premiums are already very high and the society as a whole is not willing to pay higher premiums/taxes, it is very likely that dentistry will be an early victim of the process of cutting costs, because dental diseases are not life threatening (see above). So it is to be expected that dentistry will develop into two parallel tracks. Basic services guarantee painless patients and the ability to chew. The goal is to provide a simple, efficient and cost-effective restorative and surgical treatment. This service is offered to all citizens in a given population or to insured patients with more-or-less mandatory insurance. On top of the basic service, there will be the dentistry focusing on high-end restorative solutions for wealthy patients. This type of dentistry, however, must be able to fulfill the highest functional and esthetic demands. It is typically dominated by implant and ceramic reconstructions and offers regular professional hygiene care to maintain the expensive work. Depending on the social structures in different countries, a level in between these extremes may be established as well. However, this dentistry is then highly dependent on the economic well-being of the society.

The consequences of these trends are that manufacturers of dental materials must strive for fast, easy and efficient procedures that can be delivered at low cost. This will probably be most of the business. Manufacturers must also be able to fulfill the needs of the 'high-end' clinician, who will probably work in well-organized group offices or small private clinics. This demanding sector will remain small in the future, but attractive because of the willingness to spend money for highly esthetic goals.

# Technology and Principles of Nature as Driving Forces for Progress and Invention

## Electronics and Computer Science

In the last century there were two very important discoveries. One was the invention of the transistor,[16] the technology of using silicon crystals to create a semiconductor. In 1947, William Shockley, John Bardeen and Walter Brattain made the first successful amplifying semiconductor device. They called it a transistor (from transfer and resistor). Shockley made improvements to it in 1950 that made it easier to manufacture.[17] The combination of pnp or npn layers produced the same functionality as a cathode ray tube to modify electrical signals, on a much smaller scale and with much less energy. This basic invention led to integrated circuits

(IC) of a micrometer scale on silicon wafers, which were able to perform various electrical functions in all kinds of apparatus, especially in computers and telecommunication. The first consumer products based on this technology were pocket radios, which were a completely new class of radio, making listening to music independent of the electrical power outlet. This changed lifestyles. The second important invention was the assembly of the first computers evolving from principles that were used for mechanical calculators (eg, Zuse Z3 in 1941).[18] The first electronic computers were still based on cathode ray tubes, such as the ENIAC (Electronic Numerical Integrator and Computer), which is considered the first programmable electronic calculating machine.[19] These machines were able to perform series of operations, based on binary codes, if programmed to do so. Both inventions were important, but not overwhelming. However, the combination of the semiconductor technology with the computer science has completely changed our world within a few decades. These changes are ongoing and have invaded every profession. With ongoing miniaturization and the batch production technology for integrated circuits, the science has driven the performance of such systems to the limits of today's physical knowledge. Computers in household appliances, in tools and business applications are as common as electrical lights worldwide. Furthermore, the technology has also boosted telecommunication, and with it data storage, leading to a global network with the instant availability of data and information anywhere in the world.

Of course, dentistry has not been spared from these developments. To begin with, computers were used for business administration in dental offices. In 1985, CAD/CAM technology was introduced for the manufacture of ceramic restorations[20,21] and later LED technology was used to build efficient curing lights for composite resins[22]. Digital photography has completely displaced analog photography in recent years.

From the innovations and developments of the last 60 years we can see that insight and knowledge that follow the principles of nature lead to successful and advantageous changes to our lifestyle. Two rules of nature are saving energy and space. Although the universe is infinite in size, at least in our world matter is condensed as far as possible. Amorphous structures tend to organize in crystalline structures to save space and energy. We have to keep these principles in mind as a basis for our vision of the future. If we manage to reduce machines, eg x-ray tubes, lasers, furnaces, computers, and tools, such as rotary instruments, to an appropriate size, they are not only energy and space saving, but also more convenient to handle and work with. It is worth remembering these principles as a concept for development.

Computing and electronics will greatly assist the clinician of the future. Generating almost any wavelength and combination thereof with LEDs in combination with the analysis of the reflected and/or transmitted light will lead to tools to enhance diagnostic capabilities. Computer controlled x-ray machines with intelligent software will allow reconstructing in three-dimensional every aspect of the oral cavity, even on a microscopic level, allowing monitoring of the progress/regress of disease, leading to better treatment decisions. Some versions of all these tools are already being constructed. In the future it will be possible to completely analyze the situation of the masticatory organ and to determine the best method for its reconstruction in an ideal functional and esthetic way. Having all the data stored in electronic form, it will be possible to create and construct the required restorations within the digital world. It is even possible that smart machines under the control of the clinician will perform the interventions in an optimal, minimally invasive way.

## Inorganic Chemistry and Ceramics

### New Materials and Technologies for Dental Restorations

Considering the literature on dental materials, it is remarkable that without exception publications as well as text books describe traditional scientific material parameters as elastic modulus, flexural strength, tough-

ness etc, and then consequently the available materials are described and qualified according to these parameters, eg as low-strength and high-strength materials, or low- and high-translucency materials. It is not commonly practiced to begin by investigating and considering the material properties of natural teeth, and to start from this viewpoint to assess artificial materials and their appropriate properties to serve as dental materials.

It is necessary to approach the subject of new materials and technologies for dental restorations under various aspects. One is to consider the biological, chemical, physical, mechanical and optical properties of natural teeth and conclude from this knowledge which material properties we really need for dental restorative materials in order to repair small destroyed areas or fill small cavities of a tooth, reconstruct the loss of larger portions of a tooth's crown, restore dentin and enamel losses, and finally replace a whole tooth by bridging or implantation.

In Table 17-1, various mechanical data of different dental materials are shown in comparison to the natural tooth material enamel and dentin. The materials chosen for comparison were hydroxyapatite, glass-ceramic, zirconia and dental alloys, including high-noble and non-noble alloys.

Hydroxyapatite is chemically the closest to natural tooth material (enamel). Early attempts to replace lost tooth substances by hydroxyapatite date back to the 18th century and even earlier. At that time, natural crowns were separated from the root and used to replace a decayed tooth of another patient by fixing it to the neighbor tooth with a splint.[23] It is still an open question why modern dental materials science follows the concept of strength for developing new dental materials, whereas nature fulfills the requirements for appropriate tooth materials with much less strength. Two facts can be offered as an answer: one is that the natural bond between dentin and enamel is in the range of 38 MPa[24] for more than 50 years under all masticatory, chemical and physical conditions, which is still not possible with artificial dental adhesives. Second, we have to admit that there is no example in nature for dental

Table 17-1  Mechanical data of human tooth enamel and dentin in comparison with other dental materials.

| Property | Tooth enamel | Tooth dentin | Hydroxy-apatite | Leucite reinforced ceramic (Empress) | Lithium disilicate ceramic (e.max) | Zirconia | Dental alloys |
|---|---|---|---|---|---|---|---|
| Density (g/cm$^3$) | 2.96 | 2.2 | 3.1 | 2.4 | 2.4 | 6.08 | 8–19 |
| Hardness (KHN) | 355–431 | 68 | 340–550 | 400–500 | 400–500 | 2000 | 80–700 |
| Elasticity modulus (GPa) | 84 | 14.7 | 34 | 60–70 | 95–100 | 210 | 100–200 |
| Flexural strength (MPa) | 10 | 105 | 59 | 160 | 350 | 1000 | 300–700 |
| Fracture toughness (MPa·m$^{1/2}$) | 0.77 | 3 | 0.6–1.0 | 1.2 | 3.2 | 6 | 60–100 |

bridges. Therefore, besides studying how nature solves problems it is necessary to look to various other technical fields to find solutions.

Thus the question arises whether these traditional concepts and strategies considering mainly strength will lead research and development to construct the optimum restorative dental materials in the future. Instead, we simply have to solve only two requirements as perfectly as nature. One is to improve adhesives and the second is to solve the gap situation after loosing teeth, eg by implantation.

However, the real demand cannot be satisfied with simply one material. For example the filling therapy, including minimally invasive treatments, bonds composite to teeth. After curing, the composite may reach enamel quality. Larger defects require partial or total replacements of natural tooth crowns by inlays, onlays, or artificial crowns. Today these restorations must be esthetic, and show excellent longevity. The same is true for bridgeworks requiring high strength or implants requiring both high strength and osseointegration.

A second aspect to discuss is the traditional, current and future techniques and technologies to form and manufacture dental materials to the shape that is necessary to fit to the natural situation. This means polymerization, casting, sintering, and CAD/CAM techniques, the current standard techniques that provide a mixture of built-up and cutting down techniques. In terms of saving material, at least the standard CAD/CAM tech-

nique will be replaced by a revolutionary class of generative techniques known as solid freeform fabrication (SFF). Such techniques use computer-controlled robotics to build 3D components in a layer-by-layer fashion. The advantages of SFF over conventional fabrication methods include spatially tailored composition, greater process control and flexibility, lower tooling costs, and improved performance/reliability. To date, several SFF techniques, including stereolithography, fused deposition of ceramics, laminated object manufacturing, computer-aided manufacture of laminated engineering materials, 3D printing, and robocasting have been developed.

Figure 17-7 shows a small tree-like structure fabricated by a generative technique out of a mineral material, which is impossible to produce using current CAD/CAM technologies. It has several features in common with natural products; not only the fine structured branching, but also material and energy savings from the applied fabrication technique.

The greater the workflow and progress in miniaturization in the product development of tools, instruments, apparatus and materials, the greater the reduction in weight, volume and energy consumption, as well as the increase in speed. In this respect, a remarkable occurrence is the exploration of the smallest nano-sized particles and their usage and application in manifold technological fields. Nanotechnology relates to particles of various sizes in the range of up to 100 nm and their

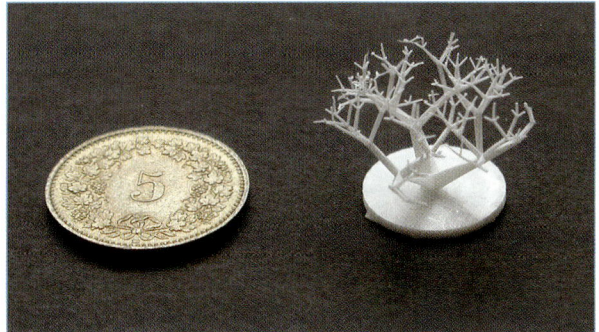

**Fig 17-7**  Solid free form fabrication (SFF) allows the efficient production of very detailed and fine structures.

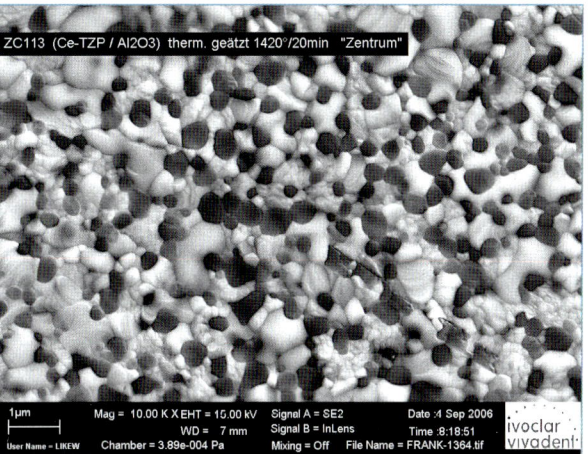

**Fig 17-8**  SEM micrograph of the thermally etched surface of Ce-TZP/Al$_2$O$_3$ nano-composite (Nanozir, Panasonic, Japan).

properties. They exhibit special chemical and physical properties that are very different from solid-state properties, especially relating to electrical and optical conductivity and chemical reactivity. The typical properties of a material during the transition from the atomic state to the solid state are generally studied. Mainly the economic areas of information and telecommunication, biotechnology, medical technology, the automobile industry and energy technology take advantage of nanotechnology. Nano particles are already widely used in surface layers of Pt and Pd as catalysts, in varnishes, creams, pastes and glue materials of any kind, and even in food. In dental materials the prefix 'nano' is mainly used for advertising purposes, without really using special properties of nano particles. A special inorganic composite consisting of alumina and zirconia is the Cer oxide stabilized material Nanozir (Fig 17-8),[25] which has higher strength and fracture toughness than the traditional yttrium-oxide-stabilized zirconia. Further developments in these directions for preferable properties, such as lower sintering temperature or higher translucency, have to be expected in the future.

We have to look again at natural procedures to see how everything is formed, whether living or non-living objects. Plants start from a seed and animals from an embryo, and even large crystals start with a small crystalline seed, and grow by building up in stages. The principles behind these methods are material and energy savings. In general, we have to understand how problems have been solved in nature. Like today's engineers, all plants and animals had to solve many technical problems during their development, such as energy production or flight.

The systems of nature demonstrate a manifold optimization, minimal energy and material consumption and an almost perfect circuit of waste recycling. With these remarkable properties, nature may provide ideas and vision for innovation and economic development. The scientific field of bionics (meaning biology and technology) delivers key innovations and improvements in various technologic fields and developing strategies, where only small steps had been made with conventional methods. Bionic means to transfer structural and functional principles of living nature for the best solution of application-oriented tasks. Because of its strong and interdisciplinary character, bionics offers great possibilities for technological development.

## Organic Chemistry and Resins

Resin composites have reached a very high degree of sophistication. Intelligent filler size distributions with an abundance of different filler materials allow the

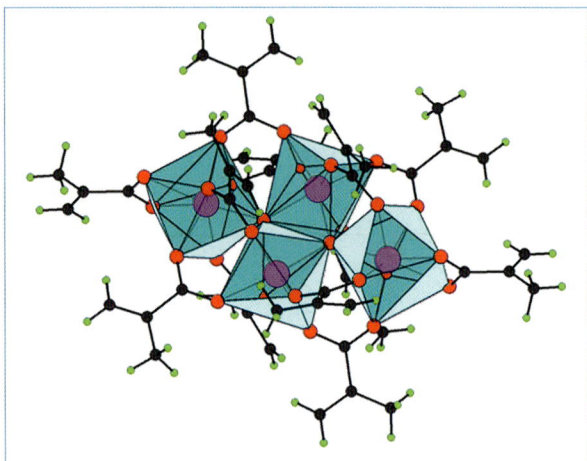

**Fig 17-9** Zirconium oxide nanocluster functionalized with acrylates.

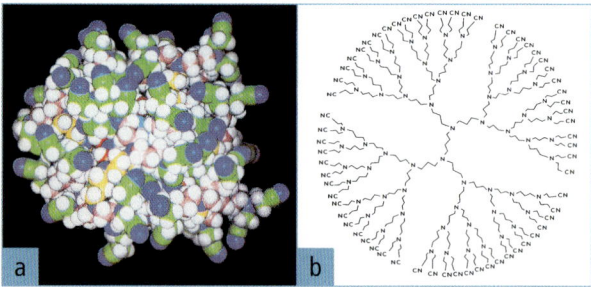

**Fig 17-10a–b** Dendrimers as an example of the bottom-up approach to produce fillers. Furthermore, such fillers can be chemically bonded to the resins because of an abundance of polymerizable groups on their surface. **(a)** Molecular model. **(b)** Structure.

developer to find optimal combinations to reach very high filler loads and excellent performance. Using nanotechnology with the bottom-up approach, functionalized fillers can be tailor made, eg Zr-O-nanoclusters (Fig 17-9) or dendrimeres (Fig 17-10). With such an approach, the boundaries between fillers and the resinous matrix can be eliminated. Such 'non-composite composites' may open new routes for creating restorative materials with multiple functions and characteristics as required. So far, the monomers used are based on acrylate chemistry. Ormocers and compomers can be seen as intelligent alternatives, but their setting reaction is still based on free-radical polymerization based on acrylate chemistry. Further composite developments are towards lower polymerization shrinkage. Epoxy-based monomers, however, require cationic polymerization. This material class poses great challenges to chemists, before the composites will perform as well as the best 'conventional' materials.

More reactive photo-initiator systems will allow for faster polymerization with better depth of cure. Varying the wavelength of the light in combination with the appropriate photo initiator may increase the ease of application for cements.

Smart application tools for restorative materials will further follow the 'convenience' trends observed in the last years.

The simple act of bonding resins to tooth hard tissue has yielded a multitude of products, which can be divided into different 'families' according to the application techniques. They require chemically demanding and complex monomers with high production costs. There are already reliable products available, and new development goals can be formulated – the trend is towards rapidity and ease. Self-repairing adhesives are conceivable, as well as more heavily filled adhesives that would be used as restorative materials. Smart materials are also possible, eg including a 'leakage indicator'. Alternatively, adhesives penetrating carious tissue could allow development of a form of dentistry that does not require mechanical caries removal or drilling.

## Biology and Medical Science

Understanding biology will open up new possibilities for dental treatment, because the intervention will use the same powerful tools as used by nature. As an example, knowing the signal factors with which the microorganisms in the plaque are communicating[26], it seems possible to create a mouthrinse containing the signal factor for becoming planctonic instead of bonded to a surface (biofilm), thus disrupting the biofilm (Fig 17-11). Understanding the biological mechanism of adhesion of microorganisms to enamel, one could create a substance that would block the adhesive sites biochemically, and therefore bacteria would still be able to live in the oral cavity, but would not be able to form biofilms on teeth. With monoclonal antibodies (MAB), specific microorganisms can be targeted. If the 'homing device' (MAB) is combined with an antimicrobial peptide, the microorganism (eg, *Streptococcus mutans*) can be selectively eliminated without harming the remaining microbial population. Taking this one step further, could salivary glands not produce only saliva, but also monoclonal antibodies to target specific microorganisms, thereby reducing the occurrence of caries or periodontal disease?

Understanding the self-aligning mechanisms nature uses to calcify enamel or dentin matrixes in order to produce dental hard tissues, 'healing' mechanisms for dental decay may be created. The 'dream' in restorative dentistry would be to create teeth instead of restoring them. This requires very deep knowledge and control of all the biological processes that lead to the complex organ, the tooth. Furthermore, to be practical one needs to be better than nature by speeding up the process. Who would wait for years to have a missing incisor replaced with bioregenerative techniques?

Intermediate goals could be bioactive interfaces. Specific implant surfaces would trigger the growth of a periodontium in order to naturally integrate the artificial root.

Another exciting route might be the combination of electronics and biological systems. Simple systems in this direction could be force sensors that diagnose bruxism and actively influence the chewing muscles towards relaxation.

However, one must consider two important things when thinking about sophisticated biological methods.
1. Common to all these potential applications of biological principles is the complexity of nature (biology). Before such methods can be applied, the involved mechanisms must be fully understood, which means that proof of efficiency and safety becomes extremely difficult and costly (also legal requirements for licensing such procedures).

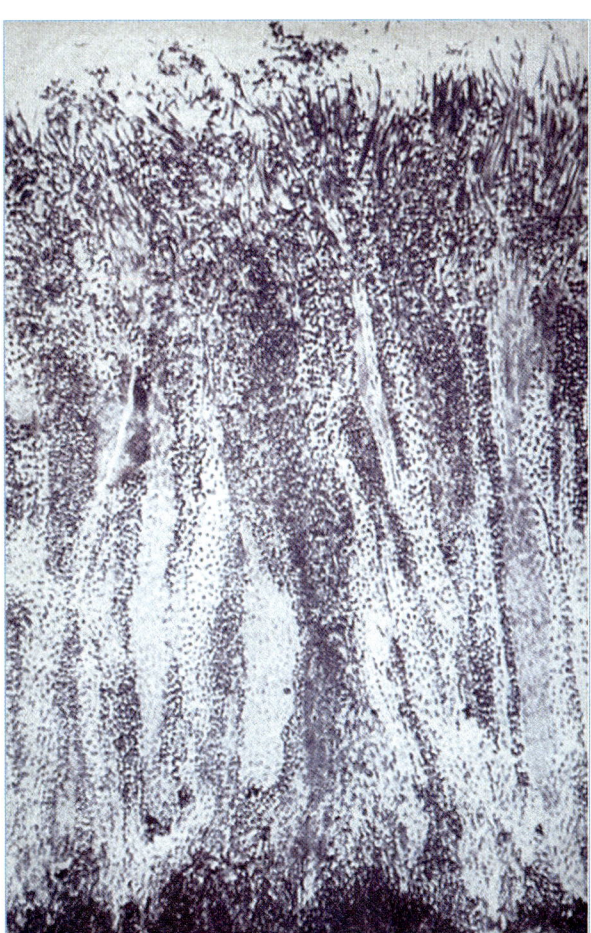

**Fig 17-11** Histological section through dental plaque. Such a biofilm is a highly organized structure, which requires communication between the different bacteria. *(reproduced with permission from Wolf K, Rateitschak K [eds]. Farbatlanten der Zahnmedizin, Band 1, Parodontologie, 3rd edition. Stuttgart: Thieme, 2004)*

2. Confronting people with extremely powerful methods generates fear and rejection. We would be dealing with genetically modified biological material. So how would you convince a patient or a mother (when it comes to prevention) to accept such technology if they are rejecting the consumption of genetically modified corn?

237

# Conclusions

The future of dentistry will be determined either by materials and technological developments or in a later phase by progress in understanding and applying biological knowledge. Furthermore, the future will be heavily influenced by social, financial, legal, and political parameters. Since changes will not occur in all countries at the same time, the transition from more traditional restorative/prosthodontic driven approaches towards more innovative, minimally invasive, preventive, biological, and energy- and material-saving approaches will be spread over many years. This will give dental materials companies time to adapt, provided that they have the right strategies to assimilate the changes needed for the future and thus stay successful.

# References

1. www.dsw-online.de/info-service/weltbevölkerungsuhr
2. Altersstruktur Wikipedia, 10 Years USA Statistic
3. Eurostatistics. Available at: http://epp.eurostat.ec.europa.eu/QueenPortletized/display.do?screen=graphicref&output=PNG&language=de&product=REF_TB_population&root=REF_TB_population/t_popula/t_pop/t_demo_mor/tps00025&zFilter=|1|
4. Statistisches Bundesamt Deutschland. Available at: www.destatis.de
5. http://www.globalchange.umich.edu/globalchange2/current/lectures/
6. Garber, D. Prosthetic gingival reconstruction within the esthetic zone. Presented at the European Academy of Esthetic Dentistry, Madrid, June 2008.
7. Aianamo A, Österberg T. Changing demographic and oral disease patterns and treatment needs in the Scandinavian populations of old people. Int Dent J 1992;42:311–322.
8. Österberg T, Carlsson GE, Sundh V. Trends and prognoses of dental status in the swedish population: analysis based on interviews in 1975 to 1997 by Statistics Sweden. Acta Odontol Scand 2000;58:177–182.
9. Mojon P. The world without teeth: demographic trends. In: Feine JS, Carlsson GE (eds). Implant overdentures. The standard of care for edentulous patients. Chicago: Quintessence, 2003:3–14.
10. Zitzmann NU, Staehelin K, Walls AW, Menghini G, Weiger R, Zemp SE. Changes in oral health over a 10-yr period in Switzerland. Eur J Oral Sci 2008;116:52–59.
11. Mojon P, Thomason JM, Walls AWG. The impact of falling rates of edentulism. Int J Prosthodont 2004;17:434–440.
12. Bundeszahnärztekammer (ed.). Statistisches Jahrbuch der Bundeszahnärztekammer zur zahnärztlichen Versorgung in Deutschland. Berlin: Quintessenz, 2008.
13. Olshansky SJ, Passaro DG, Hershow RC, Layden J, Carnes BA, Brody J, et al. A potential decline in life expectancy in the United States in the 21st Century. N Engl J Med 2005;352:1138–1145.
14. Preston SH. Deadweight? The influence of obesity on longevity. N Engl J Med 2005;352:1135–1137.
15. Palla S. Aesthetic, cosmetique or natural appearance? Presented at the European Academy of Esthetic Dentistry, Madrid, June 2008.
16. Lilienfeld EJ. Method and apparatus for controlling electric currents. US Patent No. 1745175, 22 October 1925.
17. Shockley W. Electrons and holes in semiconductors. New York: Van Nostrand, 1950.
18. Rojas R. Konrad Zuse's legacy: the architecture of the Z1 and Z3. IEEE Ann Hist Comput 1997;19:2.
19. Eckert JP Jr, Mauchly JW, Goldstine HH, Brainerd JG. Description of the ENIAC and comments on electronic digital computing machines. University of Pennsylvania: Moore School of Electrical Engineering, 1945.
20. Mörmann W, Brandestini M. Verfahren zur Herstellung medizinischer und Zahntechnischer, alloplastischer endo- und exoprothetischer Passkörper. Euro Patent No. 81 110 135.1, 1985.
21. Brandestini M, Mörmann W, Ferru A, LutzF, Kreici I. Computer machined ceramic inlays: in vitro marginal adaptation. J Dent Res 1985;64:208(Abstract 305).
22. Kennedy J. US Patent: No 005420768A: Portable LED Photocuring Device. 30 May 1995.
23. Alt KW. Die historische Entwicklung der zahnärztlichen Prothetik. In: Strub JR, Türp JC, Witkowski SWJ, Hürzeler MB, Kern M (eds.). Curriculum Prothetik, Bd. 1. 2. Aufl. Berlin: Quintessence, 2005;S37–S64.
24. Pioch Th, Staehle HJ. Experimental investigation of the shear strength of teeth in the region of the dentinoenamel junction. Quintessence Int 1996;27:711–714.
25. Fischer J, Stawarczyk B. Compatibility of machined Ce-TZP/Al2O3 nanocomposite and a veneering ceramic. Dent Mater 2007;23:1500–1505.
26. Donlan RM, Costeron JW. Biofilm: survival mechanisms of clinically relevant microorganisms. Clin Microbiol Rev 2002;15:167–193.

# INDEX